ADVANCED GYNECOLOGIC ENDOSCOPY

Edited by **Atef Darwish**

Advanced Gynecologic Endoscopy
Edited by Atef Darwish

Published by InTech
Janeza Trdine 9, 51000 Rijeka, Croatia

Publishing Process Manager Niksa Mandic

Technical Editor Teodora Smiljanic

Cover Designer InTech Design Team

Additional hard copies can be obtained from orders@intechopen.com

Advanced Gynecologic Endoscopy, Edited by Atef Darwish
p. cm.
ISBN 978-953-307-348-4

For EU product safety concerns:
IN TECH d.o.o., Prolaz Marije Krucifikse Kozulić 3, 51000 Rijeka, Croatia,
info@intechopen.com or visit our website at intechopen.com.

Meet the editor

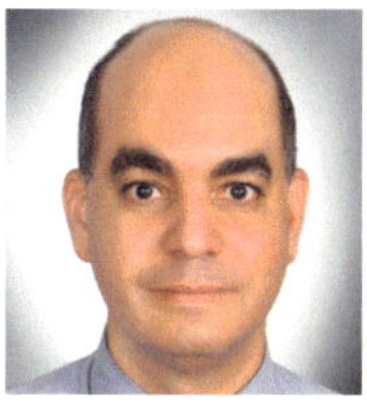

Dr. Atef Darwish graduated from Assiut School of Medicine in 1985 with an excellent grade with first class honors. He got his Master degree in 1989 with Excellent degree. Between 1992-1994, he spent 2 years at the Endoscopic Unit of Ulm University, Germany. Thereafter, he received his Medical Doctorate in 1995 through a combined program between the University of Ulm, Germany and the University of Assiut, Egypt with Excellent degree. He joined the Endoscopy Unit of Villach University Hospital in Austria, the Assisted Reproduction Unit in Düsseldorf University Hospital in Germany and the reproductive biology and minimally invasive surgery unit in the Cleveland Clinic Foundation, Clevland, Ohio, USA. Currently, he is a Professor of Obstetrics and Gynecology, Faculty of Medicine, Assiut University since July 2005. Moreover, he is a consultant of Obstetrics and Gynecology in three hospitals and he is the moderator and lecturer of many endoscopic societies. He authored an internationally registered undergraduate book, presented 59 presentations in national and international meetings, delivered a lot of lectures in Egypt, some Arabian countries and the USA and published more than 40 papers in international medical journals, and 7 papers in national journals. He received some congress prizes and awards due to his work in the field of reproductive medicine since 1995. He is a reviewer of many international journals and an associate editor of two of them. In 2009, he got a PhD degree in the reproductive medicine at the University of Utrichet, The Netherlands.

Contents

Preface

Text books on gynecologic laparoscopy are too many and really well- illustrated. This makes editing a new book in the same field a matter of challenge. The main purpose of this book is to address some important issues related to gynecologic laparoscopy that were thought to be poorly covered by other authors. We meticulously selected the authors based on their extended experience and frequent publications. Since the early breakthroughs by its pioneers, laparoscopic gynecologic surgery has gained popularity due to developments in illumination and instrumentation that led to the emergence of laparoscopy in the late 1980's as a credible diagnostic as well as therapeutic intervention. Performing reconstructive gynecological surgery is appreciated as it is cosmetically acceptable to patients. Nevertheless, the adage that no surgery is without risk also applies to laparoscopic surgery. That's why we included chapters on complications and patient selection to avoid such complications.

Along the road of refinement of endoscopic reconstructive gynecologic surgery, robotic technology, more specifically telerobotic surgical systems, has been used to bridge this gap between laparotomy and laparoscopy by enabling minimally invasive surgery with three-dimensional vision, ergonomically optimal positioning, tremor filtration, and laparoscopic instruments with intra-abdominal articulation. This remarkable technology facilitates suturing and dissection. You'll find some interesting chapters on this exiting topic.

This book is unique in that it will review common, useful information about certain laparoscopic procedures, including technique and instruments, and then discuss common difficulties faced during each operation. We also discuss the uncommon and occasionally even anecdotal cases and the safest ways to deal with them. We are honored to have a group of world experts in laparoscopic gynecologic surgery valuably contribute to our book.

This book is medium sized and includes a good number of illustrative pictures, drawings, and images that aim to make reading it informative, educational, and interesting. This book is a good preoperative reading that will remind the surgeon about important steps and possible difficulties. We hope that this book will continue to accumulate experiences of difficult conditions in laparoscopic surgery and add to the literature in a more instructive way in the future. This illustrated book is a reference text for laparoscopic gynecologic surgery. It includes all the theoretical knowledge that someone wishing to embark on training in laparoscopic surgery needs to know. It also provides information for those who perform intermediate laparoscopic surgery and who wish to learn more about advanced techniques. It provides information on why and how we perform safe laparoscopic surgery.

Prof Atef Darwish
Woman's Health University Center, Assiut,
Egypt

Part 1

Evolution of Laparoscopy

1

Evolution of Operative Laparoscopy in Gynecology: A Mirage or a Challenge?

Enakpene Christopher A[1] and Ajayi Olukunle[2]
[1]*State University of New York Medical Center, New York*
[2]*Royal Derby Hospital, Derby*
[1]*USA*
[2]*United Kingdom*

1. Introduction

The first successful surgical treatment of ectopic pregnancy was described in 1883 by Tait [1]. It was not until over a century after this (1973) that Shapiro and Adler described treatment of ectopic pregnancy by laparoscopy, the emergence of laparoscopy as a credible therapeutic intervention in the early 1980s heralded a new surgical age and today it is fast replacing most of the traditional gynaecological abdominal operations[2, 3, 4].

Technical developments in optics, illumination, video technology and instrumentation has further extended the frontiers from diagnostic to operative laparoscopy[5]. As the list of laparoscopic procedures grows, many of the traditional abdominal or pelvic surgical procedures can be done via minimal invasive approach using the laparoscope[6]. Advanced laparoscopic surgery is gradually evolving and may become the mainstay of operative management in gynaecologic oncology such as staging, lymphadenectomy, and radical surgery as well as in advanced endometriosis. Laparoscopic surgery contributes to remarkable improvement in cancer patients care, allows for quicker recovery and faster initiation of chemotherapy when indicated. The short hospital stay and recovery time have a positive impact in a cancer patient's quality of life, as they return to normal activities rapidly[7]. Furthermore, the advent and expanding roles of robotics in minimally invasive gynaecologic surgery, the future of laparoscopy promises to be brighter as this provides a means to overcome the limitations of conventional laparoscopy through the use of 3-dimensional imaging and more dextrous and precise instruments. Current studies clearly demonstrate the feasibility and safety of applying robotics to the entire spectrum of gynecologic procedures[8]. Laparoscopic surgery has gained ground due to its many advantages over laparotomy. To the patient; avoidance of the discomfort of a large abdominal incision, reduction of post-operative pain, reduction of wound complications and better cosmetic effect. Others are early mobilization, early discharge from the hospital, early resumption of routine activities and less adhesion formation[4, 7, 8]. It thus minimizes the burden on patients, their employers and their families [9]. On the part of the surgeon, improved visualisation offers the opportunity of more precise and accurate surgery [10].

As the shift of minor treatment to day, ambulatory or even office care is becoming inexorable, and major surgeries performed via laparoscopy, the resultant reduced length of hospital stay has the potential to release many more resources, thus, harnessing the advantages of laparoscopic surgery as appropriate can alleviate the problems of rising hospital costs and hospital-acquired infections[11]. Although the magnitude of saving resulting from the shorter hospital stay has been controversial, it is difficult to place a monetary value on the reduction in pain and discomfort, a shorter convalescence in an economically active group[12,13,14,15,16,17,18]. Although, steep learning curve and cost of training continue to limit universal usage of laparoscopy, the above benefits outweighs the limitations of laparoscopic surgery in addition. Vascular and bowel injuries continue to be obstacles to universal uptake of laparoscopic surgery.

2. Over viewing of the previous studies

The growth of laparoscopic surgery and its widespread acceptance into the mainstream of gynaecological practice have been faced with many challenges and pessimism. There was a great deal of opposition and pessimism of adopting laparoscopy at the inception which some antagonist termed " Foreveroscopy " because it took longer to perform than open surgery [10, 19, 20]. Some recent studies such as; the eVALuate study [20] also concluded that there is an increase in the risk of major complications associated with laparoscopic hysterectomy as compared with abdominal hysterectomy. Like many innovative and groundbreaking technologies of modern day medical practice, the introduction of laparoscopy into contemporary gynecology continue to evolve and develop. With the advances in laparoscopic surgery, potential risks of complications are no longer accepted as argument against using laparoscopic surgery rather than laparotomy for gynaecological surgeries when indicated [21 - 25]. (Level A evidence).

The current trend is towards an increasing adoption of laparoscopic surgery by gynaecologists in a number of conditions such as hysterectomy (total laparoscopic hysterectomy, supra-cervical hysterectomy and laparoscopic assisted vaginal hysterectomy), endometriosis, adhesiolysis, adnexal surgery, laparoscopic pelvic floor repair, laparoscopic urogynecology[26]. Increasingly, gynecologic oncologists are adopting the laparoscopic approach for the treatment of endometrial and cervical and ovarian cancer. Laparoscopy facilitates lymphadenectomy by providing an excellent view, haemostasis and lymph node harvest.[27,28,29]. The Royal College of Obstetricians and Gynaecologists (RCOG) as part of the list of competencies to be gained by trainees include various laparoscopic surgeries as part of the sub-speciality modules in obstetrics and gynaecology training. An important aspect of training, should be the performance of the surgical technique under the supervision of an experienced advanced laparoscopic surgeon which is at the moment a challenge to an average gynaecology training program since a significant learning curve exists with learning laparoscopic surgery [31, 32].

3. Evidenced based studies on laparoscopic surgeries

Vaginal hysterectomy should be performed in preference to abdominal hysterectomy, whenever possible. Where vaginal hysterectomy is not possible, a laparoscopic approach may avoid the need for an abdominal hysterectomy. Risks and benefits of different approaches may however be influenced by the surgeon's experience. More research is needed, particularly to examine the long-term effects of the different types of surgery [33]. (Level A evidence). A recent Cochrane review found no evidence to help quantify the value of laparoscopy for the management of early stage ovarian cancer as routine clinical practice [34]. (Level A evidence). Current available data and worldwide interest clearly demonstrate that laparoscopic techniques must now be part of the armamentarium of the gynaecologic oncologist. Postoperative morbidity and recurrence risk do not seem to be affected. Cost-effectiveness of laparoscopic procedures is based on the reduction of hospital stay and recovery time, although operating room time is increased in some procedures. Combined training in gynaecologic oncology and in laparoscopic and/or vaginal surgery is more than ever mandatory to avoid the risk of inadequate staging or management of pelvic malignancies [35].

4. Preoperative preparation

Patients selections: Appropriate patients selection for laparoscopic surgery is paramount. Ascertain a suitable indication, no contraindication for the proposed route, consideration should be given to other routes and coexisting pathologies such as pelvic organ prolapse, medical co-morbidities, expertise and equipment availability. In addition to the traditional routine of ensuring patient is of optimal health, pre operative assessment in operative laparoscopy should take cognizance of previous abdominal or pelvic surgeries or conditions that could predispose to intra-abdominal adhesions such as diverticulitis, pelvic abscess, ruptured appendix.
Body habitus of patients: This should be considered before any elective procedures. Obese patients should be encouraged to loose weight in order to reduce the risk of complications.
Assessment of abdominal and pelvic masses: This is to decide best approach to entry techniques, gas insufflations, consideration to open technique or the use of palmers point entry and gasless laparoscopy.
Anesthetic assessment: This is very essential because with the head down tilt of Lloyd Davies position or steep Trendelenburg positioning , it is not uncommon to have anaesthetic problems due to pressure of bowels on the diaphragm. Hence, communication with anaesthetic is vital. General anesthesia is the most favored as compared with regional anesthesia in laparoscopy. Operative laparoscopy necessitates optimal surgical condition, steep Trendelenburg positioning, muscle relaxation, a large pneumoperitoneum and multiple incisions all make general anesthesia the safest and most comfortable choice of anesthesia. Consent for operative laparoscopy should always include conversion to open laparatomy in case of technical difficulty or intra-operative complication.

5. Decision-making, anatomy, and key steps in the operations

Veress needle check for spring action, free gas flow in addition to laparoscopic stack check and trouble shooting know-how are important to any laparoscopic surgeon to avoid delays and complications. The click heard on piercing the rectus sheath and then again on entering the peritoneum (**double click test).** The **palmer's test** is when saline placed at veress' outer end is sucked into the peritoneal cavity due to the negative intra-abdominal pressure, and the **saline test** describes 5 ml of normal saline injected through veress needle and then withdrawn, there should then be no aspirate if the needle is in the peritoneal cavity. An opening pressure of less than 8 mmHg and loss of hepatic dullness are the other means of confirming intra-peritoneal placement of veress needle. These tests are not absolute but may be taken as an indication of intra-peritoneal entry and placement of the needle. Obviously, if one inadvertedly sticks the Veress needle into a major vessel such as the aorta, it should be left and immediate vascular surgeon's help summoned in addition to conversion to laparotomy.

Entry points: The periumbilical veress placement and gas insufflations; intra-umbilical or sub-umbilical are the most common sites for primary port placement in laparoscopy. The **Palmers point** entry , the least likely point to have adhesions, is in the mid-clavicular line 3 cm below the costal margin is useful in the presence of large pelvic mass or suspected periumbilical adhesion.

Open laparoscopy, first described by Hasson, a gynaecologist in 1970, is favoured by most surgeons. There is no difference in the risk of vascular or bowel injury using either of the above entry techniques. In a recent Cochrane review of the entry techniques by Ahmad et al, 17 included randomised controlled trials concerned 3,040 individuals undergoing laparoscopy. Overall there was no evidence of advantage using any single technique in terms of preventing major complications [36]. Insufflations pressure of 20 to 25 mmHg is recommended as it offers more room for intra-peritoneal manipulations and pushes away the gut. Other ports should be inserted under direct visualization, avoiding the blood vessels, especially inferior epigastric arteries.

6. Gasless laparoscopy

The use of gasless laparoscopy eliminates need for carbon dioxide gas for pneumo-peritoneum to create space in the intra-peritoneal cavity for surgery. The physiological problems associated with carbon dioxide pneumoperitoneum are: hypothermia, cardiac arrhythmia, cardiovascular collapse, pulmonary insufficiency, gas embolism, venous thrombosis, cerebral edema / ischemia, ocular hypertension, extra-peritoneal insufflations such as subcutaneous emphysema, and pneumomediasternum [37, 38]. Gasless laparoscopy is a cost effective procedure which offers enormous benefits for the patients, surgeons, hospitals and health care system. Several devices have been used to carry out gasless laparoscopy. I am more familiar with the "Abdo-Lift Laparoscopy" which combines the use of the abdo-lift device to lift the anterior abdominal wall and modification of other ancillary laparoscopic instruments to adapt to use of abdo-lift device. These ancillary instruments are short, strong, re-usable and durable for several years.

The ancillary instruments with abdo-lift device are: flexible silicone cannula, Metzenbaum and double jointed scissors, sponge holder, needle holder, Bozeman-Douglas clamps, tenaculum forceps, claw forceps, atraumatic clamp, knot tier and myoma fixation instrument. These re-usable, appropriate, acceptable, available, accessible and affordable instruments reduce the cost of minimal access surgery when compared with both standard laparoscopy and Da-Vinci. The problems and complications associated from iatrogenic insufflations of carbon dioxide are also completely eliminated so that minimally invasive operations can also be performed in high risks patients such as cardiac insufficiency, obstructive lung disease or during pregnancy.

7. Specific laparoscopic surgical techniques

Cross bag techniques: This was first developed by Jim Kondrup and it is used for big ovarian cystectomy without spillage of the cyst contents inside the peritoneal cavity. The ovarian mass is freed completely and carefully placed inside the endo-catch bag. The cyst is aspirated while inside the endo-catch bag and the cyst wall is completely excised without spillage of the cyst contents.

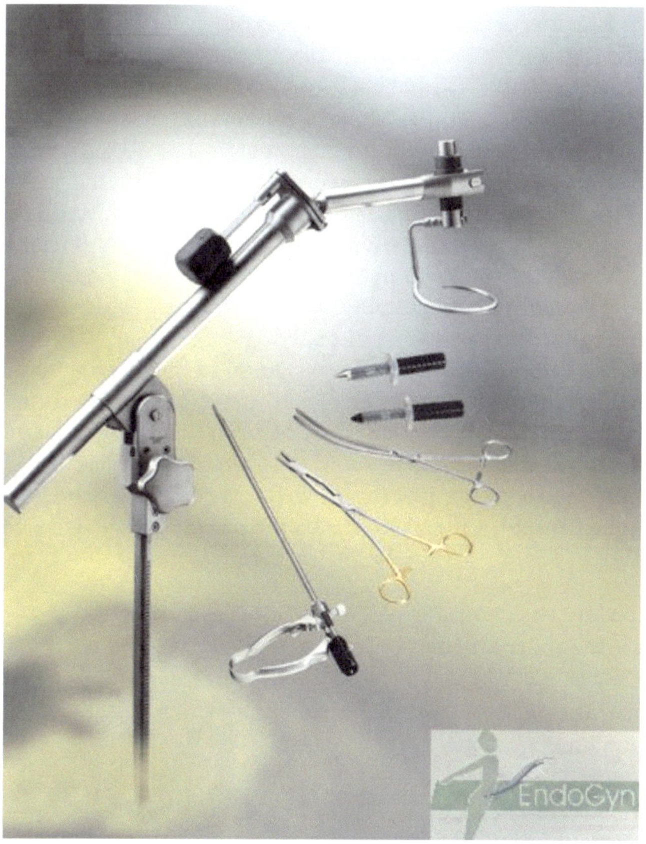

Permission obtained from EndoGyn, Germany.

Fig. 1.

Snag and bag: The cyst wall is snagged with help of negative pressure from the suction and a needles is passed through the same pot to aspirate the cyst content without spillage. Thereafter, the cyst wall is excised preserving the ovarian tissues and preventing spillage of cyst contents.

Simplified laparoscopic abdominal morcellation (SLAM): This is the use of number 11 surgical blade to cut into pieces surgical specimens and remove them in piece-meal through the 10 mm port. This is a better and faster technique than the mechanical or electrical morcellators.

8. Anatomical challenges in laparoscopy

Challenges of Obesity: The umbilicus may be displaced downward thus reference points of the aorta is distorted making injury more likely. Also one may need a longer Veress needle and trochar and cannula for entry. Insufflation through the uterus has been describes as well. Technical obstacles associated with open pelvic surgery in the obese patients are primarily those related to exposure of the operative field and access to deep pelvic structures. These obstacles present similar challenges when laparoscopy is attempted [39, 40], and there is unique difficulty of establishing pneumoperitoneum in obese patients [41]. These limitations place the obese patient undergoing laparoscopy at an inherently increased risk of conversion to laparotomy [17 - 19]. In a review of 2,530 attempted gynecologic laparoscopic surgeries, Sokol et al determined that a BMI greater than 30 kg/m2 placed patients at a more than 2-fold increased risk of unintended laparotomy [42] . Eltabbakh et al noted similar findings in a review of 47 obese patients who underwent operative gynecologic laparoscopies [43].

Challenges of Adhesions: Patients with previous pelvic and abdominal surgeries or when extensive adhesions are envisaged as in severe endometriosis, the use of Palmer's point entry or open laparoscopy is advisable. Adnexal masses and cancers or severe endometriosis may distort the pelvic anatomy and alter the course of ureters making it more liable to damage. Extended hysterectomy may pose a challenge as well. The use of trans-illuminating ureteric stents such as Uriglow ™ placed cystoscopically allows ureters to be easily identified and reduce risk of damage at surgery [44] .

The ancillary ports are most usually placed well lateral to the inferior epigastric vessels, and should be inserted high enough so that any instrument can be used on both sides of the pelvis. If there is to be anything more than the occasional suturing, a 10 mm port will allow the insertion of curved needles. Tricks to avoid the epigastric vessels at insertion of ancillary ports are trans-illumination before inserting the trochar ensures no vessel in the path and also injection of saline through a needle confirms the path when visualised in the abdomen.

Key steps

1. Appropriate patient selection
2. Pre operative assessment and consent
3. Equipments check
4. Personnel: Anaesthetist, assistants and scrub nurse
5. Positioning and ergonomics
6. Entry techniques
7. Surgery: prevent complications
8. Closure and prevention of adhesions
9. Immediate post operative
10. Discharge and Follow up

Positioning: Laparoscopy may take longer to perform in comparison to laparatomy. It is crucial to ensure optimal patients positioning and equipments set to make operators comfortable and ergonomically surgeon friendly. We preferred Lloyd Davis position to modified lithotomy, (Trendelenburg) during laparoscopic surgery because, the flexed thigh does not restrict movement during manoeuvres of the instruments. it is important to position the patient correctly on the operating table. Again, this means ensuring that the buttocks are over the edge of the table to allow full uterine ante-version. The legs are ideally placed in hydraulic leg supports with the thighs at about 45° to the horizontal while ensuring that the hips can be extended sufficiently to bring the thighs in line with the trunk should the need arise for any abdominal surgery. In addition, the legs would not interfere with manipulation of the instruments. The height of the bed should be such that surgeon should be comfortable. The visual display unit should be at the eye level in front of the surgeon and the assistants screen should be so adjusted to his or her specifications. I personally supervise the positioning of patients and ensure that operators are comfortable in order to avoid unnecessary strain. I ensure the bottom juts over the edge of the bed to allow adequate manipulation of the uterus by the second assistant.

While most gynecologists use the sub-umbilical approach , we prefer to use the vertical incision, about 10mm long to accommodate the primary port. Transverse sub umbilical or intra-umbilical incisions are used by various gynaecologists.

Virtually all the major abdominal operations described in Operative Surgery books have been performed with laparoscopic access or assistance. "What was advanced laparoscopic surgery yesterday is routine today."
Different operation room set ups are described (figure 2) as shown.

Operation room set up

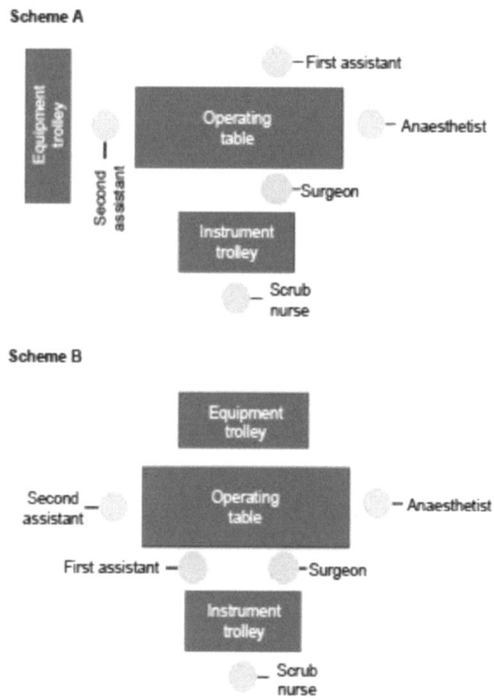

Fig. 2. From Dewhurst's Textbook of obstetrics and gynecology.

1. Lyses of adhesions
2. Appendicectomy
3. Investigations for infertility
4. Cholecystectomy
5. Ovarian/fallopian tube surgery
6. Ectopic pregnancy
7. Investigation of abdominal/pelvic pain (sub-acute intestinal obstruction and chronic pelvic inflammatory diseases) and intestinal surgery
8. Laparoscopic staging of cancer, biopsy and lymphadenectomy.
9. Myomectomy (removal of fibroids)
10. Hysterectomy
11. Morbid obesity surgery
12. Endometriosis
13. Hernia repair
14. Ovarian cysts

Table 1. Common indications of laparoscopy

1. Smaller incisions
2. Improved anatomical view to the surgeon and better visualization
3. Less collateral tissue handling and damage
4. Less internal scar (adhesions) formation
5. Less external scar formation like keloids or hypertrophic scars
6. Less general anaesthesia
7. Less post-operative pain and analgesia usage
8. Early ambulation
9. Less hospitalization time
10. Early return to normal activities and work

Table 2. Advantages of endoscopic surgeries

9. Impact of these techniques on modern practice

Laparoscopy is considered one of the first truly consumer-driven medical advances [45].
In the light of the various advantages of laparoscopic surgeries catalogued above, increased access to health information and increasing participation of patients in decision making; it is just a matter of time before we start experiencing demand for laparoscopic surgery by patients. The need for organised training and retraining of gynaecologists can therefore not be over emphasised in the interim. Laparoscopic surgical training and perfection of various techniques are influenced by: Patients demand, cost of healthcare, cost of training, length of training and increasing application of laparoscopy for most gynecological abdominal and pelvic procedures.

Recommendations and conclusions:

- Every gynaecologist should be trained in laparoscopy
- Laparoscopy should be available for all and sundry
- It is the main surgical technique of the future
- Robotic surgery development and introduction should be introduced gradually into mainstream gynecology
- Gasless laparoscopy should be part of the surgical armamentarium in any gynaecological laparoscopic surgical unit. Severe criticism that embroiled the adoption of standard (Straight stick) laparoscopy has also been melted down to the introduction of gasless laparoscopy. This important technique of minimal invasive surgery will also overcome many of the hurdles that often confront introduction of new technologies. Training and acquisition of knowledge and skills of its use should be encouraged as part of comprehensive training in minimal access surgeries in gynaecology. Its inexpensiveness, ease of use and short learning curve may eliminate most of the barriers that hinder widespread adoption of laparoscopy in gynaecological surgeries

10. References

[1] Tait RL. Five cases of extra-uterine pregnancy operated upon at the time rupture. BMJ. 1884;1:1250.
[2] Togas T, Ahmed S. Surgical Management of Ectopic Pregnancy. Clinical Obstetrics & Gynecology 1999, 42(1):31-38.
[3] Berci G, Sackier JM, Paz-Partlow M: Emergency laparoscopy. Am J Surg 1991, 161(3):332-335.
[4] Warren O, Kinross J, Parasceva P, Darzi A. Emergency laparoscopy - Current Best Practice. World Journal of Emergency Surgery 2006, 1:24.
[5] Semm K, Mettler L. Technical progress in pelvic surgery via operative laparoscopy. Am. J. Obstet. Gynecol 1980, 138: 121–7

[6] Howard, F.M. Breaking new ground or just digging a hole? An evaluation of gynecologic operative laparoscopy. J. Gynecol. Surg 1992, 8: 143–158

[7] Theodoros DT, John NB. Laparoscopy and Oncology: Where Do We Stand Today? Annals of the New York Academy of Sciences 2006, 997 (1).

[8] Arnold PA, Karen W. Evolving Role and Current State of Robotics in Minimally Invasive Gynecologic Surgery. Journal of Minimally Invasive Gynaecology 2009, 16 (3): 291-301.

[9] Nezhat CR, Nezhat FR, Metzger DA, Lucíano AA. Adhesions formation after reproductive surgery by video-laparoscopy. Fertility and Sterility 1990, 53: 1008.

[10] Gitsch E, Vytiska-Binstorfer E, Skodler W. Various effects of abdominal and vaginal hysterectomy in benign diseases. European Journal of Obstetrics, Gynecology, and Reproductive Biology 1990, 36: 259-63

[11] Paraiso MF. Laparoscopic Burch colposuspension and the tension-free vaginal tape procedure. Current Opinion in Obstetrics & Gynecology 2006, 18(4):385 - 390.

[12] Ray G. Laparoscopic surgery Best Practice & Research Clinical Obstetrics & Gynaecology, Volume 20, Issue 1, February 2006, Pages 89-104

[13] Trehan AK. Hysterectomy: Towards an Overnight Stay. Gynaecological Endoscopy 2002, 11 (4).

[14] Scrimgeour JB, Ng KB, Gaudoin MR. Laparoscopy in vaginal hysterectomy Lancet 1991, 338: 1465-6.

[15] Summit RL, Stovall TG, Lipscomb GH, Ling FW. Randomised comparison of laparoscopy assisted vaginal hysterectomy with standard vaginal hysterectomy in an out patient setting. Obstetrics and Gynecology 1992, 80: 895-901.

[16] Hill DJ. Complication of hysterectomy. Baillière's Clinical Obstetrics and Gynaecology 1997, 11: 181-97.

[17] Hulka J, Brown Levy BS, Parker WH, Phillips JM. Laparoscopic assisted vaginal hysterectomy. American Association of Gynecologic Laparoscopists' Membership Survey. J Am Assoc Gynecol Laparosc 1997, 4: 167-71.

[18] Nezhat, F., Nezhat, C., Gordon, S. and Wilkins, E. Laparoscopic versus abdominal hysterectomy. J. Reprod. Med 1992, 37: 247–250.

[19] Raju KS, Auld BJ. A randomised prospective study of laparoscopic vaginal hysterectomy and bilateral salpingo-oöphorectomy with conventional abdominal hysterectomy, each with bilateral salpingo-oöphorectomy. BJOG 1994, 101: 1068-71.

[20] Bronitsky C, Payne RJ, Stuckey S, Wilkins D. A comparison of laparoscopically assisted vaginal hysterectomy versus traditional total abdominal and vaginal hysterectomies. Journal of Gynecologic Surgery 1993, 9: 219-24.

[21] Shushan A, Mohamed H, Magos AL. How long does laparoscopic surgery really take? Lessons learned from 1000 operative laparoscopies. Hum Reprod 1999, 14 (1): 39-43.

[22] Ray G, Fountain J, Mason S, Hawe J, Napp V, Abbott J, Clayton R, Phillips G, Whittaker M, Lilford R, Bridgman S, Brown J. The eVALuate study: two parallel randomised trials, one comparing laparoscopic with abdominal hysterectomy, the other comparing laparoscopic with vaginal hysterectomy. BMJ 2004, 328:129.

[23] Chapron C, Fauconnier A, Goffinet F, Bréart G, Dubuisson J.B. Laparoscopic surgery is not inherently dangerous for patients presenting with benign gynaecologic pathology. Results of a meta-analysis, Hum Reprod. 2002, 17 (5): 1334-1342.

[24] Simon WA. Results of eVALuate study of hysterectomy techniques: Conversion to open surgery should not be regarded as major complication. BMJ 2004, 328: 642.

[25] Stephen MFS. Results of eVALuate study of hysterectomy techniques: Degree of pain cannot be commented. BMJ. 2004, 328: 642.

[26] Canis MJ, Wattiez A, Mage G, Bruhat MA. Results of eVALuate study of hysterectomy techniques: Laparoscopic hysterectomy may yet have a bright future BMJ 2004, 328: 642-643.
[27] Donnez J, Squifflet J, Jadoul P, Smets M. Results of eVALuate study of hysterectomy techniques: High rate of complications needs explanation. BMJ 2004, 328: 643.
[28] Lin, Lawrence La; Ho, Mat Ha; Haessler, Alexandra La; Betson, Lance Ha; Alinsod, Red M b; Liu, CY c; Bhatia, Narender Na. A review of laparoscopic uterine suspension procedures for uterine preservation. Current Opinion in Obstetrics & Gynecology 2005, 17(5):541-546.
[29] Pittaway DE, Takacs P, Bauguess P. Laparoscopic Adnexectomy: A Comparison With Laparotomy. AJOG 1994, 171(2):385-391.
[30] Leblanc E, Sonoda Y, Narducci F, Ferron G, Querleu D. Laparoscopic staging of early ovarian carcinoma. Current Opinion in Obstetrics & Gynecology 2006, 18(4):407-412.
[31] Burnett AF. Radical trachelectomy with laparoscopic lymphadenectomy: review of oncologic and obstetrical outcomes. Current Opinion in Obstetrics & Gynecology 2006, 18(1):8-13.
[32] Rosen D, Cario G. The learning curve for laparoscopic hysterectomy. Gyn Endosc 1998, 7:289–294.
[33] Wattiez A, Soriano D, Cohen SB, et al. The learning curve of total laparoscopic hysterectomy: comparative analysis of 1647 cases. J Am Assoc Gynecol Laparosc 2002, 9:339–345.
[34] Nieboer TE, Johnson N, Lethaby A, Tavender E, Curr E, Garry R, van Voorst S, Mol BWJ, Kluivers KB. Surgical approach to hysterectomy for benign gynaecological disease. *Cochrane Database of Systematic Reviews* 2009, Issue 3. Art. No.: CD003677. DOI: 10.1002/14651858.CD003677.pub4.
[35] Medeiros LRF, Rosa DD, Bozzetti MC, Rosa MINES, Edelweiss MI, Stein AT, Zelmanowicz A, Ethur AB, Zanini RR. Laparoscopy versus laparotomy for FIGO Stage I ovarian cancer. *Cochrane Database of Systematic Reviews* 2008, Issue 4. Art. No.: CD005344. DOI: 10.1002/14651858.CD005344.pub2.
[36] Querleua D, Leblanc E, Ferrona G, Narduccib F. Laparoscopic surgery in gynaecological oncology. European Journal of Surgical oncology 2006, 32 (8): 853-858.
[37] Ahmad G, Duffy JMN, Phillips K, Watson A. Laparoscopic Entry Techniques. *Cochrane Database of Systematic Reviews* 2008, Issue 2. Art. No.: CD006583. DOI: 10.1002/14651858.CD006583.pub2
[38] Wolf J S, Stoller ML. The physiology of laparoscopy: basic principles, complications and other considerations. J Urol. 1994; 152: 294-302
[39] Chiu AW, Chang LS, Birkett DH, Babayan RK. The impact of pneumoperitoneum, retroperitoneum, and gasless laparoscopy on the systemic and renal hemodynamics. J Am Coll Surg. 1995; 181: 397-406.
[40] Holtz G. Laparoscopy in the massively obese female. Obstet Gynecol 1987;69:423-4.
[41] Halpern NB. Access problems in laparoscopic cholecystectomy: postoperative adhesions, obesity, and liver disorders. Semin Laparosc Surg 1998;5:92-106.
[42] Loffer FD, Pent D. Laparoscopy in the obese patient. Am J Obstet Gynecol 1976;125:104-7.
[43] Sokol AI, Chuang K, Milad MP. Risk factors for conversion to laparotomy during gynecologic laparoscopy. J Am Assoc Gynecol Laparosc 2003;10:469-73.
[44] Eltabbakh GH, Piver MS, Hempling RE, Recio FO. Laparoscopic surgery in obese women. Obstet Gynecol 1999;94:704-08
[45] Phipps JH. Laparoscopic hysterectomy and oophorectomy a Practical Manual and Color atlas. Churchill livingstone 1993
[46] Geier WS. An overview of consumer-driven ambulatory surgery: operative laparoscopy. Nurse Pract 1995, 20 (36): 46 - 51.

Part 2

Anesthesia for Laparoscopy

2

Anaesthetic Considerations During Laparoscopic Surgery

Maria F. Martín-Cancho, Diego Celdrán,
Juan R. Lima, Maria S. Carrasco-Jimenez,
Francisco M. Sánchez-Margallo and Jesús Usón-Gargallo
Minimally Invasive Surgery Centre Jesus Usón,
Spain

1. Introduction

Laparoscopic surgery has improved greatly during the last years, mainly thanks to advances in both anaesthetic and surgical techniques (Llagostera-Pujol et al., 2002). Abdominal laparoscopy is normally perceived to be associated with few risks. However, clinicians should be aware of inherent dangers such as gaseous embolism, a potential inability to control haemorrhage, an increase in carbon dioxide arterial partial pressure, and changes in arterial blood pressure and heart rate. The hemodynamic and respiratory alterations associated with abdominal laparoscopy are caused by the high intra-abdominal pressure brought over by pneumoperitoneum creation. The most relevant hemodynamic changes are a decrease in venous return secondary to Inferior Vena Cava compression and increases in central venous pressure and arterial blood pressure in absence of heart rate changes. Regarding respiratory adjustments, cranial displacement of the diaphragm causes a restrictive respiratory syndrome with decreased pulmonary compliance and increased pulmonary pressures and inspiratory peak (Carrasco et al., 1998; Joris et al., 1999).

Anesthesia in laparoscopic procedures it's complicated by the pathophysiologic changes developed because of the pneumoperitoneum creation and the required positioning of the patient. It's also considered a potentially high risk procedure because of other inherent conditions: The duration of procedures is usually longer, there is a risk of visceral injury and it's difficult to estimate the amount of blood loss when hemorrhage occurs.

The anesthesiologist must have a deep understanding of the pathophysiological consequences derived from the pneumoperitoneum, to be prepared to prevent, detect and address the possible alterations that can occur during the intervention.

The physiological changes and complications derived from the pneumoperitoneum are the first topics described. The postoperative benefits of laparoscopy regarding some postoperative aspects will be described in second place. A lot of studies have been published about the advantages and effects of laparoscopic surgeries during the last 35 years, but anaesthetic techniques and laparoscopic conditions have change a lot during the last 15 years, so this review we'll be focused on those modern techniques and conditions.

2. Hemodynamic alterations in laparoscopic surgery

In abdominal laparoscopy procedures, hemodynamic and respiratory alterations are both derived from the same three origins: the first one is the intra-abdominal pressure created by the pneumoperitoneum; the second one is the existence of an insufflation gas that is absorbed by the blood; the third one is the Trendelemburg or anti-Trendelemburg positioning of the patient.

The pneumoperitoneum increases the abdominal pressure, elevates the diaphragm and can compress both small and big blood vessels. The intra-abdominal pressure obtained during these procedures, which is usually 12mmHg (Fig. 1), increases central venous pressure (CVP), heart rate (HR), systemic vascular resistances (SVR) up to a 65%, and the pulmonary vascular resistances can rise up to a 90%. Cardiac output (CO) can increase on a healthy patient in Trendelemburg position, but can also decrease to a 50% on patients in anti-Trendelemburg position or with a low cardiovascular reserve. All those changes are usually well tolerated in healthy patients but it can be different in patients with systemic diseases.

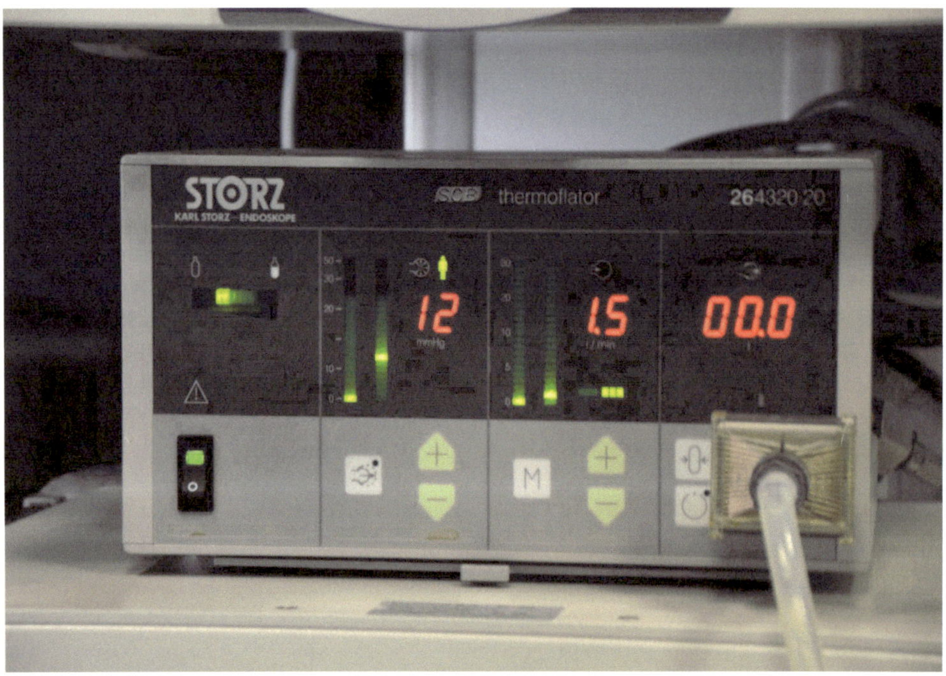

Fig. 1. CO_2 Insufflator showing normal working pressure.

When intra-abdominal pressure riches 15mmHg, because of excessive insufflations or because the patient activates the abdominal wall muscles (due to a lack of muscle relaxants that causes an increase of the abdominal wall resistance to the insufflations, cough or tube rejection), a compression of the cava vein can occur, causing a blood return reduction and a decrease in the cardiac output. The diaphragm elevation will raise intra thoracic pressure and will reduce the cardiac output. The lower CO can be compensated in a healthy patient by increasing the heart rate and arterial pressure, obtaining a stable hemodynamic status; but if an acute hemorrhage occurs, the patient turns fast in to an unstable status. Arrhythmia and bradycardia often appear in non atropinized patients during insufflation.

All the reported studies describe an increase in systemic vascular resistance during pneumoperitoneum. This increase in afterload can't be considered as a simple sympathetic reflex response to decreased cardiac output (Joris et al., 1993; Cunningham et al., 1993; As cited in Miller's Anesthesia 2005). Systemic vascular resistance also increased in studies in which no decrease in cardiac output was reported (Odeberg et al., 1994; Cunningham et al., 1993; As cited in Miller's Anesthesia 2005). Whereas the normal heart tolerates increases in afterload under physiologic conditions, the changes in afterload produced by the pneumoperitoneum can result in deleterious effects in patients with cardiac diseases and may lead to further decrease in cardiac output (Harris et al., 1996 as cited in Miller's Anesthesia 2005). The increase in systemic vascular resistance is affected by patient position. Whereas the Trendelemburg position attenuates this increase, the head up position aggravates it (Odeberg et al., 1994; Gannedahl et al., 1996; Hirvonen et al., 1995; Hirvonen et al., 1997; As cited in Miller's Anesthesia 2005)

Cardiovascular collapse and asystole cases in healthy patients have been described previously and attributed to deep vagal reflexes due to sudden insufflations.

The carbon dioxide pneumoperitoneum induce the gas absorption leading to a hypercapnia tendency. If pulmonary ventilation is not enough to eliminate the CO_2 absorbed from the pneumoperitoneum, then hypercapnia appears and the resultant acidosis can depress myocardial function and predispose to arrhythmia and cardiovascular collapse. Carbon dioxide has also direct effects on the heart; it causes arrhythmia and probably decreases contractibility. It is because of that reasons that Helium has been recommended as insufflation gas in patients with cardiac risk or respiratory disability to eliminate CO_2.

Gaseous embolism through an open vessel can produce severe hemodynamic alterations, which can produce a cardiovascular collapse by venous return blockade. Anti-Trendelemburg position increases the severity of the embolism and its repercussions delaying its treatment.

Positioning is essential for the final hemodynamic result during laparoscopy. On superior abdomen procedures, where patients are on anti-Trendelemburg position, the venous return decreases because of the remaining blood on the inferior extremities.

In healthy patients hemodynamic stability use to be maintained, just with the exception of hemorrhage, which can suddenly decompensate that stability. It's highly recommended the pre- hydration of the patient with 500-1000ml of saline solution before the beginning pneumoperitoneum. Patients that underwent intestinal cleaning use to suffer a loss of liquids, which shows up when they are positioned on anti-Tredelmburg, combined with the pneumoperitoneum and the vasodilators effects of the anaesthetic drugs.

When laparoscopic surgery is performed on the inferior abdomen, like in gynecology or pelvic surgeries, Trendelemburg position is required; it increases the venous return and compensates blood loss. However, heart patients can dramatically increase the cardiac preload. Moreover, the respiratory changes produced by the diaphragm's elevation, caused by an excessive intra abdominal pressure on Trendelemburg position, will raise intra thoracic pressure. That fact, in combination with the higher inspiratorty pressures required, will increase the cardiac impedance, or in other words the cardiac after load; At least four renal insufficiency cases have been described associated with an increase of the intra abdominal pressure due to a post surgery hemorrhage. In contrast with respiratory postoperative complications, hemodynamic complications don't seem to increase with surgery duration.

3. Respiratory alterations in laparoscopic surgery

Pathological respiratory changes occurring during laparoscopic surgery are induced by the pneumoperitoneum and the patient position (Trendelemburg or anti Trendelemburg).

The rise of the intra abdominal pressure elevates the diaphragm, decreasing that way the intra thoracic volume and interfering with the ventilation mechanisms. Those changes will be increased by the Trendelemburg position.

A maximum pressure of 10-15mmHg is recommended because respiratory alterations are well tolerated on that level. Over 15mmHg an airway pressure increase occurs together with a rise of the intra thoracic pressure, those changes compress the great and small vessels and initially show up with tachycardia and hypertension, but can produce tachycardia, hypotension and a lower cardiac output at higher pressures.

Many gases can be use to create the pneumoperitoneum, such as Helium, Argon or even nitrogen dioxide, but CO_2 still the most used. The phisyopathological alterations produced by the carbon dioxide are in relationship with the amount of gas insufflated and the insufflation's time (Surgery duration).

Pneumoperitoneum decreases thoracopulmonary compliance. Compliance is reduced by 30% to 50% in healthy (Bardoczy et al., 1993; Hirvonen et al., 1995; Kendall & Bhatt., 1995; Oikkonen & Tallgren., 1995; Fahy et al., 1995; Fahy et al., 1996; As cited in Miller's Anesthesia 2005), obese (Dumont et al., 1997; Casati et al., 2000; Sprung et al., 2002; As cited in Miller's Anesthesia 2005), and American Society of Anesthesiologists (ASA) class III or IV patients, but the shape of the pressure-volume loop does not change. After the pneumoperitoneum is created and kept constant, compliance is not affected by subsequent patient tilting (Rauh et al., 2001; As cited in Miller's Anesthesia 2005) or by increasing the minute ventilation required to avoid intraoperative hypercapnia. Reduction in functional residual capacity due to elevation of the diaphragm (Mutoh et al., 1992; As cited in Miller's Anesthesia 2005) and changes in the distribution of pulmonary ventilation and perfusion from increased airway pressure can be expected. However, increasing IAP to 14mmHg with the patient in a 10 to 20 degree head up or head down position does not significantly modify physiologic dead space or shunt in patients without cardiovascular problems (Tan et al., 1992; Bures et al., 1996; Odeberg-Wernerman & Sollevi., 1996; As cited in Miller's Anesthesia 2005).

CO_2 spreads in to the blood and it's eliminated during the expiration. But it's also accumulated in the fat tissue and muscle, which explains the high carbon dioxide expirated rate during some minutes after the end of insufflation.

Many works have been published to evaluate the increase in the carbon dioxide arterial pressure ($PaCO_2$) during laparoscopic surgery, and it have been shown that in ASA I patients with constant minute volume mechanical ventilation have an average increase in $PaCO_2$ from 4.5 to 10mmHg in conventional procedures. It has also been shown that in ASA II and ASA III patients the death space is bigger, so the reliability of the carbon dioxide measurement it's lower and the increase in $PaCO_2$ can be misdetected by capnography. In $PaCO_2$ rises above 14mmHg associated with acidosis, which are not resolved with a 20% minute volume increase, use to require the transformation of laparoscopic surgery in to open surgery.

The high diffusion of CO_2 can originate gaseous embolism, suspicious sigs are the usual ones: Third sound auscultation, expirated CO_2 reduction, arterial pressure decrease, increase of the pulmonary vascular resistance, arrhythmia and finally right heart failure.

Capnography and pulse oximetry provide reliable monitoring of $PaCO_2$ and arterial oxygen saturation in healthy patients and in the absence of acute intraoperative disturbances (Bures et al., 1996; Nyarwaya et al., 1994; Baraka et al., 1994; As cited in Miller's Anesthesia 2005). There is a lack of correlation between PaCO2 and end-tidal carbon dioxide tension ($PEtCO_2$) in sick patients, particularly those with impaired CO_2 excretion capacity, and otherwise in healthy

patients with acute cardiopulmonary disturbances. Arterial blood sampling is recommended when hypercapnia is clinically suspected, even in the absence of normal $PEtCO_2$.
In summary, during CO_2 pneumoperitoneum, the increase of $PaCO_2$ may be multifactorial: absorption of CO2 from the peritoneal cavity; impairment of pulmonary ventilation and perfusion by mechanical factors such as abdominal distention, patient position and volume-controlled mechanical ventilation; And also a depression of ventilation by premedicant and anaesthetic agents in the case of spontaneous breathing (Table 1).

<table>
<tr><td colspan="2">1.- CO_2 Absortion from the peritoneal cavity.</td></tr>
<tr><td colspan="2">2.- Ventilation / perfusion mismatch: increase dead space.</td></tr>
<tr><td>- Abdominal distension.
- Possition of the patient.</td><td>- Controlled mechanical ventilation.
(e.g., steep tilt)
- Reduced cardiac output.</td></tr>
<tr><td colspan="2">All these mechanisms are accentuated in sick patients (e.g., Obese, ASA II or III)</td></tr>
<tr><td colspan="2">3.- Increased metabolism. (e.g., insufficient plane of anesthesia)</td></tr>
<tr><td colspan="2">4.- Depression of ventilation by anaesthetics. (e.g., spontaneous breathing)</td></tr>
<tr><td colspan="2">5.- Accidental events.</td></tr>
<tr><td colspan="2">- CO_2 emphisema (i.e., subcutaneous or body cavities).
- Capnothorax.
- CO_2 embolism (Selective bronchial intubation)</td></tr>
</table>

Table 1. Causes of increased $PaCO_2$ during laparoscopy procedures (Miller, 2005).

3.1 Carbon dioxide subcutaneous emphysema

CO_2 subcutaneous emphysema can develop as a complication of accidental extraperitoneal insufflation (Hall et al., 1993; As cited in Miller's Anesthesia 2005) but can also be considered as an unavoidable side effect of certain laparoscopic surgical procedures that require intentional extraperitoneal insufflation, such as inguinal hernia repair, renal surgery, and pelvic lymphadenectomy (Mullet et al., 1993; Wolf et al., 1995; As cited in Miller's Anesthesia 2005). During laparoscopic fundoplication for hiatal hernia repair, the opening of the peritoneum overlying the diaphragmatic hiatus allows passage of CO_2 under pressure through the mediastinum to the cervicocephalic region. In these three circumstances, VCO_2, $PaCO_2$ and $PEtCO_2$ increase (Mullet et al., 1993; As cited in Miller's Anesthesia 2005). Any increase in $PEtCO_2$ occurring after $PEtCO_2$ has plateaued should suggest this complication.

3.2 Pneumothorax, pneumomediastinum and pneumopericardium

Movement of gas during the creation of a pneumoperitoneum can produce pneumomediastinum (Spielman et al., 1989; As cited in Miller's Anesthesia 2005), unilateral and bilateral pneumothorax (Whiston et al., 1991; As cited in Miller's Anesthesia 2005), and pneumopericardium (Knos et al., 1989; As cited in Miller's Anesthesia 2005). Defects in the diaphragm or weak points in the aortic and esophageal hiatus may allow gas passage into the thorax. Pneumothorax may also develop from pleural tears during laparoscopic surgical procedures at the level of the gastroesophageal junction (e.g.,fundoplication for hiatal hernia). Pneumothorax during fundoplication is more frequently located on the left side. These complications are potentially serious and may lead to respiratory and hemodynamic disturbances. Capnothorax reduces thoracopulmonary compliance, and airway pressures increase. VCO_2, $PaCO_2$ and $PEtCO_2$ also increase (Joris et al., 1995; As cited in Miller's

Anesthesia 2005). Diagnosis must be confirmed by auscultation of the chest and roentgenography.

When capnothorax develops during laparoscopy, we follow several guidelines (Joris et al., 1995; As cited in Miller's Anesthesia 2005).

- Stop CO_2 administration.
- Adjust ventilator settings to correct hypoxemia.
- Apply positive end-expiratory pressure (PEEP).
- Reduce IAP as much as possible.
- Maintain close communication with the surgeon.
- Avoid thoracocentesis unless necessary, because pneumothorax spontaneously resolves after exsufflation.

4. Changes related to patient positioning

The patient positioning on the surgery table for laparoscopic procedures must follow the same general principles than in any other surgery under general anesthesia. Hemodynamic situations leading to hypo perfusion can occur during the procedures, which can affect skin areas compressed over rigid elements. Must be considered as a general rule, that laparoscopic procedures are usually longer than open surgery procedures, so the deleterious elements will be acting more time.

The most vulnerable areas to friction or bad positioning must be protected firstly (Cornea and conjunctiva, lips, tongue and penis). It's useful to ask the patient to stay in the surgery position before the deep sedation, to indicate the anesthesiologist where does he feel uncomfortable or slight pain in order to correct the position or to protect that areas.

During the patient positioning it's also recommended to take special care of the electrosurgical scalpel plate or any other electrical device close to the patient. If the plate is not properly placed attached to the skin, the patient would be in risk of burn injuries.

When the patient is positioned in lateral recumbency perfusion is higher in the lower lung, but ventilation is more effective in the upper lung, that's because of the functional residual capacity (FRC) present in every anesthetized patient. The diaphragm relaxation leads to the lost of the inspiration's favorable curve; the abdominal mass pressures the lower lung in relaxed patients and the pressure is also transmitted to the mediastinum, contributing to reduce the FRC.

In summary, the ventilation perfusion quotient will be altered and reduced. In this case, positive end expiratory pressure (PEEP) will elevate the lower lung in to a better position at the volume-pressure curve, increasing the FRC and reestablishing the initial values.

All these are general factors to keep in mind during any laparoscopic procedure, but there are specific factors to be considered depending on the particular procedure. The specific factors are mainly related with the required patient's position: Upper abdomen procedures, lower abdomen procedures, hysteroscopy and urologic procedures.

4.1 Upper abdomen procedures

In upper abdomen laparoscopic procedures the patient use to be positioned in different anti Trendelemburg degrees, besides it favors ventilation by descending diaphragm and requires lower inspiratory pressures, it causes a reduction in the venous return and therefore in the cardiac output that can reach a 50%. A young and healthy patient can compensate it by increasing the heart rate and vascular resistances, avoiding the apparition of hypotension.

But in elderly patients or patients with systemic disease the compensation mechanisms may not be that effective and hypotension or even heart collapse can occur.
Those hemodynamic alterations can be extreme in patients presenting dehydration, when myocardial depressing drugs or vasodilator drugs are used (High propofol dosage, halogenated drugs) and in cases when excessive intra-abdominal pressure compress the cava vein (Lew et al., 1992).
Hypotension has also a pulmonary shunt effect that impairs CO_2 elimination promoting hypercapnia's cardiovascular effects. Anti-Trendelemburg position favors gas embolism and its consequences (Rock & Brown, 1994; Soper, 1994).

4.2 Lower abdomen procedures

In lower abdomen procedures (pelvic gynecology) Trendelemburg position is used, sometimes in a exaggerated degree, like in pelvic laparoscopy. That makes ventilatory condition worse, but improves venous return and increase cardiac output in healthy patients. Fortunately most of the gynecology procedures made in marked Trendelemburg position and performed in healthy young patients. However, in patients with low cardiac reserve, that CO increase can even produce a heart failure. When lithotomic position is associated, like in pelvic gynecology or intestinal procedures, the rise in the venous return is higher.
A long and pronounced Tendelemburg, together with the intra abdominal pressure can produce a reflex tachycardia that may be caused by the development of a moderate cerebral edema. Maintenance of this position requires shoulder holders, and if they are not properly placed produce brachial plexus lesions, especially when associated with arm abduction and rotation.
When arms are placed against the body during all the procedure, which can be long, intravenous catheter mast be protected, anaesthetic monitoring probes must be ensured, as well as fingers or any other part susceptible of being pinch or stocked if position changes are needed.
During procedures, surgeon's assistants must hold optics and instruments during long periods of time, which make them lean on the patient. It's the anesthesiologist responsibility to avoid that it hurts the patient.

4.3 Hysteroscopy and urologic procedures

On those two groups of interventions the positions used are the dorsal decubitus and the lithotomy position, which don't use to cause any hemodynamic or respiratory alterations, just with the exception of extremely obese patients. But in transurethral resections or hysteroscopy procedures the irrigation solution can pass in to the intra vascular space or abdominal cavity, if urinary bladder or uterus respectively is perforated. That's the reason to have a good monitoring and take some precautions like: limiting the resection time to one hour, limiting the height of the irrigation bags to 1.2 meters, checking patient's clinical symptoms (for this the patient use to be awake with loco regional anesthesia), being careful with the abdominal distension and checking often the liquid balance (incomes and outcomes).Hypothermia used to be a complication in that surgeries, but it's avoided by monitoring patient's temperature and using warm intravenous and irrigation liquids.

4.4 Positioning nerve injury

Neural enlargement must be prevented in order to avoid neurapraxia. Arm's abduction and external rotation, extreme hip abduction and knees in lithotomic position can all produce

neuropathies, despite they are transitory, they require a neurological examination, rehabilitation and postoperative care that can be avoided by prevention. It must be kept in mind that neuromuscular blockade lead to unnatural stances. (Kaplan & Rogers, 1994)
To prevent the nervous compression we must take a special care of the areas where nerves pass close beneath the skin, like the elbow, the knee, the feet or the face. The typical nervous lesion produced during the anesthesia on the brachial plexus and the lower extremities nerves are typically by combination of two mechanisms: Bony compression and enlargement.

5. Monitoring

Laparoscopic surgery is associated with a better postoperative condition (Less pain, less time to heal wounds) making the back to normal life easier to patients, but that doesn't mean a decrease in intra operative stress, especially in patients with systemic diseases. The monitoring techniques and its characteristics are the same as for open surgeries.

5.1 ASA I and II patients monitoring

Minimal standard monitoring includes: ECG, non invasive arterial pressure, auscultation, pulse oxymetry, temperature and oxygen concentration. Ventilatory monitoring is always essential (volumes, inspiratory pressure, oxygen concentration).
The ECG value is higher if it's possible to monitoring two derivations at the same time: DII for detecting arrhythmia and V5 lead to be able to detect ischemia.
It's highly recommendable to check often the non invasive arterial pressure devices, because they use to be positioned in the arm, and surgeon movements or changes in patient position can originate false data from the devices.
End-tidal concentration of carbon dioxide ($EtCO_2$) it's a part of standard monitoring in regular surgery, but it is essential in laparoscopy procedures. $EtCO_2$ determination help's in controlling the CO_2 absorption-elimination equilibrium. In healthy patients, the $EtCO_2$ is correlated with the $PaCO_2$ from 4 to 8 mmHg, but this gradient can be increased in shock or increased dead space cases. Any deep fall of $EtCO_2$ must make us think about an embolism, hypotension or heart collapse. Intra abdominal pressure and CO_2 absorption obliges the anesthesiologist to make ventilation adjustments in order to guarantee carbon dioxide elimination. The $EtCO_2$ allows these maneuvers to be quick and safe when changes appear. (Fig.2)
The shape of the capnography wave gives a lot of additional information about the patient's physiologic status. The diagnoses of a gas embolism or an intra operative bronchospasm are facilitated by the observation of $EtCO_2$.
During one lung ventilation, if alveolar ventilation remains the same, the $EtCO_2$ doesn't changes significantly and still keeping a good correlation with $PaCO_2$.
It's essential to control patient's temperature, because hypothermia is a danger in long procedures due to irrigation fluids, and the anesthesia recovery will be more soft and quick if hypothermia has been avoided.
The $EtCO_2$ and temperature allow the anesthesiologists to detect estrange but possible complications like malignant hyperthermia.
High inspiratory pressures on the ventilator can change the intra thoracic dynamic and cardiovascular function, but it can also create a piston like movement of the tracheal tube causing pharyngeal discomfort and changes in the voice tone that can be a problem during patient's recuperation process.

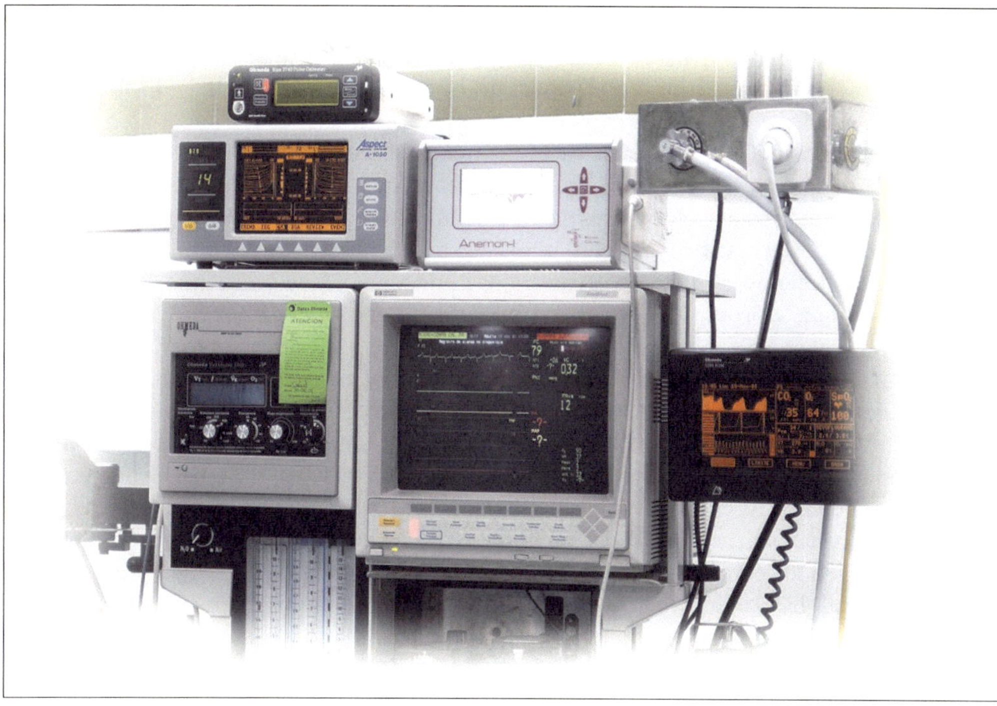

Fig. 2. Anesthetic monitoring during laparoscopic surgery.

Subcutaneous emphysema is always a laparoscopy associated risk. That makes mandatory to examine the patient for emphysema at the cervical, thorax and abdomen areas after surgery. It's also recommended to perform thorax radiography to rule out possible pneumothorax or pneumomediastinum complications.

5.2 ASA III, IV and V patients monitoring

There are no general rules regarding monitoring of systemic disease patients. Depending on the previous cardiovascular and respiratory status and depending on the expected complications as well, different techniques will be added to the standard monitoring.

There are no fixed rules about the use of the invasive arterial pressure monitoring, but it gives valuable information in every heart beat. That makes it very useful, considering also its low morbidity. On patients suffering heart disease, hypertension cases and or when important intravascular volume changes are expected, the arterial pressure value and its curve shape are essential.

Patients suffering ischemic myocardial injury or under arrhythmia risk are also ideal candidates to establish an invasive arterial pressure monitoring, same as morbid obesity patients where the non invasive measurements can be inexact. During thoracoscopy procedures with compression or distortion of the mediastinum structures risk, arterial pressure monitoring must be present to be able to detect the consequences of these compressions.

On patients with lung disease it's convenient to establish frequently a $PaCO_2$- $EtCO_2$ gradient because the elimination can be impaired. Arterial catheterization provides a source for arterial blood gasometry (ABG).

The Central venous pressure (CVP) monitoring is the most widely used method to determine and treat intravascular volume loss, but its use in laparoscopic procedures is controversial. The increased intra abdominal and intra thoracic pressure can interfere and cause false readings. When laparoscopy is performed in upper abdomen in anti Trendelemburg position CVP monitoring is use full, even knowing that the readings may be false, the tendency r orientates to address the consequences of the volume alterations. Anyway low intravascular volume changes are produced in laparoscopic procedures.
The pulmonary artery catheterization allows estimating the ventricular after load by determining the pulmonary capillary pressure or pulmonary artery occlusion pressure; it also allows performing a complete hemodynamic study and managing the hemodynamic treatment. Its advantages are controversial, but in many anesthesiologist opinions it is very useful to manage patients with left ventricle disease, severe ischemic myocardial disease, hypertrophic myocardial disease, sub aortic idiopathic hypertrophic stenosis or pulmonary hypertension. The pulmonary artery catheter in one lung ventilation patients during thoracoscopic procedures has limitations, because it can be placed on the collapsed lower lung and don't reflect directly the left ventricle pressure. On the other hand, it results essential in heart diseases patients that to be able to stand the one lung ventilation and the pneumothorax, because they need to be treated with pre load increases and/or with ionotropic drugs.
Transesophageal ECG allows an early diagnosis when monitoring heart function and ischemia, more early than pulmonary artery catheterization. However it requires an uncommon high experience level to be useful.

6. Systemic disease patients

Different precautions must be taken in systemic disease patients depending on the particular disease.

6.1 Heart disease

The selection criteria for heart disease patient are multiple. It's important to remember that heart disease patients don't have to proposed to laparoscopic procedures just with the pretext of the lower postoperative care required, because that have been proved true just in healthy patients. Because of that reason, heart disease patient need to be managed by experienced anesthesiology teams. The hypertension risk, the hemorrhage risk after improper homeostasis and the hemodynamic modifications caused by the insufflation can derivate in to life-threatening complications easily on those patients.
It must be remembered that patients having a pacemaker should be treated with special care because monopolar electrosurgical scalpel can interfere with it. Plate must be placed properly and with caution, and heart mechanical activity should be monitored. In a surgery team with a good knowledge of technical equipment selection criteria can be different and only determinate by hemodynamic modifications risks.
It's prudent to reject patients with severe alterations of diastolic function on congestive heart failure. Controlled arterial hypertension or stabilized coronary insufficiencies are not considered contraindication, but it's basic to have them under control before surgery in order to decrease the perioperative mortality.
Cardiovascular complications incidence doesn't differ from open surgery procedures. An important factor is the perioperative cardiovascular monitoring in order to detect and treat any complication presented.

6.2 Respiratory disease

Respiratory complications after laparoscopic surgery are significantly lower than open surgery (Rose, 1992; Rothwell et al., 1992; Schwed et al., 1992).

Positioning and intra peritoneal pressures raise alveolar death space; witch can be already increased by diseases like in obstructive bronchopneumonia. The $EtCO_2$ contributes to underestimate the $PaCO_2$ in patients suffering chronic respiratory insufficiencies if we compare with healthy ones. A 20% of the intra peritoneal hypertension is transmitted to the thorax during controlled ventilation procedures, that fact increases the respiratory airways pressures, what is so harmful to patients suffering bullous emphysema.

The postoperative respiratory benefits it's a very important factor to keep in mind when indicating a laparoscopic procedure to patients suffering chronic respiratory insufficiency, because during postoperative period exists a lower diminution of the pulmonary volumes with a lower diaphragm dysfunction limited to the posterior region (Rothwell et al., 1992). A quicker recovery of pulmonary function is developed during postoperative period (Putensen-himer et al., 1992; Shear et al., 1992; Armengaud et al., 1992; Cooney et al., 1992; Mahul et al., 1992) achieving normal spirometry values in 72 hours in comparison with the 8 days that it takes to recover from laparotomy procedures. Those times are both increased in elderly patients.

Thoracoscopic procedures are recommended in patients suffering restrictive respiratory insufficiency without a significant increase in airways pressure. In patients suffering bullous emphysema and obstructive chronic respiratory insufficiencies insufflation pressures must be reduced as much as possible. Any serious respiratory complication like pneumothorax should stop the surgery. Recuperation must be smooth, avoiding tremors and agitation that may increase oxygen consumption. Anesthesia is maintained until an acceptable $PaCO_2$ is reached comparing with preoperative values; extubation is performed when early signs of tube rejection are observed.

6.3 Pregnant patients

Laparoscopy is the most common surgery performed on the first semester of pregnancy (Mazzo & Källen, 1989) and there are more advanced pregnancy cases described in literature.

The most common nonobstetric surgical procedures during pregnancy are adnexal surgery, appendectomy, and cholecystectomy, and they are amenable to laparoscopic surgery (Visser et al., 2001; As cited in Miller's Anesthesia 2005).Laparoscopy during pregnancy raises several concerns. Abdominal surgery increases the risk of miscarriage or premature labor. However, all the reports in the literature of laparoscopy carried out between 4 and 32 weeks of estimated gestational age have resulted in uncomplicated pregnancies (Lemarie & van Erp, 1997; Affleck et al., 1999; Barone et al., 1999; As cited in Miller's Anesthesia 2005).

The effects of increased IAP and hypercapnia on the human fetus were also investigated. CO_2 pneumoperitoneum induced significant fetal acidosis. Fetal heart rate and arterial pressure increased, but these changes were minimal (Hunter et al., 1995; As cited in Miller's Anesthesia 2005).

Hemodynamic changes induced by pneumoperitoneum are similar in pregnant and non-pregnant women (Steinbrook & Bhavani-Shankar, 2001; As cited in Miller's Anesthesia 2005).The following recommendations (Lemarie & van Erp, 1997; As cited in Miller's Anesthesia 2005)are for safe laparoscopy in pregnant patients:

1. The operation should occur during the second trimester, ideally before the 23rd week of pregnancy, to minimize the risk of preterm labor and to maintain an adequate intra-abdominal working room.
2. Tocolytics are beneficial to arrest preterm labor, but their prophylactic use is debatable.
3. Open laparoscopy should be used for abdominal access to avoid damaging the uterus.
4. Fetal monitoring may be performed using transvaginal ultrasonography.
5. Mechanical ventilation must be adjusted to maintain a physiologic maternal alkalosis.

6.4 Laparotomy

Patients that recently underwent laparotomy surgery or patients that have suffered peritonitis used to be considered as non indicated patients. Nowadays those conditions are not considered contraindicated anymore, but special care must be taken, especially regarding ectopic insufflation.

6.5 Urological disease

There are some indications in urology laparoscopies, like in other medical specialties, perfectly known and accepted coexisting with others that still need to be accepted.
Varicocele treatment has the advantage of avoiding postoperative pain, facilitating the back to normal active life in young patients.

6.6 Obesity

Morbid obesity has respiratory and cardiovascular risks that need to be addressed and controlled during laparoscopic surgeries. The Palmer needle and trocar insertion can be difficult, requiring the use of an open laparoscope, what increases the risk of carbon dioxide diffusion in the peritoneum. Moreover, the weight of the abdominal wall is an important factor increasing the abdominal pressure. The most important benefits for these patients are: the quick recovery, the decrease of thromboembolism risk and the early alimentation begin after surgery (Bromberg et al., 1992).

6.7 Glaucoma

The intra abdominal pressure rise is accompanied by an intraocular pressure rise, which is increased by Trendelemburg position (Hvidbreg et al., 1981) but is not always harmful in short periods of time. Laparoscopy is totally contraindicated in closed angle glaucoma patients.

6.8 Intracraneal hypertension

Insufflation and Trendelemburg positioning contribute to increase intracranial rise. Laparoscopic procedures are contraindicated in patients suffering important and acute (traumatic, tumor, hydrocephalus) cranial hypertension. Pharmacological treatment or temporal shunting can be performed to control the hypertension. If a recent ventriculoperitoneal shunt has been performed there is no contraindication because a non return valve is present. The leakage tests of these valves are not totally reliable when they are suspended in cephaloraquideum liquid. A diffusion of carbon dioxide occurs along the subcutaneous way of the valve (Schwed et al., 1992).Cerebral and retinal vascular accidents can occur.

7. Summary

Advantages derived from laparoscopic surgeries are multiple and well know: Minimal trauma is produced; it reduces postoperative pain and provides a quicker recovery shortening the hospital stay. Pneumoperitoneum induces intraoperative cardiorespiratory changes. $PaCO_2$ increases because of CO_2 absorption from the pneumoperitoneum. In systemic disease patients, cardiorespiratory disturbances aggravate this increase in $PaCO_2$. Improved knowledge of the pathophysiologic hemodynamic changes in healthy patients allows for successful anaesthetic management of cardiac patients, by optimizing preload before pneumoperitoneum and through judicious use of vasodilating drugs. Alternative insufflation gases don't seem to reduce hemodynamic changes; gasless laparoscopy is more helpful in that concern, but unfortunately increases technical difficulty. General anaesthesia with controlled ventilation seems to be the best technique for operative laparoscopy. The knowledge of the pathophysiologic changes occurring during pneumoperitoneum allows a safe management of the patients, even in those with systemic disease or cardiorespiratory complications.

8. Key points

The most remarkable facts regarding anaesthesia in laparoscopic procedures are (Miller, 2005):

- CO_2 pneumoperitoneum results in ventilatory and respiratory changes. Pneumoperitoneum decreases thoracopulmonary compliance. $PaCO_2$ increases (15% to 25%) by CO_2 absorption from the peritoneal cavity. Capnography reliably reflects this increase, which plateaus after 20 to 30 minutes.
- In compromised patients, cardiorespiratory disturbances aggravate the increase in $PaCO_2$ and enlarge the gradient between $PaCO_2$ and $EtCO_2$.
- Any increase in $EtCO_2$ larger than 25% and/or occurring later than 30 minutes after the beginning of peritoneal CO_2 insufflation should suggest CO_2 subcutaneous emphysema, the most frequent respiratory complication during laparoscopy.
- Peritoneal insufflation induces alterations of hemodynamics, characterized by decreases of cardiac output, elevations of arterial pressure, and increases of systemic and pulmonary vascular resistances. Hemodynamic changes are accentuated in high-risk cardiac patients.
- The pathophysiologic hemodynamic changes can be attenuated or prevented by optimizing preload before pneumoperitoneum and by vasodilating agents, α_2-adrenergic receptors antagonists, high doses of opioids, and β-blocking agents.
- Similar pathophysiologic changes occur during pregnancy and in children. Laparoscopy can be safely managed in pregnant women before the 23rd week of pregnancy provided by that hypercapnia is prevented. The open laparoscopy approach should be considered to avoid damaging the uterus.
- Gasless laparoscopy may be helpful to reduce pathopysiologic changes induced by CO2 pneumoperitoneum but unfortunately increases technical difficulty.
- Laparoscopy results in multiple postoperative benefits allowing for quicker recovery and shorter hospital stay. These advantages explain the increasing success of laparoscopy, which is proposed for many surgical procedures.
- Improved knowledge of the intraoperative repercussions of laparoscopy permits safe management of patients with more and more severe cardiorespiratory disease, who may subsequently benefit from the multiple postoperative advantages offered by this technique.

9. References

Armengaud MH, Pipien J, Trevoux-Paul J, Alexandre JH, Cousin MT. Fonction pulmonaire après cholécystectomie par laparoscopie. Annales Françaises d'Anesthésie et de Réanimation. 1992; 11:R84

Bromberg N, Matuszak JP, Delecluze Ph, Atat I, Prevot JM, Krivosic-Horberor. Fonction pulmonaire après cholécystectomie par voie laparoscopique chez l'obèse. Ann Fr Anesth Réanim 1992;11:R20

Carrasco MS, Gomar C, Jiménez MJ, Martín MF & Lima JR. Consideraciones anestésicas en la cirugía endoscópica en humanos. In: Carrasco MS, Usón J, eds. Aprendizaje y Aplicación de la Anestesia en Cirugía Toracoscópica. Edika Med. 1998; 132–135

Cooney CM, Lyons JB, Hennigan A, Blunnie WP, Moriarty DC. Ventilatory function following laparoscopic cholecystectomy. (Abstract). Canadian Journal of Anaesthesia. 1992; 39: A54

Hvidberg A, Kessing SV, Fernandes A. Effect of changes in PCO_2 and body positions on intraocular pressure during general anaesthesia. Acta Ophthalmologica (Copenhagen). 1981 Aug; 59(4):465-75.

Joris JL, Hamoir EE, Hartstein GM, Meurisse MR, Hubert BM, Charlier CJ & Lamy ML. Hemodynamic changes and catecholamine release during laparoscopic adrenalectomy for pheochromocytoma. Anesthesia and Analgesia. 1999; 88:16-21.

Kaplan MB, Rogers R. Laparoscopic Surgery: A View From the Head of the Table. Seminars in Laparoscopic Surgery. 1994 Dec; 1(4):207-210.

Lew JK, Gin T, Oh TE. Anaesthetic problems during laparoscopic cholecystectomy. Anaesthesia and Intensive Care. 1992 Feb; 20(1):91-2.

Llagostera-Pujol S, Dilme-Muñoz J, Yeste-Campos M, Escudero-Rodríguez JR & Viver-Manresa E. Cirugía laparoscópica del aneurisma abdominal. Angiología. 2002; 54(3):252-258.

Mahul PH, Bou B, El Khoury, Riffat J, Massardier N, Guillot B. Fonction respiratorie et cholécystectomie par coelioscope digestive. Annales Françaises d'Anesthésie et de Réanimation. 1992; 11: R83.

Mazze RI, Källén B. Reproductive outcome after anesthesia and operation during pregnancy: a registry study of 5405 cases. American Journal of Obstetrics and Gynecology. 1989 Nov; 161(5):1178-85.

Miller RD. Miller's Anesthesia, 6th ed. Philadelphia, Elsevier, 2005, p 2287.

Putensen-Himmer G, Putensen C, Lammer H, Lingnau W, Aigner F, Benzer H. Comparison of postoperative respiratory function after laparoscopy or open laparotomy for cholecystectomy. Anesthesiology. 1992; 77(4):675-80.

Rose DK, Cohen MM, Soutter DI. Laparoscopic cholecystectomy: the anaesthetist's point of view. Canadian Journal of Anaesthesia. 1992 Oct; 39(8):809-15.

Rothwell BC, Katagiri M, Young RN, Nixon JA, Easton PA. Costal and crural diaphragm function after laparoscopic cholecystectomy. American review of respiratory disease. 1992; 145:A152

Schwed DA, Edoga JK, McDonnell TE. Ventilatory impairment during laparoscopic cholecystectomy in a patient with a ventriculoperitoneal shunt. Journal of Laparoendoscopic Surgery. 1992; Feb; 2(1):57-9.

Shear JM, Holtmann B, White PF. Pulmonary function following laparoscopic cholecystectomy [abstract]. Anesthesia and Analgesia. 1992; 74: 5286.

Part 3

Benefits and Indications

3

Laparoscopy in Gynecology - How Why When

A.Daniilidis, P.Hatzis, G.Pratilas,
P.D.Loufopoulos and K.Dinas
University Department Of Obstetrics And Gynecology,
Aristotle University Of Thessaloniki,
Greece

1. Introduction

Laparoscopy is a surgical procedure that has been used widely in medicine over 30 years. The faster recovery time, the minimizing of pain, hospitalization and the better aesthetic result are some of the advantages which made laparoscopy very popular among patients and surgeons. Also some technical parameters such as the magnification offered by the endoscope during the procedure and the small risk of complications resulted to the wide use of laparoscopic surgery in gynecology. Laparoscopy has gained a leading role and appears to be the gold standard method for a quiet wide range of gynecologic procedures such as tubal ligation, removal of ovarian cyst or adnexa, treatment of ectopic pregnancy, hemorrhagic rupture of a cyst, exploration of chronic pelvic pain, sterility, treatment of endometriosis, removal of fibromyomata , hysterectomy, and lately for treatment of pelvic organ prolapses, urinary incontinence and even in gynecologic cancers. Despite the advantages of laparoscopic procedures, they do not come without risk and complications for the patient. As with laparotomy there is always danger for deep vein thrombosis, inflamation and creation of adhesions. It should be noted though that compared to laparotomy there is a higher risk of injury to the major blood vessels positioned in the pelvis and the urinary system, and that is why patients considered to be subjected to laparoscopy should be carefully chosen.

2. Limitations of laparoscopy

In the case of patient selection previous abdominal surgery is the most common reason to exclude a laparoscopic approach, because of the risk of adhesions. For the same reason, patients that have a medical history of appendicitis , rupture of ectopic pregnancy, rupture of an ovarian cyst, or pelvic inflammatory disease should be selected very carefully. Also morbid obese patients (BMI >45) are in a higher risk group for laparoscopy. This is firstly because of the increased adipose tissue, so initial access to the peritoneal cavity is more difficult and also there is a need for longer trocar ports and instruments, and secondly because obese patient will have greater peak airway pressures and often cannot sustain prolonged Trendelenberg position.

3. Instruments used

As with all laparoscopic procedures the basic tool used is the endoscope-laparoscope. There are many variations in diameter size : 10 mm, 5 mm, and even 2 mm ,and laparoscopes with a 0 or 30 degrees angle of view. Trocars of 5mm and 10mm are usually used in order to gain access and insert instruments into the peritoneal cavity. Veress needle is the preferred method of a lot of surgeons in creating the pneumoperitoneum , but there are also optical-access trocars available for the same task. As with all laparoscopic procedures we use an CO2 endoflator to provide the gas needed to create the pneumoperitoneum and an imaging unit that is generaly composed of a light source, a camera head that attaches to the endoscope, it's camera control unit and an display screen. While performing the operation there are a lot of different instruments that can be used (IMAGE 1). Concerning the manipulation of tissue there are different kind of forceps: dissecting and grasping, single or double action, traumatic or atraumatic depending on the design of the distal tip. The same variety can be found in scissors, with them having straight or curved blades, with some of them being also serrated, as well as the hook-like scissors. The next basic set of tools are those used to perform electrosurgery, and they consist of unipolar tools in the shape of needle,hook or spatula shaped electrodes, and of bipolar forceps and scissors. Alternative methods to electrosurgery are the use of laser and ultrasound dissection and coagulation systems. Other tools used are suction and irrigation cannulas, aspiration needles, extraction bags, needle holders for intracorporeal suturing techniques and knot tiers for extracorporeal knotting,uterine manipulators and finally morcellator systems for the removal of large tissue specimens like fibroids or the uterus.

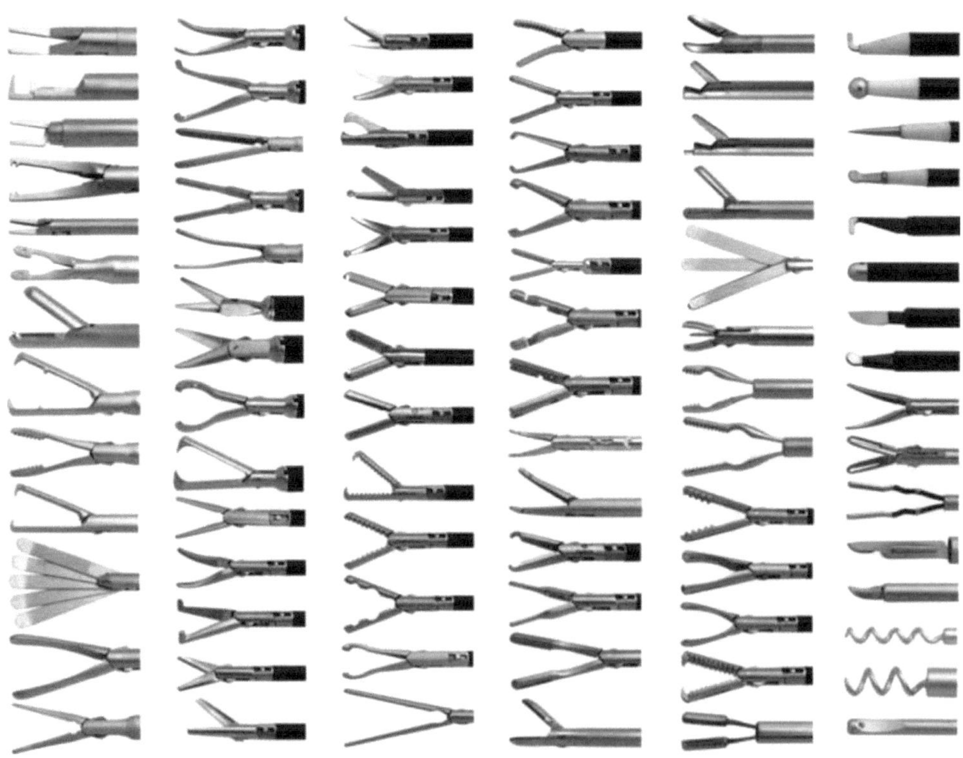

Fig. 1. Instruments for laparoscopy in gynecology

4. Patient preparation, positioning and procedures

In preparation for surgery, bowel preparation is useful as it empties the small intestine, thus facilitating vision and manoeuvrability by flattening the intestinal loops and pushing them out of the way. It must be commented that when the case is associated with an increased risk of intestinal injury, as in endometriosis of the rectovaginal septum or in major adhesiolysis, the bowel preparation must be more complete, similar to that applied prior to major bowel surgery.
Concerning the position of the patient, her arms should be padded and carefully tucked to the side and after the anesthesia and the intubation she is placed in a low lithotomy position (IMAGE 2). The legs are held in position, supported by padded obstetric knee braces or Allen stirrups.

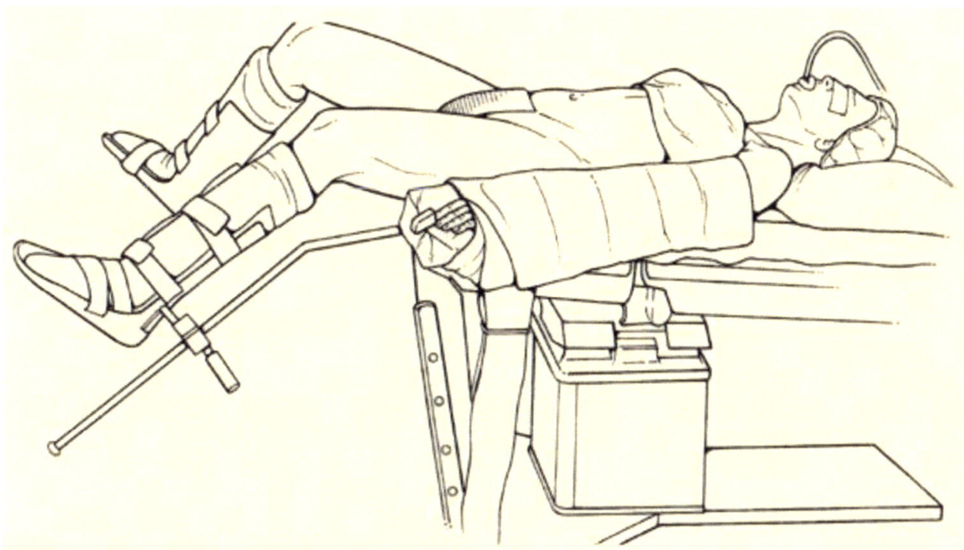

Fig. 2. Position of the patient

Abdominal and vaginal preparation follows, and afterwards a Foley catheter is placed, as is also a uterine manipulator with sterile technique.
The surgeon is placed on the left side of the patient with the first assistant on the right side and the second between the legs to use the manipulator. In cases where the surgeon is left handed he occupies the right side of the patient. The operation begins usually with an intra- or infraumbilical incision from where the Veress needle is inserted creating the pneumoperitoneum. Afterwards the main (10mm) trocar is inserted trough the same incision, after removing the Veress neddle, and the laparoscope is positioned through it. An alternative is open laparoscopy using a Hasson trocar, and is recommended for patients who have had prior abdominal surgery as it provides safe and easy access to the peritoneal cavity with minimal complications (0.5%). Types of trocars and placement methods are widely variable and are well described in both academic and industry literature. Usually two to three extra trocars (5mm usually or 10mm) are placed for most operative gynaecologic laparoscopic surgeries, two lateral and in some cases one suprapubic (IMAGE 3). The suprapubic port should be placed 3 to 4 cm above the symphysis pubis to avoid bladder injury. The lower

quadrant ports should be placed at the level of the iliac crest lateral to both the rectus muscle and inferior epigastric vessels, which are visible with the laparoscope through the peritoneum.[1]

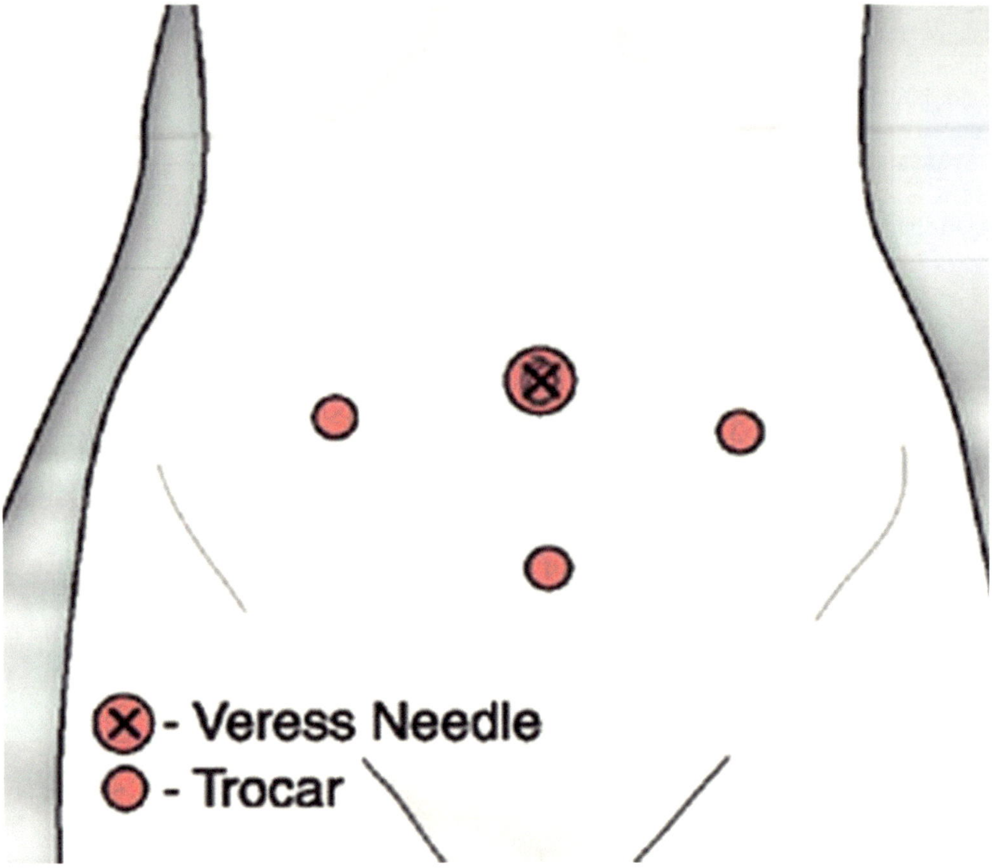

Fig. 3. Position of trocars in gynecologic operations

5. Tubal ligation

Tubal ligation is a popular and reliable method of contraception for women usually over 30 years old who have completed their family (IMAGE 4). The procedure can be executed by creating either one single umbilical port hole, if using an operative laparoscope, or usually by creating two port holes, one umbilical and one suprapubic. The general rules of gynaecological laparoscopic operations apply here also : creation of pneumoperitoneum, use of a manipulator to control the uterus and recognise well the anatomic structures of the adnexa. It is important to accuretly recognise the fallopian tube and not to avoid mistaking the round ligament for it. Once recognised there are different methods for lingation : use of bipolar or monopolar current, use of metallic clips or falop ring bands, and resection with the use of sutures to ligate. When complications occur they are most commonly haemorrhage from the fallopian tube or the mesosalpinx, and they rate from 0,1 to 4,6 % . [3-7]. The occurrence of major complications (0,6 %) like vascular injury, bowel perforation or damage to the genitourinary tract is really rare. It must be commented that depending on the technique used there are different rates of failure with the greater appearing in ligation with bipolar current and the best result when resection is used.[2,3,4]

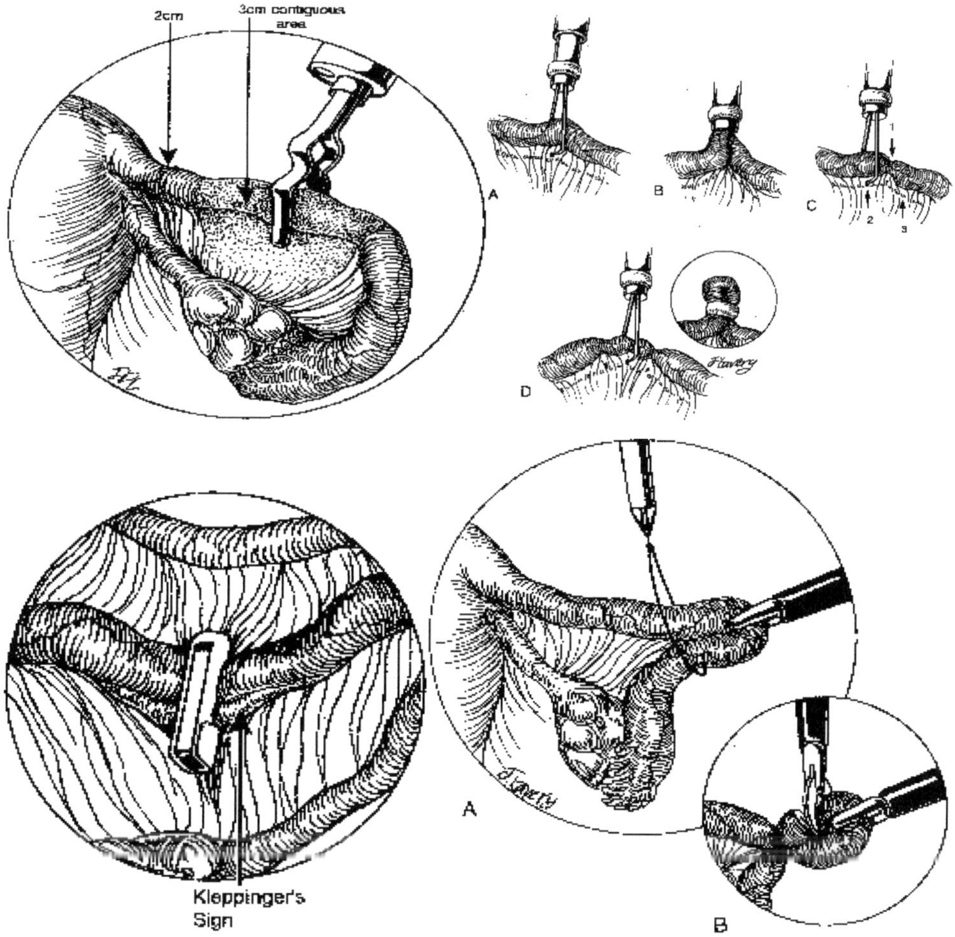

Fig. 4. Tubal ligation

6. Diagnostic laparoscopy

Another area where laparoscopy is thought to be the gold standard method is when performing a diagnostic operation. It is a minimal invasive procedure with the use of one only umbilical port that allows to visualize the lower pelvis in a great extent. Also with the introduction of more than one ports and the use of the proper instruments and technique to treat the problem that is discovered. Diagnostic laparoscopy is used for the investigation of chronic pelvic pain and infertility. In cases of women with chronic pelvic pain, various pathology might be discovered like endometriosis, adhesions, pelvic inflammatory disease, or other kind of urinary tract or bowel pathology. The first three findings are a major factor in the occurrence of female infertility, and can be explored or treated with laparoscopy. [8]

Adhesions are treated by the use of electrosurgery, CO2 laser ablation and if they are in a great proximity to structures like bowel or bladder with the use of dissecting scissors, always taking care not to damage these structures. In the case of pelvic inflammatory disease the fallopian tubes are checked for patency with the infusion of a colour agent like methylene blue from the uterus manipulator and the observation if the colour agent appears from the end of the fallopian tube. In cases of fimbrial phimosis surgical repair can be performed by inserting a closed fine atraumatic grasping forceps into the area of the phimosis and gradually opening it's jaws. This manipulation must be done very gently to avoid bleeding. [1]

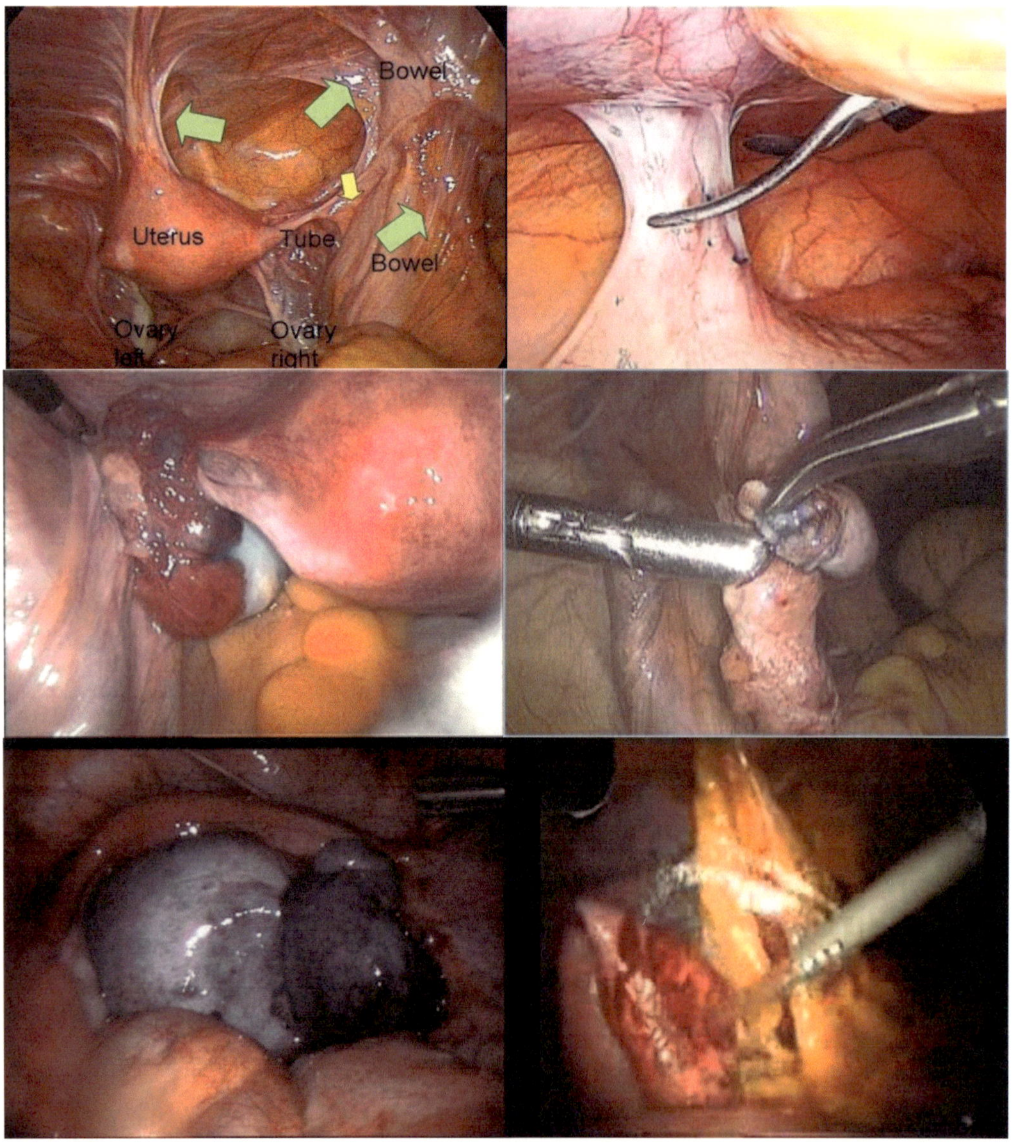

Fig. 4. Findins of diagnostic laparoscopy-adhesions, pid, tubal fimosis, ovarian absess

In the case of tubo-ovarian abscess it can also be treated laparoscopicaly by perforating the wall of the abscess, then draining it's content with an aspiration device and then irrigating it until the aspired fluid it completely clear
Endometriosis is described more thorough in the next paragraph and is treated depending on the stage it is. At early stages ablation with current or with CO2 laser is used, or if endometriotic cysts are found they are removed as described in adnexal syrgery.

7. Endometriosis

Endometriosis seems to be responsible for most pathological cases of chronic pelvic pain and also for the highest percentage of cases who are referred with primary and secondary infertility[9] . Laparoscopy holds a special place in the diagnosis of this problem as it is the gold standard diagnostic test in clinical practice for the accurate diagnosis of endometriosis [10]. Compared with laparoscopy, transvaginal ultrasound (TVS) has limited value in diagnosing peritoneal endometriosis, but it is a useful tool to make or exclude the diagnosis of an ovarian endometrioma [11]. At present, there is insufficient evidence to indicate that magnetic resonance imaging (MRI) is a useful test to diagnose or exclude endometriosis compared to laparoscopy [10]. A number of markers for endometriosis have been proposed, and probably the most commonly used is the glycoprotein CA-125, an oncofetal celomic epithelium differentiation antigen. It has been suggested that 35 U/ml could be used as a cut-off serum concentration for CA-125, below which endometriosis is unlikely to be present. Unfortunately CA- 125 measurements do not correlate well with either the progression of the disease or the response of endometriosis to treatment. Compared with laparoscopy, measuring serum levels of CA-125 has no value as a diagnostic tool. The test's performance in diagnosing all disease stages is limited, since it has about 28% sensitivity [12]. The test's performance for moderate to severe endometriosis is a bit better with a sensitivity reaching 47% [12].

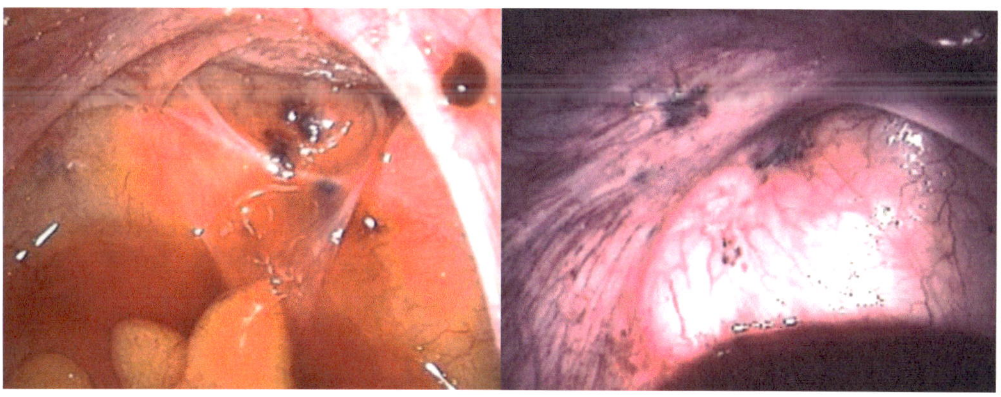

Fig. 5. Endometriosis

8. Adnexal surgery

It is important in the case of treatment of adnexal pathology, to have a full preoperative evaluation and estimation of the probability of malignancy because the manoeuvres done during laparoscopy could create peritoneal dissemination altering the stage and thus the afterwards treatment. This evaluation includes bimanual pelvic examination, sonography, a CT scan, a full blood count, tumor markers, and a pregnancy test. Surgery of the adnexa includes ectopic pregnancy and benign cysts and tumors of the ovaries.

In the case of ectopic pregnancy the indicated methods include salpingostomy of salpingectomy. Salpingostomy is done by creating a linear incision on the dilated part of the fallopian tube and then using forceps to remove the ectopic pregnancy tissue. The fallopian tube does not need to be closed afterwards. In some occasions the fallopian tube is totally removed in order to exclude the ectopic pregnancy.It is important to use and irrigation-aspiration system to remove as much blood as possible from the peritoneal cavity in order to avoid adhesions and pain post op.

An other possibility is the removal of the tumor/cyst (hemorrhagic corpus luteum, cystadenoma, teratoma, endometrioma while maintaining the rest of the ovarian tissue. This is done with careful dissection of the cyst, by using forceps for traction on both the cyst and the ovary and then using scissors, electrosurgery or blunt dissection to separate the cyst fron the ovary tissue.

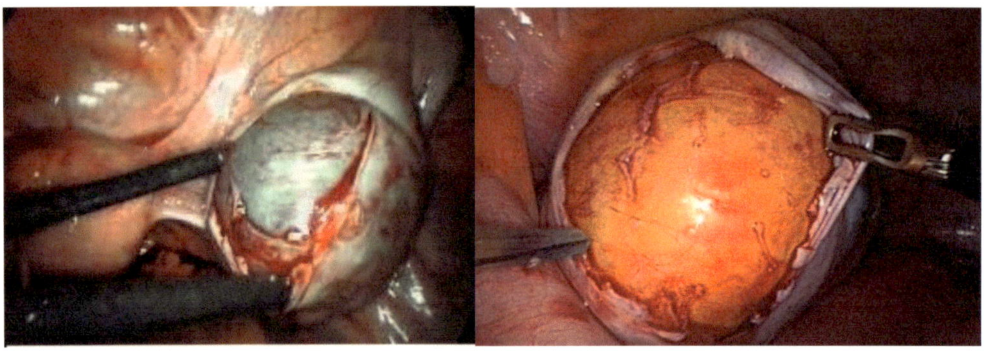

Fig. 6.

In women of older age or if excision of the cyst is not feasible , an alternative is laparoscopic salpingo-oophorectomy. In this case, the ovary is hold by an grasper atraumatic or Babcock forceps , the peritoneum is incised lateral to the ovary from the round ligament to the pelvic brim. The ureter is visualized, and the infundibulopelvic ligament is ligated and divided. The remainder of the broad ligament is dissected to the utero-ovarian ligament, which is ligated securely.

In both of the previous cases the dissected tissue is securely placed in endo bag and is usually removed via a10 mm trocar port. There are different kind of cases in this phase of the operation : The cyst being small enough to be removed directly from the trocar port, or the the cyst being too large, but then we can aspire it's content through the trocar port shrinking it enough so it can exit more easily. Lastly in cases where the cyst is too large and has a great solid portion we can perform a mini lap by extending the incision of a trocar port and removing it through there. It is important that this is our last step after inspecting carefully the endoperitoneal cavity and irrigating and aspiring any blood, because after the mini lap is performed it is difficult to maintain the pneumoperitoneum any more.

Lastly laparoscopy can be used for only aspiring the content of cysts, or taking only biopsies with the use of a true-cut sampler. These patients are selected cases where we are almost sure of the mass being benign and have a persistent (about 6 months) unilocular ovarian cyst on ultrasound and desire both ovarian preservation and immediate return to daily activities.

9. Myomectomy

Laparoscopic myomectomy constitutes a satisfying solution especially for women who wish to maintain fertility potential. The technique looks similar to laparotomy and is used in cases of myomas larger than 5 cm. Pedunculated uterine myomata usually are removed safely with either electrosurgery or harmonic scalpel. The removal of subserosal and intramural fibroids seem to be more challenging and requires surgical skills . The uterine incision is performed with electrosurgery and the myoma capsule is dissected in its entirety. Electrosurgery, sharp dissection and laser have been successfully performed for myomectomy. The myometrium should be closed with 0 or 2-0 absorbable suture and the serosa with 4-0 suture. Endometrial cavity's integrity can be evaluated by injecting indigo carmine dye after myomectomy. The results of myomectomy in an oncoming pregnancy or delivery are still under discussion.

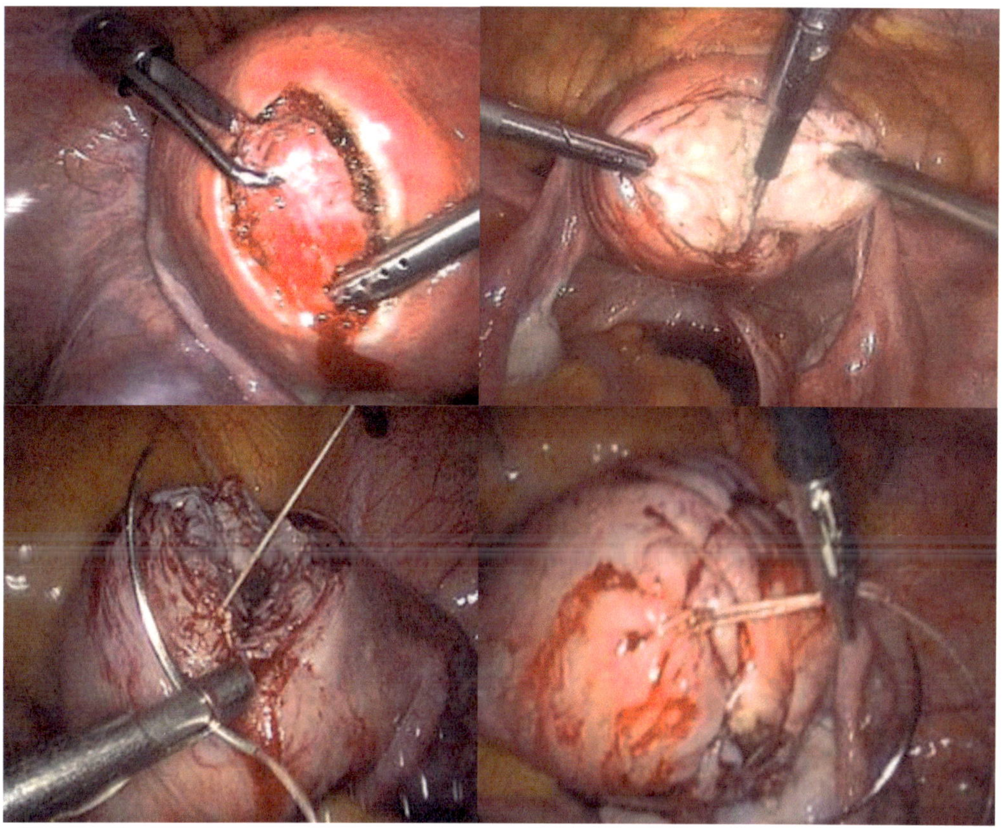

Fig. 7.

10. Hysterectomy

Hysterectomy is the commonest surgical operation in non-pregnant women. Laparoscopy was firstly performed in order to assist vaginal hysterectomy. Laparoscopic assisted vaginal hysterectomy (LAVH) increases the visualization of the upper pelvis and allows difficult operations to be performed, where extended adhesions or large ovaries consist.

Additionally, this technique has been documented by prospective, randomized, multicenter studies to be safer and more efficacy in blood loss, operative complications, postoperative pain and hospital stay than LAVH. Electrosurgical technologies, such as harmonic scalpel, Ligasure, bipolar cautery, have been developed to perform uterial artery ablation safely.
The laparoscopic hysterectomy (LSH) has a significantly shorter operative time than LAVH or total abdominal hysterectomy, shorter hospital stay and fewer complications. Essential supposition is a normal cervical cytology of the patient. Total laparoscopic hysterectomy (TLH) is a similar technique to LSH, which additionally uses a colpotomizer in order to facilitate the vaginal incision. Data by the Cochrane database have analyzed differences between TAH, TVH, and LH. Meta-analysis compared LH to TAH and found LH to be associated with reduced blood loss, shorter hospital stay, more rapid return to normal activity and fewer infections. LH had longer operating times and more frequent injuries of ureter and bladder. No difference between TVH and LH were mentioned.[14-20]

11. Laparoscopy in cancer

Endometrial cancer

Laparoscopic surgery of endometrial cancer involves resection of the uterus, cervix, tubes, ovaries and pelvic and para-aortic lymph nodes. The surgery is both diagnostic (staging) and therapeutic (80% cure). Laparoscopic pelvic and para-aortic lymph node sampling and pelvic cytology are added to the previously described hysterectomy procedures.The operative staging procedure usually includes total extrafascial hysterectomy, bilateral adnexectomy, intraperitoneal exploration, cytological washing and lymphadenectomy. Laparoscopic approach is a longer operation but involves less blood loss, a shorter hospitalization, and fewer intraoperative and postoperative complications.[21-23]

Cervical cancer

Early cervical cancers are treated surgically, by radical abdominal hysterectomy and pelvic lymphadenectomy (RAH). The main difference between RAH and TAH is that during RAH, lymphatic tissue is removed lateral to the uterus. Mobilizing the ureter makes surgeon's movements safer. Lymph nodes usually removed are common iliac, external and internal iliac. A few reports for laparoscopic radical hysterectomy and lymphadenectomy show that it is combined with larger operative time (even for experienced surgeons), less blood loss, fewer complications and a shorter hospital stay.[24,25]

Ovarian cancer

The rate of confirmed malignancy in patients with adnexal masses ranges between 0,3 to 1,2% and the publication of case histories describing undetected ovarian cancers treated by laparoscopy has given rise to criticism of this type of procedure. Ovarian cancer staging includes removal of the affected ovary and fallopian tube, pelvic and para-aortic lymph nodes, infracolic omentectomy, pelvic and subdiaphragmatic washings, and multiple peritoneal biopsies (anterior, posterior, right, and left pelvis; right and left para-colic spaces; beneath the diaphragm; and any suspicious areas). Uterus should be excised except of the cases that patient wishes to maintain fertility potential (only for Ia to Ic stage of disease). Additionally to these, laparoscopy can be performed for checking possible recurrence of disease, especially in cases of women with ovarian cancer who have a moderate elevation in the biomarker CA-125 postoperationally.

12. Training

Training for laparoscopic surgery in gynecologic oncology takes place at most fellowship programs. Dry labs can provide familiarity with instrumentation, practice with pelvic simulators, and, sometimes, realistic teaching with advanced computerized simulators. Porcine labs may allow novice surgeons an opportunity to train and learn to manage surgical complications with the laparoscope. As with most surgical procedures, confidence is gained through mentorship, careful patient selection, and repetition. Laparoscopic techniques are gaining popularity and probably will become the standard of care for endometrial cancer, because the newly trained gynecologic oncologists are well versed in these techniques.

13. Conclusions

Laparoscopic gynecologic surgery has become common place in today's gynecologic practice. As a method it provides many benefits for the patient as a minimal invasive procedure, either it is performed as a purely diagnostic procedure or as a surgical treatment. It is considered the gold standard method for exploring infertility or chronic pelvic pain as the gynecologist can explore with direct view the pelvis and the hole peritoneal cavity without subjecting the patient to the extent trauma of laparotomy. It also has a unique value in the diagnosis of endometriosis as it is the only mean of setting a sure diagnosis through direct view. Today more and more classic gynecologic operations are being replaced by laparoscopy, like tubal lingation, adnexal surgery, myomectomy, hysterectomy, and even cases of gynecologic cancer. Despite the numerous advantages it provides, it should not be considered a panacea, as it remains a surgical procedure and has the risk of complications as every other procedure. It is also important to consider that the first steps of the laparoscopic procedure are done in a "blind" way, so the selection of which patients are suitable for the procedure is something that must be done correctly, excluding patients that might be classified as high risk.

14. References

[1]Luka Mencaglia, Luka Minelli, Arnaud Wattiez, Manual of gynecological laparoscopic surgery

[2] Schwartz DB, Wingo PA, Antarsh L, et al. Female sterilization in the United States, 1987. Fam Plann Perspect 1989;21:209–12.

[3] Peterson HB, Xia Z, Hughes JM, et al. The risk of pregnancy after tubal sterilization: findings from the U.S. Collaborative Review of Sterilization. Am J Obstet Gynecol 1996;174: 1161–8.

[4] Peterson HB, Xia Z, Wilcox L, et al. Pregnancy after tubal sterilization with bipolar electrocoagulation.Obstet Gynecol 1999;94:163–7.

[5] Huber AW, Mueller MD, Ghezzi F, et al. Tubal sterilization: complications of laparoscopy and minilaparotomy. Eur J Obstet Gynecol Reprod Biol 2007;134:105–9.

[6] Chaovisitsaree S, Piyamongkol W, Pongsatha S, et al. Immediate complications of laparoscopic tubal sterilization: 11 years of experience. J Med Assoc Thai 2004;87:1147–50.

[7] Jamieson DJ, Hillis SD, Duerr A, et al. Complications of interval laparoscopic tubal sterilization: findings from the United States collaborative review of sterilization. Obstet Gynecol 2000;96:997–1002.

[8] Christopher P. DeSimone, MDa,Frederick R. Ueland, Mda, Gynecologic Laparoscopy, Surg Clin N Am 88 (2008) 319–341
[9]A. Daniilidis & H. Giannoulis & T. Tantanasis &K. Papathanasiou & A. Loufopoulos & J. Tzafettas Diagnostic laparoscopy, infertility, and endometriosis – 5 years experience Gynecol Surg DOI 10.1007/s10397-007-0357-7
[10] Royal College of Obstetricians and Gynecologists (2006) Greentop guideline no 24. The investigation and management of endometriosis. RCOG, London
[11] Moore J, Copley S, Morris J, Lindsell D, Golding S, Kennedy S (2002) A systematic review of the accuracy of ultrasound in the diagnosis of endometriosis. Ultrasound Obstet Gynecol 20: 630–634
[12] Mol BW, Bayram N, Lijmer JG, Wiegerinck MA, Bongers MY, van der Veen F et al (1998) The performance of CA-125 measurement in the detection of endometriosis: a meta-analysis. Fertile Steril 70:1101–1118
[13] Marana R, Busacca M, Zupi E, et al. Laparoscopically assisted vaginal hysterectomy versus total abdominal hysterectomy: a prospective, randomized, multicenter study. Am J Obstet Gynecol 1999;180:270–5.
[14] Muzii L, Basile S, Zupi E, et al. Laparoscopic-assisted vaginal hysterectomy versus minilaparotomy hysterectomy: a prospective, randomized, multicenter study. J Minim Invasive Gynecol 2007;14:610–5.
[15] Bojahr R, Raatz D, Schonleber G, et al. Perioperative complications in 1706 patients after a standardized laparoscopic supracervical hysterectomy technique. JMinim Invasive Gynecol 2006;13:183–9.
[16] Milad MP,Morrison K, Sokol A, et al. A comparison of laparoscopic supracervical hysterectomy versus laparoscopic assisted vaginal hysterectomy. Surg Endosc 2001;15:286–8.
[17] El-Mowafi D, Madkour W, Lall C, et al. Laparoscopic supracervical hysterectomy versus laparoscopic vaginal hysterectomy. J Am Assoc Gynecol Laparosc 2004;11:175–80.
[18] Sarmini OR, Lefholz K, Froeschke HP. A comparison of laparoscopic supracervical hysterectomy and total abdominal hysterectomy outcomes. J Minim Invasive Gynecol 2005;12: 121–4.
[19] Cheung VY, Rosenthal DM, Morton M, et al. Total laparoscopic hysterectomy: a five-year experience. J Obstet Gynaecol Can 2007;29:337–43.
[20] O'Hanlan KA, Dibble SL, Garnier AC, et al. Total laparoscopic hysterectomy: technique and complications of 830 cases. JSLS 2007;11:45–53. 340 DESIMONE & UELAND
[21] Zapico A, Fuentes P, Grassa A, et al. Laparoscopic-assisted vaginal hysterectomy versus abdominal hysterectomy in stages I and II endometrial cancer: operating data, follow up and survival. Gynecol Oncol 2005;98:222–7.
[22] Obermair A, Manolitsas TP, Leung Y, et al. Total laparoscopic hysterectomy versus total abdominal hysterectomy for obese women with endometrial cancer. Int J Gynecol Cancer 2005;15:319–24.
[23] Malur S, Possover M, Michels W, et al. Laparoscopic-assisted vaginal versus abdominal surgery in patients with endometrial cancer- a prospective randomized trial. Gynecol Oncol 2001;80:239–44.
[24] Frumovitz M, Reis R, Sun C, et al. Comparison of total laparoscopic and abdominal hysterectomy for patients with early-stage cervical cancer. Obstet Gynecol 2007;110:96–102.
[25] Ghezzi F, Cromi A, Ciravolo G, et al. Surgicopathologic outcome of laparoscopic versus open radical hysterectomy. Gynecol Oncol 2007;106:502–6.

Part 4

Difficulties, Risks and Complications

4

Inappropriate Circumstances for Laparoscopic Surgery

Atilla Şenaylı[1] and Yeşim Şenaylı[2]
[1]*Pediatric Surgery, T.C.S.B. Etlik İhtisas Education and Research Hospital*
[2]*Anesthesiology and Reanimation, T.C.S.B. Health Education General Directorate*
Turkey

1. Introduction

Laparoscopy is increasingly selected instead of the laparotomies at the last three decades. The earliest indications of laparoscopies were mostly for gynaecological treatments and cholecystectomies (Cunningham, 1998). Since then, spectrum has been expanding. Increasing laparoscopy experience caused expansion of the indications and, contrary to this, declining the contraindications. So, it can actually be accepted that, in the near future, there will be trace contraindications for laparoscopic procedures. Gastrointestinal operations, especially bowel obstruction treatments are attentive for this trend, thus increased surgical experience and improved surgical instrumentation changed opinions about the most emphasized contraindications for laparoscopic surgery (Reissman & Spira, 2003). Consequently, surgeons who are willing to learn and develop their skills have to observe changes efficiently as laparoscopy indications, contraindications and risks definitions has been changing fast.

In a lot of studies, it was proved that surgeons' experience is the important factor for successful laparoscopies and many obstacles like laparoscopy-related complications, conversion rate, morbidity and mortality rates decreased with increasing experience (Tekkıs et al, 2005). As Jansen et al explained, technical improvement and increasing experience in laparoscopy will probably continue to reduce the incidence of surgical complications (Jansen et al, 1997). Soot et al also reported significant decreases in the rates of the problems like conversions and they experienced that conversions rates changed from their first 25 patients to last 25 patients sharply in fundoplication cases (Soot et al, 1999).

Problems detected after gaining experience are usually the issues of technical problems and patient-related problems. Contraindications, in other words: not performing laparoscopy and conversions are main aspects of technical and patient related problem that interfere using laparoscopy or completing the laparoscopic attempts. We can easily put forward by evaluating the literature that contraindications will be minimized but if conversions are not focused on, the presence of this aspect may prevent authors from reaching successful laparoscopic results. Therefore, conversions must be evaluated in great attention. Conversion means changing laparoscopic procedure to open procedure because of intraoperative difficulties. Conversions, as mentioned above, can be related to experience but also to technical and patient's problems. Conversion is not a defeat but choosing the most appropriate way of treating the patient (Agresta et al, 2004). Simopoluos et al also considered the conversion as an alteration, not a failure, of the operative plan due to anatomic problems to avoid further complications (Simopoluos et al, 2005). In our opinion, conversions are not complications but should rather be considered as salvage for preventing more serious problems. Surgeons convert laparoscopies to prevent patients from possible injuries (Reissman & Spira, 2003). If there is a doubt for safety and efficiency of the operative procedure, the surgeon should convert the procedure immediately to an open procedure (Cucinotta et al, 1998).

The entity, conversion, confused authors for laparoscopic operations. Thus, there are still controversies about performing laparoscopy for some conditions. These controversies are prolongation of the hospital stay and conversion related complications. From the patients' view, it can be said that they are disappointed with spending more time in hospital, facing complications related to conversion and consuming more money consequent to a laparoscopic operation converted to an open procedure. From the surgeons' view, conversions have not only been a failure in decision-making but also have been a disappointment and discouragement (Marusch et al, 2001). Significantly increased postoperative morbidity and mortality because of the conversions may be recognized for the disappointment of the surgeon (Marusch et al, 2001). Therefore, this situation forced surgeons through laparotomy particularly in private practice or in non-teaching hospitals which interrupt the expansions of the procedure (Dubuisson et al, 2001).

Delis et al stress that a correct preoperative decision making for operation style can only be made with preoperative prediction of postoperative morbidity for each patient (Delis et al, 2010). It was pointed out that knowing the variables associated with the risk of conversion would avoid wasteful laparoscopic attempts by proceeding directly to an open operation. (Simopoluos et al, 2005). Schmidt et al defined this entity as knowledge of the factors associated with success or failure of the laparoscopic approach and surgeon who has this knowledge will be cautious for preoperative preparation and counseling of patients (Schmidt et al, 2001).

According to all these considerations, conversions can be determined as perfect situations for a surgeon to face with patients' circumstance defining a real unsuitable factor for laparoscopy. Therefore, based on the above information, in our study, we expected to highlight the variable kind of situations forces surgeons to change their intraoperative plan and so, we try to structure a description for the inappropriate circumstances of the diseases for laparoscopy. For this, we evaluated conversions to find clues of predictive factors and to lighten surgeons for systematized decision-making of operations.

2. Evaluation method for the conversions

Some retrospective studies have already been taken their places in literature for predictability of conversions. For instance, Shen et al shared their experience with laparoscopic adrenalectomy to evaluate the reasons for conversion and to identify the high risk patients requiring conversion (Shen et al, 2004). We evaluated the English literature and detected a lot of articles mentioned about conversions. We focused on different types of articles like case reports, prospective and retrospective studies, reviews and meta-analysis. Among these reports we pay attention on complications, contraindications and especially on conversions. Our main purpose is to understand the operations that were converted to laparotomy and "Results" sections of the selected articles were especially evaluated. The situations of these patients figured out that patients could be operated with laparoscopy but for some reasons the operations were ended as laparotomies which meant that something interfere the surgeons' laparoscopy success. After the formation of this article subgroup, we sought for the reasons of conversions. Conversions occurred during the *"laparoscopic approach"*, which meant to be at the very beginning of the operations, were excluded because they were usually caused by accidental processes like Veress needle accidents. Some conversions were because of the *"laparoscopic techniques"* which meant to be operating difficulties of the surgeon. Since surgeons' technical difficulty is a kind of personal subject, we also excluded this factor. As a result, we only evaluated the anatomical and physiopathological events that changed the way of surgery. Tekkis et al defined conversion reasons in three parts as patient-specific, procedure- specific and surgeon-specific factors (Tekkis et al, 2005). According to this classification, we can define that, we evaluate the patient-specific factors. Then, detailed reasons of conversions were tried to be found to put forward a solid definition of the conversion reason. As Schmidt et al clarified, by understanding the reasons for conversion, laparoscopic success may be improved via modifying standard preoperative medical management or using additional technological capabilities (Schmidt et al, 2001).

3. Gall bladder operations

Laparoscopic cholecystectomy is the most reported operation in literature for conversions. After developed in France, laparoscopic cholecystectomy expanded to United States in 1988 (Shea et al, 2004). Higher interest in the subject subsequently caused higher conversion rates at the beginning periods and because of the accumulated data conversions reasons can be evaluated more clearly (Shea et al, 2004). Yun et al determined the rates of conversion to open surgery in earlier studies as high as 10% (Yun et al, 2010). After continuation the laparoscopic cholecystectomies conversion rates reduced to 3.3% (Yun et al, 2010). It was defined that acceptable conversion rate for elective laparoscopic cholecystectomy is 3-5% and for emergent laparoscopic cholecystectomy because of acute cholecystitis is 6-35% (Simopoluos et al, 2005). There is still a high rate of conversion for emergency cholecystectomies (Yun et al, 2010). Unfortunately, uniform definitions of the risk factors indicating conversion laparoscopic to open cholecystectomy have not been formulated by authors (Simopoluos et al, 2005). Karayiannakis et al defined the conversion criteria as risky adhesiolysis, inadequate exposure of operative field and definition problem for anatomy (Karayiannakis et al, 2004). In the meta-analysis of Shea et al, conversion reasons were figured out as dense adhesions, inflammation, common bile duct stones, acute cholecystitis and gangrenous gallbladder (Shea et al, 2004). They reported 1,400 patients for the conversion of 25,763 patients by evaluating 75 cholecystectomy articles in a meta-analysis and among these patients, dense adhesions (n = 290 (%20.7)), inflammation (n = 146(%10.4)), common bile duct stones (n=95(%6.8)), acute cholecystitis (n=96(%6.9)) and gangrenous gallbladder (n=15(%1.1)) were operative problems for conversion (Shea et al, 2004). Cucinotta et al also introduced that adhesions and insufficiently visualized biliary anatomy were their main problem to perform conversion (Cucinotta et al, 1998). In Akyürek et al series, patients without a history of laparotomy had more conversions than the patients with histories of upper or lower laparotomies and the most reason was dense adhesion in Calot's triangle (4 patients), uncertain anatomy (2 patients), friable gallbladder (1 patient) and thick cystic duct 1 patient (Akyurek et al, 2005). Simopoluos et al also reported the inability to define the anatomy in Calot's triangle as the most common reason for conversion and among these patients 24 (1.5 %) had no inflammation and 46 (16.9%) had an inflamed gallbladder (Simopoluos et al, 2005). In literature, two reports investigated the conversion reasons in details for laparoscopic cholecystectomy (Akyurek et al, 2005), (Simopoluos et al, 2005). Therefore, these literatures can be defined as two samples for throughout evaluation of predictors. Akyürek et al defined adhesions to decide the way of operation after entering the abdominal cavity and used 3-point grading system for this purpose (Akyurek et al, 2005). Grade 1 adhesions had filmy thickness, avascular, grade 2 had moderate thickness with limited vascularity and grade 3 adhesions had dense thickness with well vascularization (Akyurek et al, 2005). However, direct correlation between this grading score and conversions were not clear in this study (Akyurek et al, 2005). Simopoluos et al found male gender, previous upper abdominal surgery, higher age, diabetes and severity of inflammation were significant predictors for conversion. Male gender with 60 year-old age was a high predictor for conversion (Simopoluos et al, 2005). Degree of inflammation was predicted for the high rate of conversion (Simopoluos et al, 2005). Detailed data for the inflammation of the gall bladder were; elevated WBC count higher than 9000/ml, fever higher than 37.5^{o} C, total bilirubin levels higher than 1.2 mg/dl, aspartate transaminase higher than 60 U/L, alanine transaminase >60 U/L (Simopoluos et al, 2005).

In addition, Smith et al suggested ultrasonography for dilated common duct, choledocholithiasis and revealed a relative contraindication to laparoscopic cholecystectomy (Smith, 1992). Ultrasonographic evaluation could be expected to be leader for the evaluation of conversions but to our knowledge, a practical and definite usage of ultrasonography about the common duct and presence of choledocholithiasis predicting conversions has not been present in the literature.

3.1 Gastrointestinal operations

Laparoscopic procedures for intestinal diseases, especially for intestinal obstructions, have been under cautious evaluations and controversies have not been solved although progressive advantages were structured in laparoscopic treatment (Strickland, 1999). Collected information about conversion in this section was classified as anatomic definition or presentation related definition to ease the evaluation. Therefore, anatomic definitions are classified as stomach, duodenum, liver, pancreas, intestinal operations and presentation related definitions were classified as intestinal obstructions, abdominal trauma, obesity, diverticular, inflammatory diseases and tumoral diseases. Spleen is not evaluation in this section.

3.1.1 Intestinal obstructions

One of the reasons of controversies for acute abdomen may be originated from discouraging conversion rates. Chung et al reported 38.2% conversion rates for emergent laparoscopic surgery for acute abdomen (Chung et al, 1998). Wullstein & Gross reported laparoscopic operations for small bowel obstruction and conversions were reported as high as (51·9 per cent) (Wullstein & Gross, 2003). Suter et al reported 43% conversion for their mechanical small bowel obstruction (Suter et al, 2000). Many authors estimated the operations for massive abdominal distension, the presence of peritonitis, highly inflamed bowel,

hemodynamic instability, and severe comorbid conditions such as heart and lung diseases as contraindication for laparoscopic operations (Szomstein et al, 2006). As seen in intestinal obstructions, suspected adhesions guided surgeon for laparotomy because of the possibility of limited visualization and risk of bowel injury (Reissman & Spira, 2003). Le Moine et al reported that patients with a known frozen abdomen must not be treated with laparoscopy and if laparoscopy was planned to be used in these patients needing emergent surgery (e.g., active hemorrhage, peritonitis, complete bowel obstruction) may be handle with great cautious (Le Moine et al, 2003). Chung et al mentioned about reasons for these conversions like advanced disease, uncontrollable fecal spill, forced exposure because of dense adhesions, debridement, abscess drainage, vascular surgery and hemodynamic deterioration (Chung et al, 1998). Obscured view due to intestinal distension with extensive adhesion and reduced field of the vision or perforations were the main reasons for conversion (Wullstein & Gross, 2003), (Suter et al, 2000).
Suter et al recognized the usage of preoperative plain abdominal film showing a small bowel diameter exceeding 4 cm might be a predictive instrument for an increased risk of conversion (Suter et al, 2000). They reported that dilation of the intestinal loops reduced the working space as expected and increased intestinal fragility with distension might be correlated the plain abdominal graphy substantially (Suter et al, 2000). Conversion in these circumstances are not surprising, because the working space in the abdominal cavity is considerably shrank (Suter et al, 2000). On the other hand, they operate patients with laparoscopy even with a diameter exceeding 5 cm but conversion should not be underestimated if any difficulty was detected during the laparoscopy (Suter et al, 2000). Some authors classified the acute bowel obstructions for the availability of laparoscopic management (Reissman & Spira, 2003). These criteria are proximal obstruction, partial obstruction, simple "single band" obstruction, and localized radiographic distension, no signs of systemic sepsis and mild abdominal distension (Reissman & Spira, 2003).

3.1.2 Abdominal trauma

Trauma is in another main part of the argument for urgent laparoscopy and authors have different opinions for emergent surgery of trauma. Contraindications are defined as hemodynamic instability, known diaphragmatic injury, obvious intraabdominal injury, overt peritonitis or evidence of intraperitoneal penetration, posterior penetrating trauma with high likelihood of bowel injury (Villavicencio & Aucar, 1999). Treatments for abdominal trauma with laparoscopy were defined as exploration of penetrating trauma in tangential gunshot wounds. It was pointed out that laparoscopy sensitivity for gastrointestinal injuries were as low as 18% but it might be used for the definition of the need of laparotomy (Villavicencio & Aucar, 1999). However, Villavicencio et al defined the laparoscopy as a therapeutic tool for traumatic abdominal injuries. In their review of the studies, including 154 patients in 4 series, they showed that laparoscopy may be performed for at least 34% (53 patients) of the trauma patients treated with laparotomy (Villavicencio & Aucar, 1999).

3.1.3 Adhesions

Adhesions lead dangerous separations of target organs and are the most seen circumstance for conversion (Schmidt et al, 2001). Le Moine et al reported that conversion related to adhesions and/or inflammatory pseudotumour was the major reason in their series and 21 of the total 24 conversion patients had these problems (Le Moine et al, 2003). Agresta et al emphasized that the entity of unclear anatomy of adhesions were the most frequent causes of conversion (Agresta et al, 2004). As a result of previous operations, adhesions might be detected in next attempts and region of the previous surgery must be evaluated as a risk factor. Prior abdominal surgery caused inability to obtain adequate exposure for the critical region of interest and this is a predictor for open conversion and complications (Karayiannakis et al, 2004). Previous upper abdominal surgery caused 19% conversion which was significantly higher than among those with previous lower abdominal surgery (3.3%) and those without previous surgery (5.4%) (Karayiannakis et al, 2004). Contrary to these opinions, Schmidt et al did not accept the number of prior abdominal procedures or the entity of previous abdominal surgery as a real predictor of conversion (Schmidt et al, 2001).

Some investigations were focused on the fact adhesion to make a classification. Tekkis et al classified their patients into three parts: patients with no adhesions, loose filmy adhesions that can be separated by blunt dissection and adhesions requiring up to 50% or more sharp dissection for separation with serosal injury or full-thickness injury. (Tekkis et al, 2005). Additionally, Karayiannakis et al reported about radiodiagnostic factors and offered using ultrasonography to explore the spontaneous or manual compression-induced visceral slide and to map the geography of dense intraperitoneal adhesions (Karayiannakis et al, 2004).

In various laparoscopic gastrointestinal operations, same predictive factors may be detected for conversions. For antireflux reoperations, Floch et al reported that adhesions were the most seen conversion reasons (4 patients in total 9 conversions) to the open procedure (Floch et al, 1999). Total conversion rate was 20% for other antireflux operation series. (Floch et al, 1999).

For colon operations, Schmidt et al reported that 44 of 110 patients (40%) underwent 45 attempted laparoscopic procedures that were converted to open procedures. (Schmidt et al, 2001). This was the conversion rate of the patients who had prior colonic anastomosis and adhesions (Schmidt et al, 2001). Eighty percent of these converted patients were operated for segmental colonic resection and 78%of the conversions were needed during the lysis of the adhesion (Schmidt et al, 2001).

For appendectomies, Ball et al reported that performing laparoscopic operations became also impossible when extensive cecal adhesions were detected during appendectomy (Ball et al, 2004). Conversion to an open procedure was required for 10 patients because the appendix could not be mobilized after extensive cecal adhesions (Ball et al, 2004).

Adhesion in detailed investigation has not been reached in literature although it was figured out as a very important conversion factor. This may be because of the absence of diagnostic tools for the direct evaluation. Ultrasonography was used for evaluation in a study which can be accepted as an objective criterion. Therefore, we believe that systematized preoperative evaluation planning may be designed in the future.

3.1.4 Obesity

Obesity is one of the main problems for conversion. Different conversion rates were described in various operations for obese patient. Tekkis et al reported conversion risks were higher when body mass index was higher than 30. Additionally, conversion was significant if body mass index was greater than 50 (Tekkis et al, 2005). Patients undergoing conversion were significantly heavier (body mass index, 26.5) than those in whom the procedure was completed laparoscopically (body mass index, 24.9; $P < 0.05$) (Marusch et al, 2001). Conversion rates for laparoscopic colorectal surgery are 7% to 25% for larger series and 2% to 41% for smaller series (Tekkis et al, 2005). Tekkis et al reported conversion of obesity for colorectal surgery in 12 patients (9.6%) in their series. In another report, Poddoubnyi et al defined that patients weighing more than 90 kg converted to open procedure up to 75% of the procedures and morbidity has been reported as 78% (Poddoubnyi et al, 1998). Increased intraoperative complications related to higher conversion rates are not surprising for obese patients in laparoscopic colorectal surgery (Poddoubnyi et al, 1998). Massive obesity is also the reason of obstacle in reaching esophageal hiatus and caused conversion. (Higa et al, 2000) (Marusch et al, 2001). Chelala et al reported some of their patients who needed conversions because of difficult and risky dissection for their gastric banding operations (Chelala et al, 1997). Also they reported that left hepatic hypertrophy was risky for conversion causing four conversions to open procedure (Chelala et al, 1997). Subxyphoid ultrasonography was performed to evaluate hepatic hypertrophy for obese patients but significant correlation was not found (Chelala et al, 1997). Instead of this, early conversion determination was offered after introduction of the laparoscope and retraction of the liver to the right. (Chelala et al, 1997). Positioning the liver retractor more to the left of the xyphoid was reported to be the solution of conversion possibility.

3.1.5 Intraabdominal tumor

Curative laparoscopic surgery has still been investigating for gastrointestinal malignancies (Moreno et al, 1998). Tumor size and anatomical definition of the disease might be important for gastrointestinal operations. Excessive tumor bulk larger than 15 cm was defined to be an important factor for conversion (Tekkis et al, 2005). Marusch et al reported that medical situation of the patient has to be clarified for the size of tumor and intraoperative problems causing conversion would not be surprising if precautionary measures are not performed (Marusch et al, 2001), (Jaroszewski et al, 2004). Jaroszewski et al evaluated diagnostic tools for pancreatic tumors and showed that transabdominal ultrasonography(US) and computerized tomography(CT) is effective lower than 50% to 60% but spiral CT is more sensible (Jaroszewski et al, 2004). Magnetic resonance imaging has 45% to 91% success for insulinoma detection but endoscopic US is the most effective tool with preoperative detection rates of 86% to 93% (Jaroszewski et al, 2004). For insulinomas, invasive techniques such as percutaneous transhepatic venous sampling and arterial stimulation with venous sampling for insulin may be used but Laparoscopic Intraoperative US (LIOUS) gives excellent results for preoperative localization techniques(Jaroszewski et al, 2004). In spite of these technical possibilities if the tumor could not be identified accurately or vascular relations could not be seen effectively, conversion to open exploration should be considered (Jaroszewski et al, 2004). For colorectal tumor cases, Kwok et al reported 100 patients of colorectal carcinoma with colon or colorectal resection and experienced that phase 1 patients had higher conversion rates than phase 2 and rates were 33.3%and 8.9%respectively (Kwok et al, 1996). The important point of low conversion rates in phase 2 patients is the strict selection of the patients in this phase for laparoscopy and careful laboratory evaluations (Kwok et al, 1996). Careful selection of patients will reduce conversions and they pointed out that patient with bulky tumors, adjacent organ invasion with tumor or neighboring tissues has to be evaluated (Kwok et al, 1996). Also unexpected complications, intra-abdominal and abdominal wall tumor seeding are important for conversions (Moreno et al, 1998). For tumor operations, hemorrhage and perforations may be seen because of the adhesions of the tumor and therefore, Marusch et al warned surgeons for these adhesions (Marusch et al, 2001). Only pancreatic leakages had prolonged hospitalization after conversions and others conversion reasons had not important affects for hospitalizations according to completed laparoscopies. (Jaroszewski et al, 2004).

3.1.6 Diverticular and inflammatory diseases

Diverticular and inflammatory diseases can be the reason of conversion. Severity of diverticular disease provoke higher incidence of conversion (Marusch et al, 2001). Overall conversion rate was 7.2% but in less severe forms like peridiverticulitis, stenosis, or recurrent attacks of inflammation, conversion rates decrease to 4.8% and in severe forms like covered perforation, abscess, fistula, or bleeding, conversion was performed in 18.2% patients (Marusch et al, 2001), (Le Moine et al, 2003). Schmidt et al reported 58% conversions for fistula (Schmidt et al, 2001). Tekkis et al had 37.6% of conversion for inflammation and 13.6% of abscess/fistula caused conversions (Tekkis et al, 2005). Fistula (excluding enterocutaneous or perirectal fistulas) as an indication of surgery may cause conversion during laparoscopic procedure (Schmidt et al, 2001).

According to Le Moine et al, obesity was the only predictive factor for diverticular diseases in their experience but they added that attention had to be paid to the presence of sigmoid stenosis or fistula and severity of diverticulitis (Le Moine et al, 2003).

Crohn's disease with colonic (extracecal) subtype had a challenging technique caused by transmural inflammation and foreshortened mesentery makes things difficult (Schmidt et al, 2001). Additionally, patients with the colonic subtype of Crohn's disease appear in general to have a higher severity of disease, making them less amenable to laparoscopic approaches. (Schmidt et al, 2001). In Crohn's disease the degree of inflammation can be variable and unpredictable, which affects the technical complexity, surgical safety and laparoscopy success. (Schmidt et al, 2001). Presence of the Crohn's disease was not a predictor itself but disease severity and technical difficulty makes the difference for the conversion rates (Schmidt et al, 2001).

As smoking is known to exacerbate Crohn's disease, it was found to be significant for the association with conversion (Schmidt et al, 2001).

Colonoscopic evaluations may progress with complication resulting operations. Thus, colonoscopy may be a predictor. Hansen et al evaluated the patients resulted with laparoscopy after colonoscopic complications (Hansen et al, 2007). In three (27%) cases conversion from exploratory laparoscopy to open laparotomy was performed and one of them had perforation appeared to be into the lesser omental bursa which was difficult to access, the other had perforation was deep in the pelvis (Hansen et al, 2007). Third case was converted for optimum management of a large segment of small bowel seen hyperemic and inflamed from fecal soilage. (Hansen et al, 2007). The mean perforation size causing conversion in their patients was 1.1 cm (range 0.2–2 cm) but Hansen et al also added that conversion might be performed on the base of doubt of the repair security.(Hansen et al, 2007).

Laparoscopic biopsies for bowel lesions can cause conversions on an already weakened wall (Atchabahian et al, 1996). Atchabahian et al reported that they had an experience for Degos' disease and they offer not to perform biopsy for certain diagnosis (Atchabahian et al, 1996). Other reasons for conversion were the usage of steroid medication and preoperative malnutrition (Schmidt et al, 2001).

3.1.7 Liver and pancreas diseases

Surgeons are under pressure of the circumstances about the laparoscopic techniques for organs like liver or pancreas because of the presence of difficulty for retractions with current instrument, decision of resection margins and potential major injuries with neighboring tissues (Fong et al, 2000). Although there are difficulties, laparoscopic liver operations have begun in recent times. Cherqui et al was one of the leaders of laparoscopic liver operations and they reported 2 conversions among their 28 patients (Cherqui et al, 2000). First patient converted for hemorrhage originating from the neighboring tissue of the focal nodular hyperplasia and the other one converted because of the insufficient sight (Cherqui et al, 2000). Dagher et al reported conversion for seven patients (10%) (Dagher et al, 2007). Diffuse bleeding during the parenchymal transection (3 patients) is the most important factor for conversion especially in segmental resections (Dagher et al, 2007). Exposure difficulties (2 patients: 1 segmentectomy V and 1 bisegmentectomy V–VI), unsatisfactory progression during parenchymal section (1 patient: trisegmentectomy V–VI–VII), and an anatomic variant of portal branches (1 patient: right hepatectomy) also caused other conversions (Dagher et al, 2007). On the other hand it was emphasized that only 2 patients were converted after the learning period (Dagher et al, 2007). Santambrogio et al used laparoscopic ultrasonography (LUS) to clarify the tumoral pathologies and only 2 patients were converted in their 15 patient series (Santambrogio et al, 2007). One of the patients had three lesions in segment 3 shown with LUS but bleeding from the adhesion between tumor and omentum caused conversion. The other patient had tumors near the portal pedicle of the left lobe caused an early conversion decision (Santambrogio et al, 2007).
Patients with pancreatic diseases reported by Jaroszewski showed that lesion in uncinate process of pancreas adjacent to superior mesenteric vein may cause conversion (Jaroszewski et al, 2004). Jaroszewski et al offered laparoscopic intraoperative ultrasonography (LIOUS) for decision-making (Jaroszewski et al, 2004). However, it can be unsuccessful and conversion may need as experienced in one of their patient (Jaroszewski et al, 2004).

3.1.8 Duodenal diseases

Treatments for duodenal diseases with laparoscopic procedures were defined. Duodenal perforations were repaired by laparoscopy and only five (17%) patients underwent conversion to an open procedure (Kathouda et al, 1996). Large perforations (diameter 6 mm) were reported to be the reasons for conversion in 3 patients. Additionally, beginning time of the symptoms was defined to be significant for conversion and if the symptoms began for more than 24 hours conversion rate detected 33% of the patients (Kathouda et al, 1996). Conversion rates were 0% when symptoms began less than 24 hours (Kathouda et al, 1996).

3.1.9 Stomach operations

Difficult dissections of posterior esophagus, identification problem of left diaphragmatic crus and hemorrhage are the main reasons of conversion during laparoscopic

fundoplication but obstacle in the view is the most important factor for experienced surgeons (Soot et al, 1999).
Laparoscopy was also used for pyloromyotomy and conversions were reported. Sitsen et al reported 3 patients with mucosal perforation with laparoscopy which converted to transverse right upper quadrant minilaparotomy (Sitsen et al, 1998). For pyloromyotomy, prolongation of hospital stay was not significant after conversions (Sitsen et al, 1998).
For laparoscopic gastric ulcer treatments, Siu et al reported 21.5% conversion rate (Siu et al, 2004). Agresta et al reported conversion rate as 12% for their operated 51 patients because of inadequate ulcer localization (Agresta et al, 2004). Ulcer perforations larger than 10 mm and nonjuxtapyloric gastric ulcers were the main group of conversion but there were patients converted for technical difficulties and unidentifiable perforations (Siu et al, 2004).
Higa et al reported hepatomegaly as an important risk factor for the conversions of gastric operations (Higa et al, 2000). Huge liver interfere the operation sight especially for esophageal hiatus procedures. Therefore, performing safe dissections are challenging (Higa et al, 2000). Additionally small abdominal cavity was determined to be a risk for conversion (Higa et al, 2000). Some patients with past abdominoplasty caused the inability to establish an adequate pneumoperitoneum preventing safe dissection and visualization (Higa et al, 2000).

3.1.10 Intestinal operations

Laparoscopic treatment of invagination reduction was evaluated and 22.4% reduction failure revealed during endoscopic treatments which lead to open procedure (Poddoubnyi et al, 1998). Most conversions in this report were seen for ileoileocecocolonic invaginations (8 in 22 cases) but ileoileal, ileocecal and ileocecocolonic invaginations were reported also (Poddoubnyi et al, 1998).
One the most performed laparoscopic procedure for intestinal treatments was laparoscopic appendectomy. So et al reported 47% of conversions which was correlated with inexperience (So et al, 2002). It was reported that at least 20 cases had to be operated for optimum laparoscopy knowledge (So et al, 2002). Difficulty of dissection is the main reason of conversion and also unclear anatomy, appendicle mass and inadequate working space for appendectomy (So et al, 2002). Mucinous appendicieal tumor is important for laparoscopic appendectomies and special effort has to be spent while grasping the tissue. Appendiceal malignancies were reported to be evaluated earlier to prevent the patient from seeding of the tumor (Moreno et al, 1998). Another aspect that has to be kept in mind to prevent from conversion is retrocecal location of the appendix (Moreno et al, 1998).

4. Spleen operations

Conversion rates in laparoscopic splenectomies were reported as 0% to 19% in different studies (Brody et al, 1999), (Kathouda et al, 1996). Performing laparoscopic splenectomy was considered to be a contraindication at first, but soon, especially for enlarged spleens, diseases involving spleen were managed successfully by laparoscopy (Targarona et al, 1998). Although the main argument for conversions has been originated from the weight of the spleen, there have been controversies related to conversions caused by splenic weight. Targarona et al reported in their series that conversions occurred because of splenomegaly, weighing 2500 g to 3500 g for the patients with spherocytosis and non-

Hodgkin's lymphoma (Targarona et al, 1998). For the enlarged spleen weighing as much as 2500 g, they foresaw that it would be difficult to obtain enough intraabdominal space to manipulate the spleen (Targarona et al, 1998). Mahon & Rhodes reported that their 6 patients among the 39 operated splenectomies were converted to open procedure whose wet spleen weights were more than 1 kg (Mahon & Rhodes, 2003). However, Glasgow & Mulvihill pointed out that the weight was not important and reported successful laparoscopies of the patients who had spleen weighting over than 3890 g (Glasgow & Mulvihill, 1997). According to Katkhouda et al lymphoproliferative disease could be recognized as having high conversion rate and spleen weight over 3800 g has to be taken into account for conversion in spite of controversy is present (Kathouda et al, 1996). They converted 4 patients because of this reason. At the beginning of their practice Kathkhouda et al used preoperative CT scan or ultrasound in defining the spleen size but later they abandoned this procedure because they revealed size dependent decision-making useless in their practice except the patients with ITP or gallstones in patients with hemolytic anemia (Kathouda et al, 1996). Therefore, we summarize these variable informations as laparoscopic splenectomy for the spleen weight higher than 2500 g may be performed in great cautious and in any period of laparoscopy, if difficulty begins, conversions must be performed.

Bleeding may be another obstacle for laparoscopic splenectomy. Targarona et al reported conversions in 2 patients caused by diffuse oozing and difficulty in handling the spleen related to idiopathic thrombocytopenic purpura and AIDS-related thrombocytopenia (Targarona et al, 1998). Bleeding was the main reason for Glasgow et al and six patients converted for this reason (Glasgow & Mulvihill, 1997). They reported the first 4 patients in their beginning period of the practice and the last 2 were in experienced periods (Glasgow & Mulvihill, 1997). They emphasized that converted patients did not have previous abdominal surgery (Glasgow & Mulvihill, 1997). Katkhouda et al reported that three patients converted for bleeding (Kathouda et al, 1996). They found conversion rates for lymphoproliferative diseases higher than idiopathic thrombocytopenic purpura (Kathouda et al, 1996). Katkhouda et al reported the hemorrhage during hilar dissection as a conversion reason in 3% of their patients (Kathouda et al, 1996).

Densely adherent abdominal structures to the spleen are one of the reasons of conversions of laparoscopic splenectomies (Brody et al, 1999). Brody et al reported one of the patients in their series with adhesive omentum on the spleen without prior operation history which was the cause of the tears as the reasons of laparotomy (Brody et al, 1999). Also splenectomy of a patient with pancreatitis had adherent pancreatic tail to the splenic hilum required conversion in their series (Brody et al, 1999). They additionally reported that after handled with experience this would not be a problem (Brody et al, 1999).

Katkhouda et al reported that splenectomies for trauma were excluded for laparoscopic procedure and in their series laparoscopies did not have priority for malignancy diagnosis (Kathouda et al, 1996).

Predictive factors are not clarified in details for laparoscopic splenectomy. Acute and/or traumatic reasons are generally accepted as the reasons of laparotomy. Bleeding and adhesions are preoperative problems that have to be recognized during the procedure but preoperative predictability is not strong enough for decision-making. Although best evaluations are focused on the weight of the spleen, defining a precise prediction is not easy even for weight measuring with these findings yet.

5. Gynaecological operations

Risk factors for gynaecological operations are not different from other operation types. Chi et al reported that laparoscopic procedures were converted to laparotomy for 3 reasons; complications during the laparoscopy, technical difficulty and change in the planned treatment of malignancy (Chi et al, 2004). Some reported predictors are obesity, previous laparotomy, coexisting medical conditions, anticoagulant use (Jansen et al, 1997). Jansen et al reported 13 of 47 patients (11.8%) converted to laparotomy because of previous operations which were the most frequently encountered association for conversion (Jansen et al, 1997).

Severe pelvic inflammatory disease and adhesions obliterating the cul-de-sac that may cause bowel perforation possibility is a risk factor for transfundal laparoscopy (Santala et al, 1999). Chi et al also reported adhesion as a predictive factor and defined the previous abdominal surgeries causing poor visualizations with dense adhesion (Chi et al, 2004). Walker et al reported 434 converted patients (25.8%) in their large series and the most seen reason for conversion was poor exposure in 246 patients (14.6%) (Walker et al, 2009). Also, cancer was found to be an important factor affecting 69 patients (4.1%) for conversion (Walker et al, 2009). Excessive bleeding was cited as the reason for conversion in 49 patients (2.9%) (Walker et al, 2009). Body mass index (BMI) was also reported to be important and a concordance was defined with the increasing conversion percentage and BMI (Walker et al, 2009). BMI of 25 kg/m2 had 17.5% conversion rate, BMI to 35 kg/m2 had 26.5% conversion rate and BMI with greater than 40 kg/m2 had 57.1%conversion rates (Walker et al, 2009).

Laparoscopic myomectomy is investigated for conversions. Conversion incidence for myomectomy varies in a spectrum from 10.7% to 41.4% (Dubuisson et al, 2001). Although subserous and intramural myomas has been treated by large number of teams, the technique is difficult, time consuming, and involve a high risk of conversion to laparotomy (Dubuisson et al, 2001). Dubuisson et al experienced that most of the patients converted to laparotomy were related to cleavage problem and suturing difficulty (Dubuisson et al, 2001). To prevent patient from this, Dubuisson et al used US examination and size at US, intramural type, anterior location of the biggest myoma were defined to be useful (Dubuisson et al, 2001). They reported that intramural myoma, anterior myoma and myoma larger than 50 mm had a higher risk for conversion (Dubuisson et al, 2001). Conversion of the intramural myoma, especially big myomas, depended on the difficulty of suturing the deep hysterotomy (Dubuisson et al, 2001). As a laboratory entity, although there is a controversy for this subject, preoperative usage of GnRH agonist, independent from the duration or dosage, is found to be a predictive factor for conversion (Dubuisson et al, 2001).

Dubuisson et al reported that systematic research for adenomyosis had to be performed and US had to be used cautiously before the operations (Dubuisson et al, 2001). Malignancy does not have a definitive surgical treatment modality for either laparoscopy or laparotomy (Sagiv et al, 2005). After the frozen section, immediate decision has to be made to complete the operation (Sagiv et al, 2005). If the laparoscopic ovarian cystectomy is performed, cyst size does not affect the plan even for the huge cyst size (Sagiv et al, 2005).

6. Retroperitoneal and urologic operations

The use of laparoscopy in urologic surgery has gained attention since 1990 (Mendoza et al, 1996). Authors evaluating the urologic and retroperitoneal laparoscopic operations reported different opinions. For instance, Fergany et al put forward that patients with multiple previous abdominal surgeries, acute intraperitoneal infectious problems and uncorrected bleeding diatheses should not be operated (Fergany et al, 2000). Mendoza et al performed 1,022 different urologic laparoscopic procedures and they converted 15 patients (Mendoza et al, 1996). These conversions were due to either suboptimal visualization, difficulty with dissection from scar tissue, excessive obesity, or bleeding (Mendoza et al, 1996). Esposito defined another perspective for conversion of retroperitoneal diseases and reported that endo- and retroperitoneal vessel lesions generally require immediate conversion which was different from endoabdominal vessels (Esposito et al, 1997).

6.1 Nephrectomy

Nephrectomy with laparoscopy has advantages according to laparotomy but when conversion performed hospital stays and complications increases. Keeley & Tolley reported that their converted patients had a longer operative duration and length of stay in hospital (Keeley & Tolley, 1998). Complication rate for both laparoscopic nephrectomy (17.5%) and nephroureterectomy (18%) was found to be similar in their series including the patients with inflammatory conditions such as pyonephrosis, staghorn calculi, xantogranulomatous pyelonephritis (Keeley & Tolley, 1998). Keeley & Tolley converted five cases to open surgery; four for failure to progress (two with staghorn calculi /pyonephrosis, one with locally advanced transitional cell carcinoma and one with xantogranulomatous pyelonephritis), and one to remove a large policyctic kidney (Keeley & Tolley, 1998).

Partial nephrectomy with laparoscopy is more difficult than total nephrectomy and needs more experience. Possible renal and extrarenal complications can cause more conversion (ElGhonemi et al, 2003). ElGhonemi et al reported that they converted 4 patients because of difficulties in completing anastomosis, two converted for kidney rotation and one had a huge pelvis (ElGhonemi et al, 2003). According to ElGhonemi et al significant peritoneal tear causes leak of the gas and this problem was also a conversion reason and one patient was converted to open surgery (ElGhonemi et al, 2003).

Matın added that the presence of any ureteric tumour is a contraindication to laparoscopic nefroureterectomy (Matın, 2005).

6.2 Prostatectomy

Bhayani et al used laparoscopy for prostatic treatments and converted 13 patients (1.9%) to open procedure (Bhayani et al, 2004). Four of their patients had dense adhesions, 2 patients had obesity BMI greater than 30 and one patient for inadequate tumor resection at the bladder neck (Bhayani et al, 2004). Periprostatic scarring and cleavage problems were the main reason of conversion (Bhayani et al, 2004). Bhayani et al added that patients with markedly enlarged prostate and patients treated with androgenic deprivation therapy should not be operated with laparoscopy (Bhayani et al, 2004).

6.3 Adrenalectomy

Adrenalectomy has been one of the most investigated operations among retroperitoneal laparoscopic operations. Advantages of laparoscopic adrenalectomy could be described as decreased operative blood loss, reduced narcotic requirements, and shorter hospital stay and recovery time have been reported in small series (Gagner et al, 1997). In one of the biggest series, Shen et al reported 8 conversion for 261 patients between 1993 and 2003 (Shen

et al, 2004). Rate of conversion for adrenalectomy ranges from 0% to 5% in the literature but reasons for conversion to open adrenalectomy was studied in a few studies (Shen et al, 2004). By retrospective evaluation of 3 converted patients, it was realized that laparotomy had to be plan according to radiographic appearance or dimension of the tumor (Shen et al, 2004). Tumor adhesions to neighboring tissue were the reason of the conversions of the 3 patients (Shen et al, 2004). These cases were right-sided adrenal tumors which effected liver and vessels like inferior vena cava and right renal vein (Shen et al, 2004). Two of the 8 converted patients in Shen et al series had tumors with 15 and 16 cm in size that caused conversion (Shen et al, 2004). Gagner et al reported three converted patients in their series. The first patient in their report had 15 cm angiomyolipoma in right adrenal gland (Gagner et al, 1997). Second case had invasion to posterior muscles and third has 12 cm right adrenal mass (Gagner et al, 1997). Gagner et al revealed that a mass in adrenal gland larger than 15 cm might be accepted as contraindication for laparoscopy (Gagner et al, 1997). It was also reported that metastatic nodes in the periaortic chain or close to the bladder detected by magnetic resonance imaging or metaiodobenzylguanidine nuclear scan desires open technique rather than laparoscopy (Gagner et al, 1997).
Shanberg et al reported that right-sided retroperitoneal laparoscopic adrenalectomy was difficult to accomplish. Right adrenal vein and the inferior vena cava were the main reasons of limitation of the process (Shanberg et al, 2001).

7. Inappropriate circumstances for anesthesia

The reports about the problems related to anesthesia as a reason of conversion of the laparoscopic procedures to laparotomy were very few (Cunningham, 1998). The reason of this situation may originate from the lower incidence of anesthesia-related complications during laparoscopy (Girish, 2001). Usually, case dependent reports were presented and most of them were determined in the surgical series. However, careful evaluations give clues in finding out some issues that can be accepted as predictors for anesthesia related conversion.
Bleeding is an important aspect for conversion. For patients with cirrhosis laparoscopy and open procedure has risks of bleeding (Delis et al, 2010). Delis et al reported 12 cases that had to be converted and five of 12 had bleeding problems (Delis et al, 2010). For these patients, MELD scorring system is used for predicting the rates of the conversions in their study and all these patients had higher scores before operations (Delis et al, 2010). One of the fields MELD scorring system is used for the evaluation of the postoperative outcome of the cirrhotic patients (Delis et al, 2010). MELD score included three laboratory test measured preoperatively: international normalized ratio (INR), serum total bilirubin (TBil), and serum creatinine (Cr) and was calculated using the following formula: MELD = 9.57 x $\log_e$ (Cr mg/dL) + 3.78 x $\log_e$ (TBil mg/dL) + 11.20 x $\log_e$ (INR) + 6.43 (Delis et al, 2010). Median MELD scores of these patients was 15 (range 11-22) described in their study and higher conversion rate was noted in patients with MELD score above 13 (Delis et al, 2010). Bleeding consists in special feature for spleen operations. Brody et al reported two patients affected from the bleeding (Brody et al, 1999). These patients had less than 50,000 mm^{-3} platelet counts and intraoperative oozing was detected (Brody et al, 1999). Authors figured out that patients with ITP and platelet counts less than 50,000 mm^{-3} undergo a preoperative bleeding time for assessment of qualitative clotting capabilities (Brody et al, 1999). It was reported

that early ligation of splenic artery through lesser sac and platelet infusion with adjunctive blood products might be suitable to interfere bleeding and to prevent the patient from conversion (Brody et al, 1999).

Pre-existing chronic obstructive and restrictive lung diseases may have challenges in laparoscopy. Hypoxemia and respiratory acidosis was documented in recent studies (Cunningham, 1998). Brody et al reported a conversion of chronic obstructive pulmonary disease (COPD) patient secondary to an extensive smoking history complicated by nocardia pneumonitis 3 months before operative intervention (Brody et al, 1999).

Intraperitoneal carbon dioxide (CO_2) insufflation and changes in patient positioning might cause hemodynamic, pulmonary, and endocrine problems (Girish, 2001). Alterations in arterial blood pressure (i.e., hypotension and hypertension), dysrhythmias, and cardiac arrest are some of the major hemodynamic complications (Girish, 2001). Bradyarrhythmias, atrioventricular dissociation, nodal rhythm, and asystole have been reported and the incidence of dysrhythmias during laparoscopy is found to be approximately 14% (Girish, 2001). Reissman & Spira reported that gas insufflation may cause altering in the cardiac output and compress the femoral veins but conversions because of this mechanism are not clear (Reissman & Spira, 2003). In a study significant cardiac performance decrease was shown after peritoneal insufflation during laparoscopic procedures especially in young patients who were operated for gynecological diseases (Harris et al, 1996). Harris et al reported that cardiovascular collapse was experienced in their patients (Harris et al, 1996). Kathouda et al reported 2 conversions for their intestine perforation operations because of cardiovascular instability (Kathouda et al, 1996).

Significant hypoxemia and hypercapnia are the major pulmonary complications during laparoscopy particularly in patients with severe pulmonary disease and limited elimination of CO_2 (Girish, 2001). $ETCO_2$ levels might not correlate with arterial CO_2 concentrations in these patients (Girish, 2001). Bhayani et al reported that two cases were converted because of hypercarbia that was unresponsive to hyperventilation and lowering of carbon dioxide gas insufflation (Bhayani et al, 2004). They treated patients with hypercarbia by increasing the minute ventilation and lowering the insufflation pressure. Bhayani et al warned surgeon and anesthesiologist for proper communication during operation against hypercarbia situations (Bhayani et al, 2004). Bhayani et al suggested conversions if hypercarbia continue in spite of hyperventilation and lowering insufflation (Bhayani et al, 2004). However increased risk of lung injury owing to increase in alveolar pressures has to be recognized particularly in patients with extensive pulmonary disease (Girish, 2001). Getting ready for possible problems, preoperative pulmonary functions and arterial blood gas analysis may be performed in significant dysfunctioning patient group (Girish, 2001). If laparoscopy is performed, operation would better be monitored by a radial artery cannula for arterial blood gas analysis (Girish, 2001).

Gas embolism might be important that could be observed with precordial Doppler gynecologic laparoscopic procedures but of the patients' evaluated, 69% CO_2 embolism diagnosed by transesophageal echocardiography for laparoscopic cholecystectomy procedures without significant cardiopulmonary changes (Girish, 2001). Six percent of patients undergoing laparoscopic nephrectomy had gas embolisms detected by transesophageal echocardiography (Girish, 2001). Clinical importance has not been detected yet.

Obesity is another factor that had to be recognized by anesthesiologist. Conversion rates vary from 14% to 36% compared with 5% to 6% in non-obese patients, depending on the type of and indication for surgery. (Lamvu et al, 2004). Simopoluos et al described obesity as a risky and hazardous factor for conversion to open cholecystectomy (Simopoluos et al, 2005). Body mass index (BMI) is important for conversion. Tekkis et al reported high rates of conversions with high BMI undergoing low pelvic surgery or left-sided colectomy. As predictors of conversion, shown in multivariate analysis, ASA grade, BMI, type of surgery, intraabdominal abscess, or fistula, and surgeon seniority has to be recognized (Tekkis et al, 2005). Suter et al reported two converted patients who were operated for small bowel obstruction (Suter et al, 2000). These patients were in ASA 4 risk category and one of them was an 80-year-old alcoholic patient with liver cirrhosis and the other one was a 53-year-old man with coronary heart disease (Suter et al, 2000).

There is a controversy for the conversions due to diabetes mellitus but Simopoluos et al reported the possibility of conversion of diabetic patients might occur for the presence of acute inflammation or changes in the wall from microvascular diseases (Simopoluos et al, 2005).

Among medications steroids were shown to be related with conversion to an open procedure (Schmidt et al, 2001). This could be accepted as an important side effect of the drug. Association of steroids, being malnourished and smoking made the conversion risk higher (Schmidt et al, 2001). Schmidt et al explain this association of the factors as the severity of the patients 'disease which subsequently hardens the operation itself (Schmidt et al, 2001).

There were demographic studies about the affect of gender on conversions (Simopoluos et al, 2005). Some authors reported male gender has a correlation whereas some does not agree with it (Simopoluos et al, 2005). It was also added by the authors that the reason of the prediction of gender was unclear.

8. Conclusion

Looking over the picture of laparoscopy, it can easily be said that expansion of the usage, indications and accesses is in a positive trend and in a fast motion. Therefore, it will not be surprising to foresee a significant decrease in the contraindication parameters in a near future. During this expansion and progression of laparoscopic procedures, literature has already begun to enhance its' difficulties, complications and conversions. According to many authors, conversions may give suitable clues for the better and easier operations, but if they are taken into account. For this reason, many reports defined conversions in all types of laparoscopic operations. Conversion, as it is figured out in literature, elongated the healing time, hospital stay and perhaps added new complications in the therapy process of the patient. Discouragement and disappointment is another dimension of the problem, as the result arise totally different from preoperative planning of the surgeon and patient because of the conversion.

So, voting out laparoscopy or completing the laparoscopy plan in success is one of the main goals in laparoscopic surgeries. For this purpose, problems interrupting laparoscopy have to be known. Definition of predicting factors of conversions are important at this point. Authors put forward previous operations to make standard definitions of predicting factors but consensus has not been maintained. Some strong predictors that all the authors agree with, consists in different parameters in details which causes controversies. Although, predicting factors like adhesions, obesity, unclear anatomy, bleeding, hypercarbia, tumor size have been figure out, it is hard to say that systematized way of decision-making has been structured by the authors that reported these predictors.

Another problem is insufficient demonstration of the reasons for conversion. By evaluating the literature of conversion for the sake of clear planning of operations, we can say that the missing part of the reports is the precise definition of the conversion reasons. This interrupts the accumulation of the knowledge. Exact and objective definitions of reasons will stimulate the accumulation of the useful information and conversion reasons will be classified after this. As a result, authors will easily understand the patients' potential conversion. Thus, it will be better to define the exact situation of the conversion reasons with measurable criteria and putting forward the exact differences of the converted patient from completed laparoscopies.

In the next step, it will be important to evaluate the diagnostic tools, invented or augmenting instruments, either laboratory or radiological, to foresee a conversion reason and to figure out the predicting factor. Usage of some diagnostic tools and laboratory instruments are reported in this chapter for this reason although it is not sufficient.

Having the data consisting in descriptions and diagnostic evaluations, one can successfully review the decision-making algorithm and may structure it in details for successful plan. We can speculate that diagnostic tools predicting the conversions may ease the surgeons' decisions and patients' expectations for healing in a schedule. Finally, we also speculate that it is time to configure international study groups for conversion investigations to organize all these data, diagnostic tools.

9. References

Agresta,F.; De Simone, P., Bedin, N. (2004). The Laparoscopic Approach in Abdominal Emergencies: A Single-Center 10-Year Experience. *Journal of the Society of Laparoendoscopic Surgeons* 8, 25-30, ISSN 1086-8089

Akyurek, N.: Salman, B., Irkorucu, O., Tascılar, O., Yuksel, O, Sare, M. & Tatlıcıoglu, M. (2005). Laparoscopic Cholecystectomy in Patients With Previous Abdominal Surgery. *Journal of the Society of Laparoendoscopic Surgeons*. 9,178–183, ISSN 1086-8089

Atchabahian, A.; Lasinu, M.J., Riche, F., Briard, C. & Nemeth J, V. (1996). Small Bowel Fistulae in Degos' Disease: A Case Report and Literature Review. *The American J of Gastroenterol* 91, 2208-11, ISSN 0002-9270

Ball,C. G.; Kortbeek, J. B., Kirkpatrick, A. W. & Mitchell, P. (2004). Laparoscopic appendectomy for complicated appendicitis An evaluation of postoperative factors. *Surg Endosc* 18, 969–973, ISSN 0930-2794

Bhayani, S. B.; Pavlovich, C.P., Strup, S.E., Dahl, D. M., Landman, J., Fabrizio, M. D. Sundaram, C.P., Kaouk, J. H. & Li-Ming, S. (2004). Laparoscopic Radical Prostatectomy: A Multi-Institutional Study Of Conversion To Open Surgery. *Urology* 63, 99–102, ISSN 0090-4295

Brody, F. J.; Chekan, E. G., Pappas, T. N. & Eubanks, W. S. (1999). Conversion factors for Laparoscopic splenectomy for immune thrombocytopenic purpura. *Surg Endosc* 13, 789-791, ISSN 0930-2794

Chelala,E. ; Cadie´re, G. B. , Favretti, F. , Himpens, J., Vertruyen, M., Bruyns, J., Maroquin,L. & Lise, M. (1997). Conversions and complications in 185 laparoscopic adjustable siliconegastric banding cases. *Surg Endosc* 11, 268–271, ISSN 0930-2794

Cherqui, D.; Husson, E., Hammoud, R., Malassagne, B., Stephan, F., Bensaid, S., Rotman, N. & Fagniez, P.(2000). Laparoscopic Liver Resections: A Feasibility Study in 30 Patients. *Annals of Surgery*. 232, 753–762, ISSN 0003-4932

Chi, D. S.; Abu-Rustum, N.R., Sonoda , Y., Awtrey, C., Hummer, A., Venkatraman, E. S., Franklin, C.C., Hamilton, F., Gemignani, M.L. & Barakat, R. R. (2004). Ten-year experience with laparoscopy on a gynecologic oncology service: Analysis of risk factors for complications and conversion to laparotomy. *American Journal of Obstetrics and Gynecology* 191, 1138-45, ISSN 0002-9378

Chung,R. S. ; Diaz, J. J. & Chari, V.(1998). Efficacy of Routine laparoscopy for the acute abdomen *Surg Endosc* 12, 219–22, ISSN 0930-2794

Cucinotta, E.; Lazzara, S. & Melita, G. (2003). Laparoscopic cholecystectomy in cirrhotic patients. *Surg Endosc* 17,1958–1960, ISSN 0930-2794

Cunningham, A. J. (1998). Anesthetic Implications of Laparoscopic Surgery. *Yale Journal Of Biology And Medıcıne* Vol 71, pp. 551-578, ISSN 0044-0086

Dagher,I.; Proske, J. M., Carloni, A., Richa, H., Tranchart, H., Franco, D. (2007). Laparoscopic liver resection: results for 70 patients. *Surg Endosc* 21, 619–624, ISSN 0930-2794

Delis, S.; Bakoyiannis, A., Madariaga, J., Bramis, J., Tassopoulos, N. & Dervenis,C. (2010). Laparoscopic cholecystectomy in cirrhotic patients: the value of MELD score and Child–Pugh classification in predicting outcome. *Surg Endosc* 24. 407–412, ISSN 0930-2794

Dubuisson, J.B.; Fauconnier, A., Fourchotte, V., Babaki-Fard, K., Coste, J. & Chapron, C. (2001). Laparoscopic myomectomy: predicting the risk of conversion to an open procedure. *Human Reproduction* 16, 1726-1731, ISSN 0268-1161

El-Ghoneimi, A.; Farhat, W., Bolduc, S., Bagli, D., Mclorie, G., Aigrain, Y. & Khoury, A.(2003). Laparoscopic dismembered pyeloplasty by a retroperitoneal approach in children. *BJU International* 92, 104-108, ISSN 2042-2997

Esposito,C. ; Ascione, G. , Garipoli, V., De Bernardo, G. & Esposito, G. (1997). Complications of pediatric laparoscopic surgery. *Surg Endosc* 11, 655–657. ISSN 0930-2794

Fergany, A.F.; Novick, A.C. & Gill, I.S.(2000). Laparoscopic urinary diversion. *World J Urol* 18, 345-348, ISSN 0724-4983

Floch,N. R.; Hinder, R. A. , Klingler, P. J. , Branton, S. A., Seelig, M.H., Bammer, T. & Filipi, C.J. (1999). Is Laparoscopic Reoperation for Failed Antireflux Surgery Feasible? *Arch Surg* 134, 733-737, ISSN 0004-0010

Fong, Y.; Jarnagin, W., Conlon, K. C. , DeMatteo, R., Dougherty, E. & Blumgart, L.H. (2000).Hand-Assisted Laparoscopic Liver Resection Lessons From an Initial Experience. *Arch Surg* 135, 854-859, ISSN 0004-0010

Gagner, M.; Pomp, A., Heniford, B. T., Pharand, D. & Lacroix, A. (1997). Laparoscopic Adrenalectomy Lessons Learned From 100 Consecutive Procedures. *Annals Of Surgery* 226, 238-247. ISSN 0003-4932

Girish, P.J.(2001). Complications of Laparoscopy. *Anesthesiology Clinics of North America* 19, 89-105, ISSN 0889-8537

Glasgow, R. E.; Yee, L. F. & Mulvihill S. J. (1997). Laparoscopic splenectomy The emerging standard. *Surg Endosc* 11, 108–112. ISSN 0930-2794

Hansen, A. J. ; Tessier, D. J., Anderson, M. L. & Schlinkert, R. T. (2007). Laparoscopic Repair of Colonoscopic Perforations:Indications and Guidelines. *J Gastrointest Surg* 11,655–59, ISSN 1091-255X

Harris, S.N.; Ballantyne, G.H., Luther, M. A. & Perrino, A.C.Jr. (1996). Alterations of Cardiovascular Performance During Laparoscopic Colectomy: A Combined Hemodynamic and Echocardiographic Analysis. *Anesth Analg* 83,482-7, ISSN 0003-2999

Higa, K. D.; Boone, K.B. & Ho, T. (2000). Complications of the Laparoscopic Roux-en-Y Gastric Bypass: 1,040 Patients - What Have We Learned? *Obesity Surgery* 10, 509- 13, ISSN 0960-8923

Jansen, F.W.; Kapiteyn, K., Trimbos-Kemper, T., Hermans, J.& Trimbos, J.B. (1997). Complications of laparoscopy:a prospective multicentre observational study. *British Journal of Obstetrics and Gynaecology* ,Vol 104, pp.595-600. ISSN 1470-0328

Jaroszewski, D. E.; Schlinkert, R. T., Thompson, G. B., Schlinkert, D. K. (2004). Laparoscopic Localization and Resection of Insulinomas. *Arch Surg* 139, 270-274, ISSN 0004-0010

Karayiannakis, A. J.; Polychronidis, A., Perente, S., Botaitis, S., Simopoulos, C. (2004). Laparoscopic cholecystectomy in patients with previous upper or lower abdominal Surgery. *Surg Endosc* 18, 97–101. ISSN 0930-2794

Katkhouda, N.; Waldrep, D., Feinstein, D., Soliman, H., Stain, S.C., Ortega, A.E. & Mouiel, J. (1996). *Am J Surg* 172, 585-590, ISSN 0002-9610

Keeley, F.X. & Tolley, D.A. (1998). A Review of our first 100 cases of laparoscopic nephrectomy:defining risk factors for complications. *BJU* 82, 615-618, ISSN 0007-1331

Kwok, S. P. Y. ; Lau, W. Y. , Declan Carey, P., Kelly, S. B., Leung, K. L. & Li, A. K. C. (1996). Prospective Evaluation of Laparoscopic-Assisted Large-Bowel Excision for Cancer. *Annals of Surgery* 223, 170-176. ISSN 0003-4932

Lamvu,G.; Zolnoun, D., Boggess, J. & Steege, J. F. (2004). Obesity: Physiologic changes and challenges during laparoscopy. *American Journal of Obstetrics and Gynecology* 191, 669-74, ISSN 0002-9378

Le Moine, M. C.; Fabre, J.M., Vacher, C., Navarro, F., Picot, M.C. & Domergue, J.(2003). Factors and consequences of conversion in laparoscopic sigmoidectomy for diverticular disease. *British Journal of Surgery* 90, 232–236, ISSN 0007-1373

Mahon, D. & Rhodes, M. (2003).Laparoscopic splenectomy: size matters *Ann R Coll Surg Engl.* 85,248–251, ISSN 0035-8843

Marusch, F.; Gastinger, I., Schneider, C., Scheidbach, H., Konradt, J., Bruch, H.P., Köhler, L., Barlehner, E., Köckerling, F. &Laparoscopic Colorectal Surgery Study Group (LCSSG).(2001). Importance of Conversion for Results Obtained with Laparoscopic Colorectal Surgery. *Dis Colon Rectum* 44, 207-216, ISSN 0012-3706

Matın, S.F. (2005). Radical laparoscopic nephroureterectomy for upper urinary tract transitional cell carcinoma: current status. *BJU International* 95, Suppl 2 , 68-74, ISSN 2042-2997

Mendoza, D.; Newman, R.C., Albala, D., Cohen, M.S., Tewari, A., Lingeman, J., Wong, M., Kavoussi, L., Adams, J., Moore, R., Winfiled, H., Glascock, M., Das, S., Munch, L., Grasso, M., Dickinson, M., Clayman, R., Nakada, S., McDougall, E.M., Wolf, S., Hulbert, J., Leveillee, R.J., Houshair, A. & Carson, C. (1996). Laparoscopic complications in markedly obese urologic patients (A multi-instutional review). *Urology* 48, 562-567, ISSN 0090-4295

Moreno, G.S.; Shmookler, B.M. & Sugarbaker, P.H. (1998). Appendiceal mucocele. *Surg Endosc* 12, 1177-1179, ISSN 0930-2794

Poddoubnyi, I.V.; Dronov, A.F., Blinnikov, O.I., Smirnov, A.N., Darenkov, I.A. & Dedov, K.A. (1998). Laparoscopy in the treatment of Intussusception in Children. *J Pediatr Surg* 33, 1194-1197, ISSN 0022-3468

Reissman, P. & Spira, R.M. (2003). Laparoscopy for Adhesions. *Seminars in Laparoscopic Surgery* Vol 10, pp 185-190. ISSN 1071-5517

Sagiv, R.; Golan, A. & Glezerman, M. (2005).Laparoscopic Management of Extremely Large Ovarian Cysts. *Obstet Gynecol* 105, 1319 –22, ISSN 0029-7844

Santala, M.; Jarvela, I. & Kauppila, A.(1999). Transfundal insertion of a Veress needle in laparoscopy of obese subjects: a practical alternative. *Human Reproduction* 14,2277-278, ISSN 0268-1161

Santambrogio, R.; Opocher, E., Pisani Ceretti, A., Barabino, M., Costa, M., Leone, S., Montorsi, M. (2007). Impact of intraoperative ultrasonography in laparoscopic liver surgery *Surg Endosc* 21, 181–188. ISSN 0930-2794

Schmidt, C. M.; Talamini, M.A., Kaufman, H.S., Lilliemoe,K.D., Learn, P. & Bayless, T. (2001). Laparoscopic Surgery for Crohn's Disease: Reasons for Conversion. *Annals of Surgery* 233, 733–739. ISSN 0003-4932

Shanberg, A.M.; Snaderson, K., Rajpoot, D. & Duel, B. (2001). Laparoscopic retroperitoneal renal and adrenal surgery in children. *BJU International* 87, 521–524, ISSN 2042 -2997

Shea, J. A.; Healey, M. J., Berlin, J. A., Clarke, J. R., Malet, P. F., .Staroscik ,R. N., Schwartz, J. S. & Williams, S.V.(2004). Mortality and Complications Associated with Laparoscopic Cholecystectomy A Meta-Analysis. *Annals of Surgery* Vol. 224, 609- 20, ISSN 0003-4932

Shen, W. T.; Kebebew, E., Clark, O.H. & Duh, Q.Y. (2004). Reasons for Conversion from Laparoscopic to Open or Hand-assisted Adrenalectomy: Review of 261 Laparoscopic Adrenalectomies from 1993 to 2003. *World J.Surg* 28, 1176–1179, ISSN 0724-4983

Simopoulos, C.; Botaitis, S., Polychronidis, A., Tripsianis, G. & Karayiannakis, A. J. (2005). Risk factors for conversion of laparoscopic cholecystectomy to open cholecystectomy. *Surg Endosc* 19: 905–909. ISSN 0930-2794

Sitsen,E.; Bax, N. M. A. & van der Zee D. C.(1998). Is laparoscopic pyloromyotomy superior to open surgery? *Surg Endosc* 12, 813–815. ISSN 0930-2794

Siu, W. T.; Chau, C.H., Law, B. K. B., Tang, C.N., Ha, P. Y. & Li, M. K. W. (2004). Routine use of laparoscopic repair for perforated peptic ulcer *British Journal of Surgery* 91, 481–484. ISSN 0007-1373

Smith, E. B.(1992). Complications of laparoscopic cholecystectomy. *Journal of the National Medical Association* 84, 880-882, ISSN 0027-9684

So, J.B.Y.; Chiong, E.C., Chiong, E., Cheah, W.K., Lomanto, D., Goh, P. & Kum, C.K.(2002). Laparoscopic Appendectomy for Perforated Appendicitis. *World J Surg* 26, 1485-1488.

Soot, S. J.; Eshraghi, N., Farahmand, M., Sheppard, B. C. & Deveney, C.W. (1999). Transition From Open to Laparoscopic Fundoplication The Learning Curve. *Arch Surg* 134, 278-281, ISSN 0004-0010

Strickland, P.; Lourie, D. J., Suddleson, E. A., Blitz, J. B. & Stain, S. C. (1999). Is laparoscopy safe and effective for treatment of acute small-bowel obstruction? *Surg Endosc* 13, 695–698. ISSN 0930-2794

Suter, M.; Zermatten, P., Halkic, N., Martinet, O. & Bettschart V. (2000). Laparoscopic management of mechanical small bowel obstruction Are there predictors of success or failure? *Surg Endosc* 14, 478–483. ISSN 0930-2794

Szomstein, S.; Lo Menzo, E., Simpfendorfer, C., Zundel, N., Rosenthal, R.J.(2006). Laparoscopic Lysis of Adhesions. *World J Surg* 30, 535–540. ISSN 0724-4983

Targarona, E. M. ; Espert, J. J., Balagu, C., Piulachs, J., Artigas, V. & Trias, M. (1998). Splenomegaly Should Not Be Considered a Contraindication for Laparoscopic Splenectomy. *Annals of Surgery* Vol. 228, 35-39. ISSN 0003-4932

Tekkis, P. P.; Senagore, A.J. & Delaney, C. P. (2005). Conversion rates in laparoscopic colorectal surgery A predictive model with 1253 patients. *Surg Endosc* 19: 47–54. ISSN 0930-2794

Villavicencio, R.T. & Aucar, J.A. (1999). Analysis of Laparoscopy in Trauma. *J Am Coll Surg* 189, 11-20, ISSN 1072- 7515

Walker, J. L.; Piedmonte, M. R., Spirtos, N. M., Eisenkop, S. M., Schlaerth, J. B., Mannel, R. S., Spiegel, G., Barakat, R., Pearl, M. L. & Sharma, S.K.(2009). Laparoscopy Compared With Laparotomy for Comprehensive Surgical Staging of Uterine Cancer: Gynecologic Oncology Group Study LAP2. *J Clin Oncol* 27, 5331-5336, ISSN 0732-183X

Wullstein, C. & Gross, E. (2003). Laparoscopic compared with conventional treatment of acute adhesive small bowel obstruction *British Journal of Surgery* 90, 1147–1151, ISSN 0007-1373

Yun, S. S.; Hwang, D. W., Kim, S. W., Park, S.H., Park, S. J., Lee, D. S. & Kim, H. J. (2010) Better Treatment Strategies forPatients with Acute Cholecystitis and American Society of Anesthesiologists Classification 3 or Greater.*Yonsei Med J* 51:540-545, ISSN 0513-5796

5

Electro-Surgery Practices and Complications in Laparoscopy

Ming-Ping Wu
The Division of Urogynecology and Pelvic Floor Reconstruction,
Department of Obstetrics and Gynecology,
Chi Mei Medical Center, Tainan
College of Medicine, Taipei Medical University, Taipei
Taiwan

1. Introduction

Operative laparoscopy is widely accepted as an efficacious technique in the treatment of gynecologic lesions. The patients, as well as the surgeons, may enthusiastically accept these new minimally invasive techniques in treating gynecologic as well as surgical diseases [1]. Since the introduction of the small medical video camera in the mid-1980s, the advent of laparoscopic surgery has brought a revolution in surgical techniques with shorter hospitalization and convalescence [2],[3]. However, surgeons who are well trained in open techniques do not automatically have that same status in laparoscopic cases. Therefore, surgeons who are skilled in open techniques may still require further training to become adapted with laparoscopic techniques. The required spatial orientation, hand-eye coordination and manipulative skills under laparoscopy are quite different [4]. All surgeons are aware of their own "learning curves", during which time complication rates may be appreciable [4],[5]. Although the complication rate may decrease when more experience is gained with the laparoscopic procedure, the increasingly advanced and difficulty procedures performed by the gynecologists via laparoscopic further potentiates the higher risk of complications [6].

The rapidity of the uptake of these procedures into routine use and numerous adverse outcomes have raised justifiable concern [7],[8]. According to Magrina *et al.* review among 1,549,360 patients, the overall laparoscopic complication rate ranges 0.2-10.3% [6]. An early learning curve with limited cases may account for the high complication rate up to 10.3% (47 of 452 patients) [9, 10]. In a Finnish national-wide study [11], the major complication rate in overall gynecologic laparoscopies was 0.4% (130/ 32,205) among total procedures, and 1.26% (118/ 9,337) in operative laparoscopies. In an American Association Gynecologic Laparoscopy (AAGL) membership survey for laparoscopic-assisted vaginal hysterectomy (LAVH) was 6.59% (983/ 14,911) [12]. In Taiwan, Lee *et al.* reported the major complication rate 1.66% (12/ 722) in LAVHs group [13]; Wu *et al.* reported 1.59% (24/ 1,507) [14] and 0.72% (31/4307) in the follow-up study [15]. Since laparoscopic surgery is highly experience-dependent, follow-up studies in different study periods deserve continuous attentions.

Urinary bladder and bowel injuries comprise the main part of the complications. **Bladder injuries** are relatively common in the gynecologic field, especially in LAVHs. The complication rate was 2.4% (22/9,337) in Finnish study [11], and 1.08% (161/14,911) in AAGL study [12]. In Taiwan, Lee *et al.* reported 0.8% (6/722) [13]; it was 0.40% (6/1,507) [14] and 0.30% (13/ 4107) in Wu *et al.* follow-up study [15]. **Bowel injuries**, although not common, is one of the most serious complications when not detected and managed promptly. van der Voort *et al.* reported, based on 29 studies, the incidence of laparoscopy-induced gastrointestinal injury was 0.13 % (430/ 329,935) and of bowel perforation 0.22 % (66/ 29,532). The incidence may be under-reported due to retrospective and complication that occurred after leaving hospital being overlooked [16].The small intestine was most frequently injured 55.8 % (227/ 407), followed by the large intestine 38.6% (157/ 407), and the stomach 3.9 % (16/ 407) [17]. The reported bowel injury rates ranged from 0.16% (15/ 9,337) [11] to 0.62% (93/ 14,911);[12] 0.28% (2/ 722) in Lee *et al.* LAVHs stud;[13] 0.33% (5/ 1,507) in Wu *et al.* study.[14], and 0.16% (7/ 4,107) in the follow-up study [15]. Nevertheless, laparoscopy-induced bowel injury is associated with a high mortality rate of 3.6% [17].

2. Electrosurgery use in laparoscopic surgery

The behavior of electricity in living tissue is generally governed by Ohm's law:

Voltage (V)= current (I) x resistance (R)

Electrical current flows through a continuous circuit. Voltage is the necessary electromotive force that mediates or drives this electron movement through the circuit. Heat is produced when electrons encounter resistance [18]. The electricity has the following characteristics, which how it works and how it associates complications: i.e. (i) electricity takes the path of least resistance, (ii) seeks ground, and (iii) must have a complete circuit to do work [18].Understanding the electrosurgical principles is essential for using appropriate currents and techniques to achieve the desired tissue effect and to avoid complication [19].

Electrosurgical units (ESUs) are the most common piece of electrical equipment in the operating room. The constant presence of the ESU in the operating room assists surgeon to achieve desired tissue effect, but also increases the potential for electrosurgical injury [20]. With electrosurgery, we can achieve tissue effects such as cutting (also called vaporization), fulguration (also called superficial coagulation, or spray coagulation), and desiccation (also called deep coagulation) [20],[21],[22]. Primary factors that determine tissue effects of electrosurgery include energy modality (monopolar or bipolar), generator power output (watts), the alternating current waveform, the current density, and surgical techniques.

1. **Energy modality**, i.e., monopolar and biopolar. In monopolar electrosurgery, the current flows starts with the active electrode, through the patient and the return electrode for the completion of the circuit [21]. With monopolar current, the instrument tip is one pole, whereas the second pole is the grounding pad. In bipolar electrosurgery, both active and return electrodes are located at the surgical field, typically within the instrument tip [21]. The electrodes are only millimeters apart, therefore relatively low power of bipolar systems are needed to desiccate the tissue [23]. The power output of bipolar instruments is one-third to one-tenth that of monopolar systems.
2. **Generator power output** is most often indicated via a digital readout on the face of the generator. Others may have a logarithmic scale from 1 (lowest) to 10 (highest), making exact settings and adjustments more difficult [20],[18],[23]. Surgeons should understand what kind of generator they use and in what scale the power is presented.

3. **Alternating current waveforms** include cut waveform (continuous, non-modulated, undamped), blended waveform (different percentage duty cycle), and coagulation waveform (interrupted, modulated, damped), which are used for different surgical aims [20],[18],[23]. However, these labels are misleading because they do not necessarily produce the tissue effects that are associated with the terms "cut" and "coagulation" [23]. In fact, "cut" waveform can coagulate, and "coagulation" waveform can cut. Moreover, "cut" waveform is often the most appropriate current to use for tissue coagulation [23]. A cut waveform incorporates higher current but lower voltage than coagulation waveforms at the same power setting. As contrast, coagulation waveform has higher voltage and lower current than a cut waveform of the same power setting [18]. Therefore, with the same wattage, coagulation waveform has a much higher voltage than cut current. Higher voltages are more likely to produce unwanted effects and injuries than lower voltages. In more simple terms, for the same power levels, cut waveform produce less charring and tissue damage [23].
4. **Current density** depends on the area of surface contact, and the shape or size of the electrode [20],[18],[23]. Current density can affect the tissue effect as well as the heat production. The greater the current that passes through an area, the greater the effect will be on the tissue. Also, the greater the amount of heat that is produced by the current, the greater the thermal damage on tissue [18]. Heat generated at the tissue is inversely proportional to the surface area of the electrode. Smaller electrodes provide a higher current density and result in a concentrated heating effect at the site of tissue contact [18]. When the contact area is decreased by a factor of 10 (e.g. 2.5 cm2 to 0.25 cm2), the current density increases by a factor of 100 (e.g. 0.01 amp/cm2 to 1 amp/cm2), and the resulting final temperature increases from 37oC to 77oC. Thus, a small contact area produces high enough temperatures to cut [24],[22].
5. **Surgical techniques** include hand-eye coordination, speed of procedure, proximity between the electrode and the tissue, and dwell time [20],[18],[23]. During the learning curve, hand-eye coordination difficulties may be encountered involve working in a two-dimension environment with their hands generally disassociated from their eyes, esp. in radically new operative skills [25]. The speed of procedure will result in either less or more coagulation and thermal spread [18]. Proximity between the electrode and the tissue can determine contact (e.g. desiccation effect) or non-contact tissue effect, e.g. fulguration effect [23]. The dwell time determines the amount of tissue effect. Too long activation will produce wider and deeper tissue damage more than the anticipated desired tissue effect [18].

3. Mechanisms of injury

The majority of laparoscopic complications happen subsequent to the followings: the entry to the peritoneal cavity, the delivery of energy to the surgical site (e.g. electrosurgery) and specific high-risk procedures [26]. A trocar or Veress needle caused the most bowel injuries 41.8% (114/ 273), followed by a coagulator or laser 25.6% (70/ 273). In 68.9 % of instances of bowel injury, adhesions or a previous laparotomy were noted [17]. Injuries during laparoscopic electrosurgical procedures can be attributed to misidentification of anatomic structures, mechanical trauma, and electro-thermal complications [12]. Misidentification and mechanical trauma can occur laparoscopically, just like that in laparotomy [27]. Moreover, surgical skills become more difficult when the surgeon's spatial orientation and hand-eye coordination have not been well established.

Electro-thermal injury may result from the following situations: direct application, insulation failure, direct coupling, capacitive coupling, etc.

1. **Direct application.** Electrosurgical injury may happen via direct application similar to open laparotomy. It may be due to unintended activation of the electrosurgical probe, e.g. moving from the intended operating area to an iliac artery or vein on the pelvic sidewall, or operating on a moving ovarian cyst [28].
2. **Insulation failure-induced stray current** occurs when damage occurs to the covering of the active electrode, allowing the current to contact non-target tissue, which is often out of view of the surgical team members. Pre-operative careful inspection of the equipment before and after use is the best means of identifying defective insulation [20]. Two major causes of insulation failure include the use of high voltage currents and the frequent re-sterilization of instruments which can weaken and break the insulation [21]. Breaks in the insulation create alternate pathways for current to flow. With a high enough concentration of current, injury to adjacent organs is possible. This occurs primarily when a coagulation waveform is used due to its high voltage output [21]. A common equipment defect is a break in insulation. The risk of a break may be increased when using a 5-mm insulated instrument through a 10-mm sleeve, or by repeated use of disposable equipment [20]. Extensive burns and operating room fires can occur from these current leaks with temperatures measured to be as high as 700 °C [29].
3. **Coupling. Direct coupling** occurs when the electrosurgical unit is accidentally activated while the active electrode is in close proximity to another metal instrument e.g. laparoscope, metal grasper forceps, within the abdomen [21]. Current from the active electrode flows through the secondary instrument through the pathway of least resistance, and potentially damages adjacent structures or organs in direct contact with the secondary instrument. Direct coupling can be prevented with visualization of the electrode in contact with the target tissue and avoiding contact with any other conductive instruments prior to activating the electrode [20]. Ito *et al.* reported a small bowel perforation after a thermal burn caused by contact with the end of the laparoscope during gynecologic laparoscopy [30]. The preventive maneuver is to activate the electrode only when it is fully visible and in contact with the target tissue [30]. However, one must keep in mind that the depth of penetration of thermal energy goes beyond that seen by the naked eye; therefore, unrecognized injuries can present later after progression of the damaged tissue [20].

   Capacitive coupling occurs when two conductive elements or instruments are separated by an insulator and form stored energy. An electrostatic field is created between the two conductors such that current through one conductor is transmitted to the second conductor once the net charge exceeds the insulator's capacity [21]. The electric current is transferred from one conductor (the active electrode), through intact insulation, into adjacent conductive materials (e.g. bowel, etc) without direct contact. For example, in a hybrid trocar sleeve, i.e. a nonconductive (plastic) locking anchor is placed over a conductive (metal) sleeve, the plastic anchor will stop the transmission into the abdominal wall over a large surface. This results in capacitive coupling. It happens to adjacent bowel, and results in bowel burns. Although the most common example of a capacitor being created is the placement of an active electrode, surrounded by its insulation, down a metal trocar, this can also occur with plastic trocars [27],[29]. Capacitor coupling may be minimized by activating the active electrode only when it is in contact with target tissues, limiting the amount of time that the coagulation setting (with its high-voltage peaks) is used, and by using metal cannulas that allow stray current to be dispersed through the patient's abdominal wall, not internal tissues [18],[23].

4. **Return electrode burns.** The primary purpose of the grounding (dispersive) pad is to prove the path of least resistance from the patient back to the generator and to ensure an area of low current density [31],[32]. To complete current circuit, the return electrode must be of low resistance with a large enough surface area to disperse the electrical current without generating heat. If the patient's return electrode not completely in contact with the patient's skin, or is not able to disperse the current safely, then the current exiting the body can have a high enough density to produce an unintended burn [21]. The quality of contact between the return electrode and the patient's skin can be compromised by excessive hair, adipose, bony prominences, presence of fluid, or scar tissue. It is important to have good contact between the patient and a dispersive pad [20]. No other object, including hair, clothes, gauzes, and so on, should be between the patient and the grounding pad
5. **Alternative site burn** can happen if the dispersive (ground) pad is not well attached to the patient's skin [20]. When the dispersive pad is compromised in the quantity or quality of the pad/patient interface, electrical circuit can be completed by some small grounded contact points, thus producing high current densities and causing a burn. Examples of such contact points include electrocardiogram (EKG) leads, towel clip, intravenous stand or stirrup, and neurosurgical head frames [31],[32]. The stray current could be intensified if the return electrode was distant from the operating site or if the grounded sites occurred in the path between the active and return electrode. In the case of ground-referenced electrosurgical units, even if the return electrode was disconnected, electrosurgery would continue with current finding alternative pathways to return to the ground. Electrocution of the patient under these circumstances was possible [21].

4. Preventive and adjuvant protective maneuvers

4.1 Pre-operative phase

1. **Knowledge of electrosurgical biophysics.** A thorough understanding of the biophysical principles of radio-frequency electrical energy is of supreme importance [20],[18],[23]. For example, when the generator output cannot accomplish tissue effects as expected, it should be suspected first that there is a defect in the ground plate or its connection, or that an alternative pathway for the current has been instituted [32].
2. **Bowel preparation** is important if it is anticipated that the large bowel is at risk [28]. It facilitates operative maneuvers by increasing intra-peritoneal free space and reducing inadvertent bowel trauma [33]. Additionally, bowel preparation reduces the severity of complications which may occur after bowel perforation. Also, the use of naso-gastric tube is recommended, esp. after several trials of endotracheal intubation, to diminish the possibility of a trocar entry into the stomach [15].
3. **To choose proper current waveform mode.** In monopolar electrosurgery, both "cut" or "coagulation" waveform can be used for either cutting effect or fulguration effect. A cutting current power setting must be between 50 and 80W to be effective. Typically, the coagulation current is effective with the power setting in the range of 30–50W. Although it is possible to cut tissue using coagulation currents at high power, the end result is greater charring and tissue damage [18]. Use bipolar instruments whenever possible [33].
4. **To improve dexterity and hand-eye coordination** through sequential phases of training, i.e. didactic phase, laboratory experience, observation and/or assistance, and

preceptorship [25]. The chances of direct trauma are greater during laparoscopic surgery because the surgeon is limited to visualize in only two-dimensions, with surgeon's hands generally dissociated from their eyes, esp. when operating on mobile organs [28],[34].

5. **Team resource management (TRM).** It is important to organize a laparoscopic team, including biomedical engineer, perioperative nurses and other operation room personnel, and promote extended education activities and participation in medical conferences. When adapting the wisdom of crew resource management (CRM) from aviation to medicine, there still some challenges. Surgical team also needs to improve team communication and coordination [35].

4.2 Intra-operative phase

1. **Safe pneumo-peritonization and entry.** The site of primary entry is usually the umbilicus, but there is a high risk of subumbilical adhesions that may contain bowel in patients with a history of previous laparotomy [26]. There is therefore a risk of injury to the bowel regardless of the entry method, and in these cases, consideration should be given to the use of an alternative site such as left upper quadrant, i.e. Palmer's point [36]. Te Palmer's entry is safe with a lower failure rate in the patients with risks of underlying adhesions and more appropriate in the presence of a large pelvic mass or a nearby hernia [36]. Contraindications to the use of this site, such as hypersplenism or a distended stomach, should be excluded before entry [26].
   The blind insertion of a Veress needle or first trocar to create the pneumoperitoneum has been shown to cause vascular and visceral injuries. No single insertion technique is universally safe and divorced from complications in establishing pneumoperitoneum. The use of the open laparoscopy method introduced by Hasson may reduce the likelihood of bowel injury in patients who are likely to have anterior wall adhesions [37]. Other techniques include a well-executed open technique with employment of digital pressure to and local adhesiolysis [38], and/or adjuvant instruments, e.g. optic access trocar [39],[40] can be offered as suggestion for reducing injuries. In addition, the radially expandable sleeve with a tapered blunt dilator and cannula has been proposed to a potential safer laparoscopic trocar access [41]. The radially expanding access system (STEP) trocar entry had less trocar site bleeding when compared with standard trocar entry [42]. The trocar-cannula systems with safety apparatus do not necessarily guarantee the safety during entrance of the abdominal wall, because the relatively thick plastic shields need extra effort push the shield through the transveralis fascia and peritoneum [31],[43].
2. **To identify individual anatomic variation.** Left and right pelvic anatomic locations are not necessarily mirror images, laparoscopically. The course of the inferior epigastric vessels can be more difficult to identify in overweight patients. The proximity of the ureter to the uterosacral and infundibulopelvic ligaments reaffirms the need to identify them before dissection [44].
3. **The adequate electrosurgical techniques,** e.g. do not activate electrode in the air, converting to laparotomy when indicted. Activating the electrode in the air, when not in use, will create an 'open circuit', which can result in a capacitive current effect, too. Capacitive coupling is increased by open circuits, use of 5-mm cannulas (versus 10 mm), and higher generator voltages [45]. This situation can be avoided by using multiple, short activation time that allows normal tissue to remain cool [27].

Meanwhile, do not activate the instrument in close proximity or direct contact with another instrument [21]. Activate the electrode only when whole tissue is in the field of vision, to minimize the chances of direct trauma. After the use of electrosurgery, keep it in view until it has cooled or removed from the body [33]. Meanwhile, surgeons should learn to operate via traditional laparotomy before progressing to laparoscopy. In order to minimize complications, trainees need to become proficient at converting to laparotomy when the procedure cannot be completed laparoscopically [25],[28] .

4. **The adequate use of current waveform and advanced biopolar facility.** By lowering the concentration of the current used, coagulating with a cutting current, and using an active electrode monitoring system, the risk of accidental burns caused by insulation failure can be reduced [21]. Advanced bipolar facility include: Ligasure (Valley Lab Covidien, Boulder, CO, U.S.A), Gyrusw Olympus Gyrus ACMI (Maple Grove, MN, U.S.A), EnSeal (Ethicon Endo-Surgery, Cincinnati, OH, U.S.A). Ligasure combined the technology of pressure and bipolar energy; Gyrus used pulsed bipolar energy; EnSeal combined high levels of pressure and temperature sensitive electrodes [46].
5. **To use electrosurgical accessory safety equipment** when possible. **A return electrode monitoring system (REM)** is a dual-padded patient return electrode system designed to monitor irregular separation of the ground pad. It can actively monitor tissue impedance (resistance) at the contact between the patient's body and the patient return electrode, and interrupts the power if the quality and/or quantity are compromised. REM can monitor and assist to avoid return electrode burn. This system inactivates the generator if a condition develops at the patient return electrode site that could result in a burn [20]. **Active electrode monitoring (AEM)** e.g. Encision, Inc, (Boulder, CO, U.S.A), was developed to minimize the risks of insulation failure and capacitive coupling, active electrode monitoring systems now exist [21]. When interfaced with electrosurgical units, these systems continuously monitor and shield against the occurrence of stray electrosurgical currents. Critical to the success of these systems are the integrated laparoscopic instruments which have a secondary conductor within the shaft that provides coaxial shielding [21]. If any stray energy is sensed, the radiofrequency generator shuts down before a burn can occur [46]. The use of an active electrode monitoring system and limiting the amount of time that a high voltage setting is used can also eliminate concerns about capacitive coupling [20].

Tissue response technology (TRT) uses a computer-controlled tissue feedback system that automatically senses resistance of the tissue and adjusts the output voltage to maintain a consistent effect across different tissue density, to achieve a consistent tissue effect. Newer generator constantly monitor impedance to maintain the preset wattage over a broad range of impedance, avoiding unnecessary higher wattage with potential hazards [28]. Improved performance can now be achieved at lower electrosurgical settings [47]. **Vessel sealing technology,** which combines with bipolar electrosurgery with tissue response generators and optimal mechanical pressure, can seal and fuse vessel walls up to 7 mm in diameter [21]. This technology delivers high current and low voltage to the targeted tissue and denatures the vessel wall protein; the mechanical pressure allows the denatured protein to form a coagulum [48]. Thermal spread appears to be reduced when compared to traditional bipolar electrosurgical systems. Valleylab, Gyrus ACMI, and SurgRx, Inc. are three companies which have developed devices for both open and laparoscopic applications

[48],[49],[50]. **Smoke evacuation scavenger system** can improve the operation field from smoggy atmosphere. It also protects patients, as well as surgical staffs, from the exposure of smoke and the byproducts during laparoscopic procedures [51].

6. **To use adjuvant protective procedure.** Some adjuvant protective procedures were suggested during laparoscopic surgeries. In addition to these preventive maneuvers, Wu *et al.* inserted a bladder retractor via urethral meatus into the bladder cavity to identify the utero-vesical space, especially in cases with dense fibrotic adhesion (Fig. 1). The bladder retractor with oval-shaped tip can mobilize the bladder and counter-act with the uterine mobilizer to expose vesico-uterine space at an adequate distance, which was not achieved easily with standard laparoscopic techniques [52]. Lin and Chou conducted a modified procedure of Laparoscopic assisted vaginal hysterectomy (LAVH) by preligating the uterine arteries, in which a pair of polydioxanone (PDS) clips were placed at the uterine artery located between the ureter and the bifurcation of the hypogastric artery before the uterine vessels were desiccated [53]. Chang *et al.* use the retrograde umbilical ligament tracking method for uterine artery ligation to prevent excessive bleeding from uterine vessels and ureterhal thermal injury, especially in huge uterine size [54]. The adjuvant protective procedures may account, at least in part, for the lower ureteral injury rate [15]. A high index of suspicion and prior visualization and/or retroperitoneal dissection of the ureter, will be helpful in decreasing ureteral injury [55].

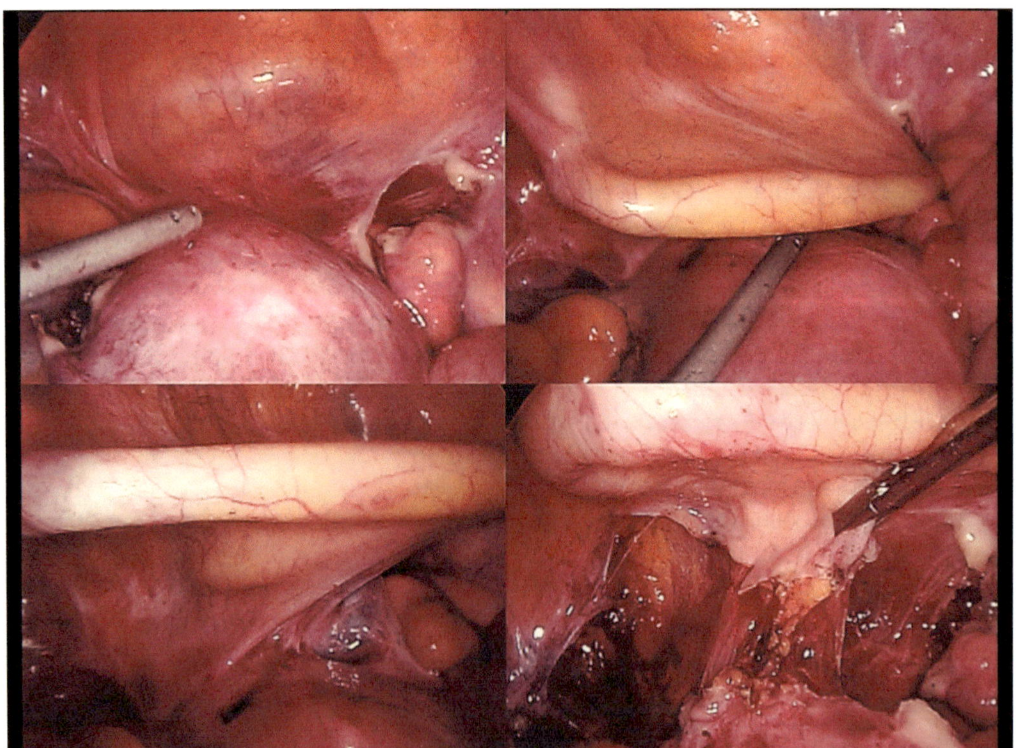

Fig. 1. A bladder retractor via urethral meatus into the bladder cavity to identify the utero-vesical space in cases with dense fibrotic adhesion.

5. Recognition of complication and salvage procedures

5.1 Intra-operative phase

1. **Entry (Veress- or trocar-) related.** The treatment of bowel injuries depends upon the extent of damage. If the Veress needle has been inserted into a hollow viscus without tearing, no further therapy is indicated, since its small diameter leaves no defect; and the muscular wall will close over this puncture spontaneously [33]. However, when the insertion of the trocar into a small intestine, leaves a large defect, e.g. one-half the diameter of the lumen, a segment resection and anastomosis should be performed through laparotomy. If the perforation has occurred, it may be beneficial to leave the trocar in situ to serve to identify the site of laceration [56].
2. **Urinary tract injury. Bladder injury** can be detected by direct visualization of either bladder mucosa or Foley balloon (Fig. 2). If a bladder injury at laparoscopy is suspected but not immediately identified, diluted methylene blue should be instilled into the bladder via a Foley catheter. The bladder will be seen to fill and the dye will leak out through any lacerations [26]. To observe the gas leakage into the urine bag intra-operatively is another detection methods [15]. When bladder injury was recognized intra-operatively, it can be repaired vaginally, laparoscopically or by laparotomy without incident (Fig. 3). Early recognition with immediate salvage procedure could overcome further sequelae [57]. The extended use of an indwelling catheter should be considered.

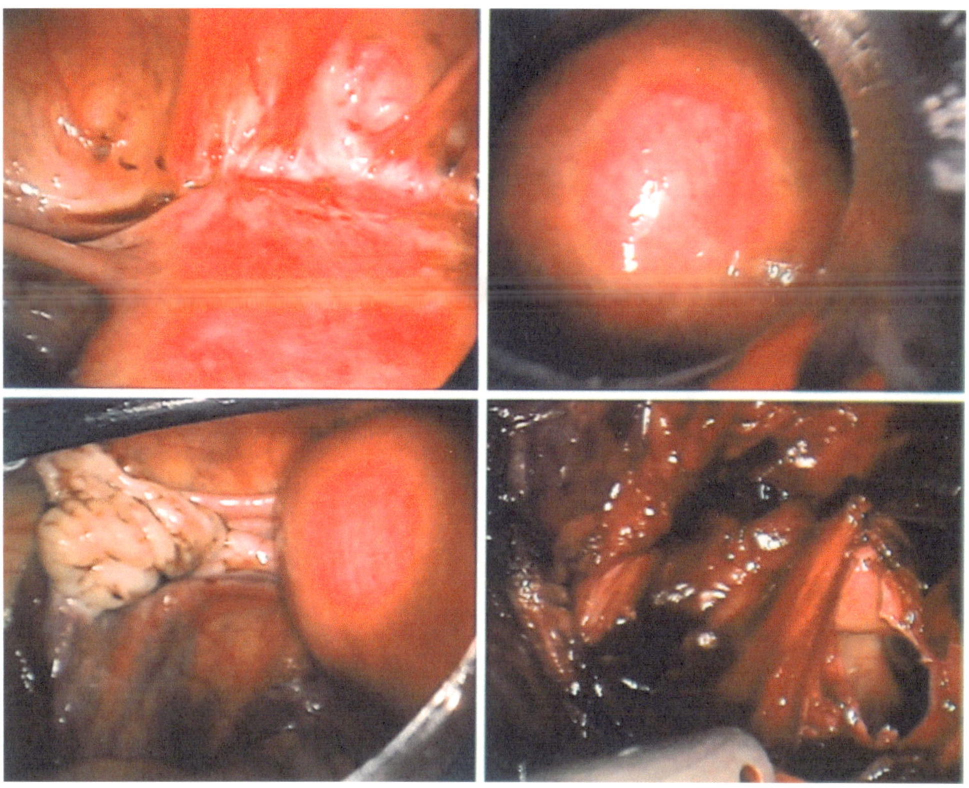

Fig. 2. Bladder injury detected by direct visualization of bladder mucosa and Foley balloon.

Ureteral injuries in gynecologic laparoscopy usually are not recognized intraoperatively, only those patients with persistent abdominal and/or flank pain, abdominal distention, and fever may raise the cautions during post-operative phase [55]. Those intra-operative recognized ureteral injuries can be solved by direct laparoscopic end-to-end reanastomosis (Fig. 4). It can be also resolved by double-J ureteral stent with or without the assistance of ureteroscopy (Fig. 5). If the initial salvage procedure fails, percutaneous nephrostomy and antegrade ureteral double-J stent is a backup procedure to avoid the subsequent ureteral fistula.

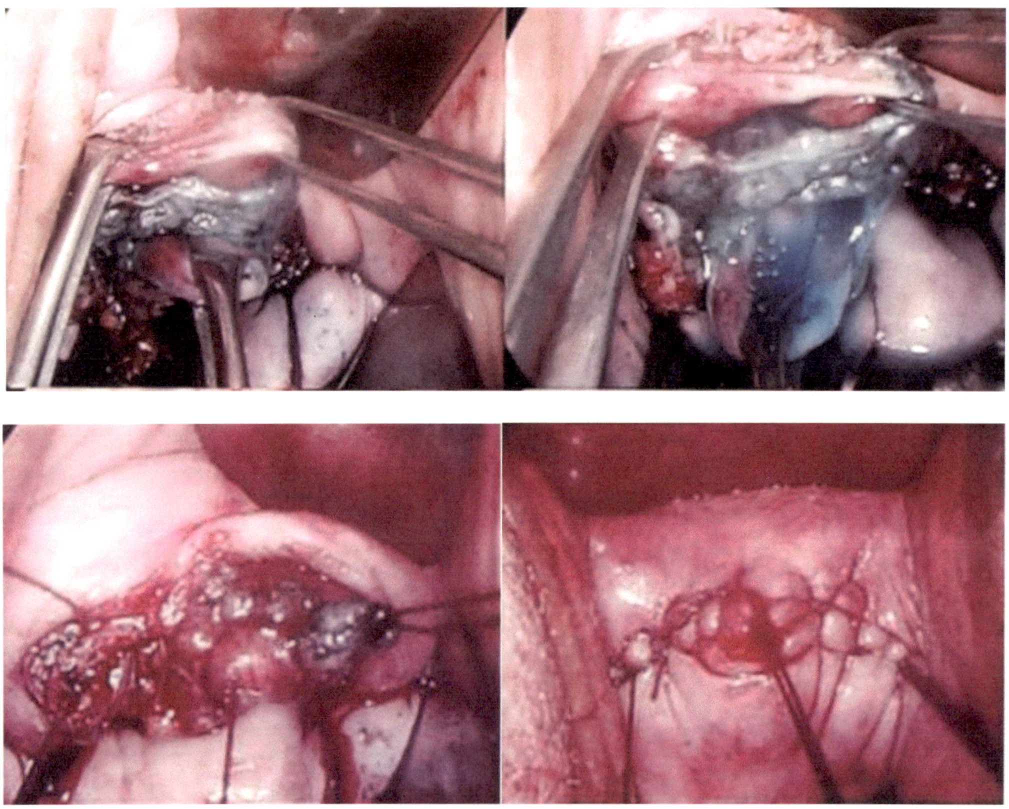

Fig. 3. Bladder injury was recognized intra-operatively, and was repaired vaginally.

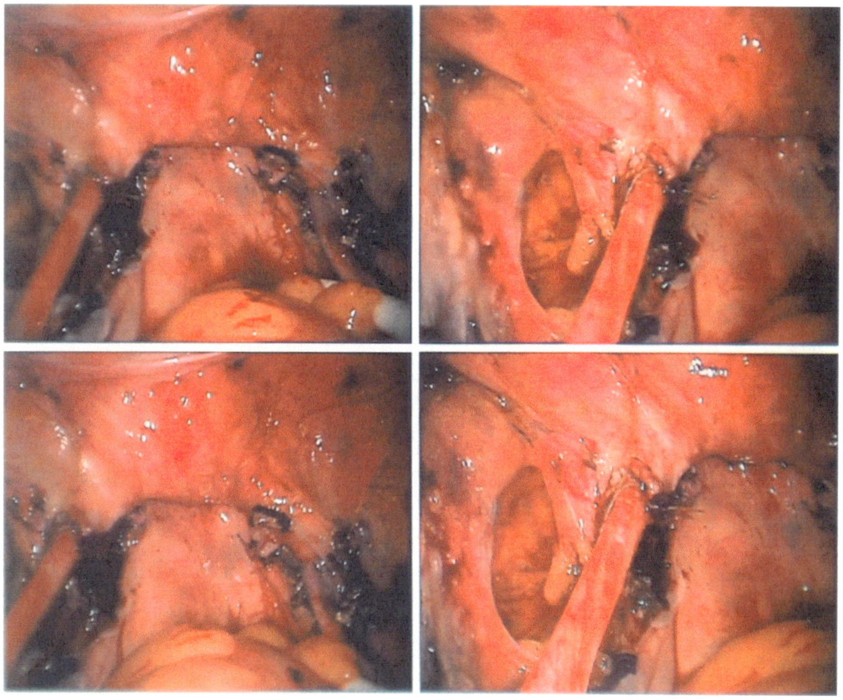

Fig. 4. Ureteral injuries recognized intraoperatively and was repaired by laparoscopic end-to-end reanastomosis.

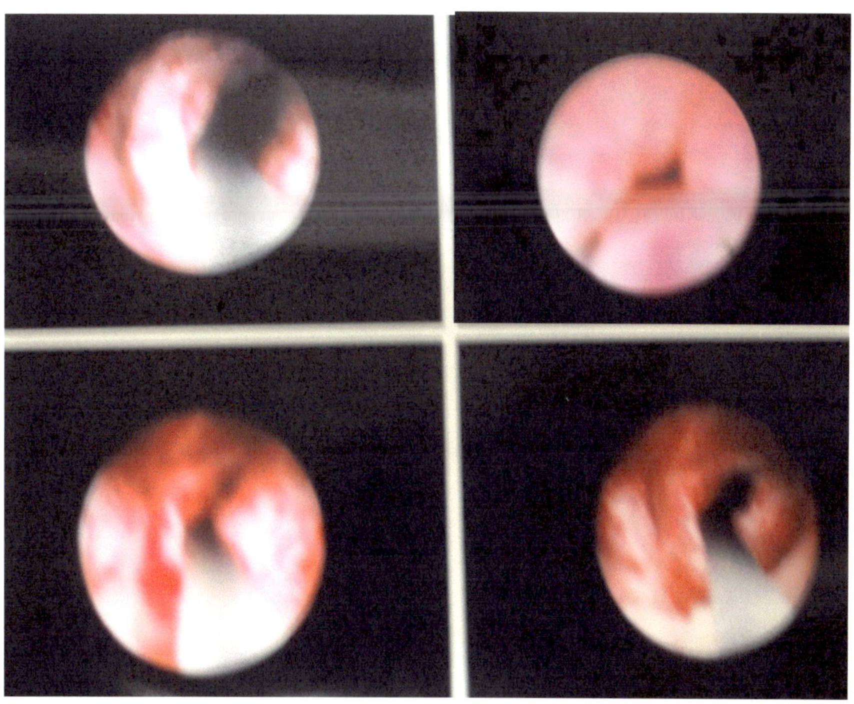

Fig. 5. Ureteral injuries recognized intraoperatively with the assistance of ureteroscopy.

3. **Bowel injury.** The time of diagnosis was reported 61.6% (154/ 250) recognized during surgery; 5.2% (13/ 250) recognized early post-operative phase within the next 48 hours; 10.4% (26/ 250) bowel injuries diagnosed late, at least on the third postoperative day or later. Another 22.8% (57/250) diagnosed after the conclusion of surgery, the number of hours elapsed was not reported [17]. A laparotomy was most frequently performed to manage the laparoscopy-induced bowel injury (78.6%). Conservative (7.0%) and laparoscopic (7.5%) treatment were used considerably less often [58],[17].

Stomach injury is a rare complication, it may be encountered after several trials of endotracheal intubations (Fig. 6). The inadvertent endotracheal intubation can cause excess gas inflated into the stomach and displaced the hyperinflated stomach as low as the periumbilical area [15]. Naso-gastric intubation for decompression is helpful to prevent gastric injury for those cases with distended stomach. **Injury to small bowel** or prepped colon, primary closure in two layers under laparoscopic guidance is recommended [33]. In selected cases with trocar-induced penetrating injuries of the bowel, institution of drainage and antibiotics can allow possible medical management of the problem, and thereby preclude conversion to laparotomy [59]. Conservative management comprised percutaneous drainage of abscesses, antibiotics or expectant treatment [17].

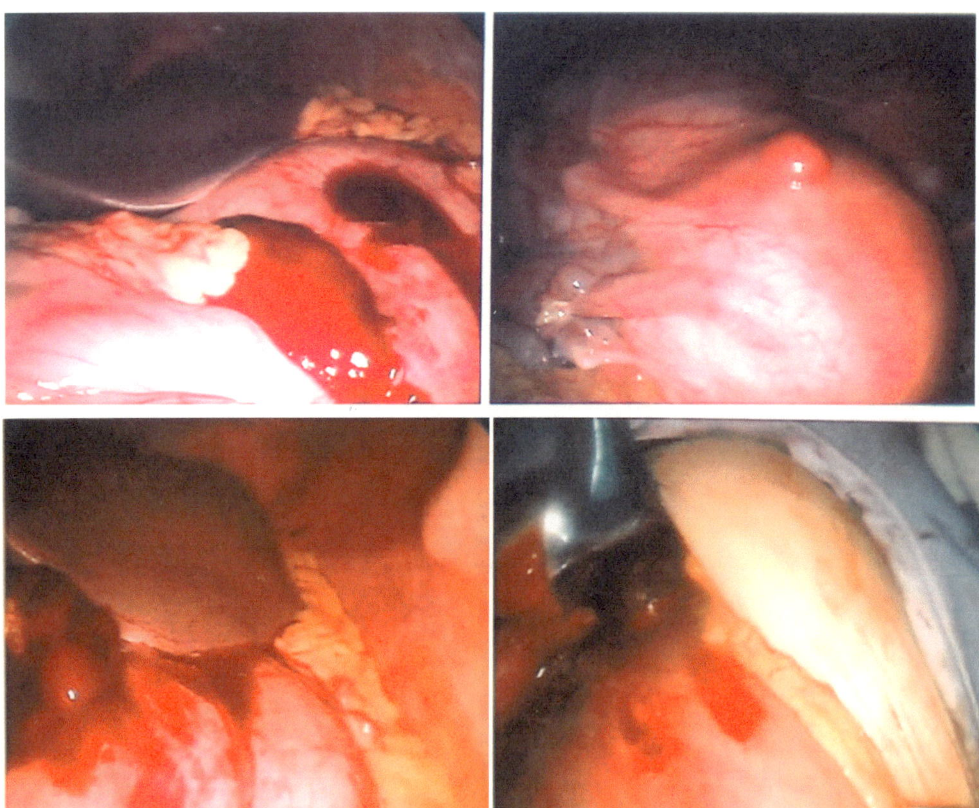

Fig. 6. Stomach injury by the introduction of primary trocar after several trials of endotracheal intubations.

When a large bowel injury is identified at the time of surgery, it is appropriate to repair this immediately, usually with the direct involvement of colorectal surgical colleagues [26]. The exact technique of repair will depend on the size of the injury, the exact site, and whether bowel preparation has been performed before surgery. As for colon injury, the transverse colon and sigmoid colon are most commonly traumatized by the trocar insertion. The spillage of foul-smelling gas through the insufflation needle is a helpful diagnostic sign [56]. The treatment options include primary repair, colostomy or segmental resection [33]. Superficial lesions can be treated with a laparoscopic purse-string suture placed beyond the margins of the thermally affected tissue or by postoperative observation alone [28]. Defects involving the full thickness of the bowel wall require direct surgical repair via laparoscopy or open lapaarotomy [56]. A suture to oversaw a lesion was performed mainly for serosal damage or burn sites, and for perforations that were discovered immediately [17]. Primary closure of the perforation trauma was reported to be a safe method, with a failure rate varying from 1.2% to 2.4 %, as an alternative to traditional colostomy if the absence of contraindication. The contraindication included more than two associated injuries, the need for blood transfusion over 4 units, significant contamination, increasing colon injury severity scores [60]. A laparoscopic suture closure followed by copious irrigation until the effluent becomes clear might be also satisfactory [61]. Suturing was the procedure most often performed at laparotomy, 63% times (61/ 97), followed by bowel resection with reanastomoses 26% (25/ 97). A diverting stoma was required 11 % (11/ 97) [17]. Full-thickness penetration of the rectum can occur during the excision of rectal endometriosis. After excision of the nodule of the recto-sigmoid colon, a single-or double-layered repaired can be done by laparoscopic assisted transvaginal approach or total laparoscopic intracorporeal technique [62]. Concerning the unprepared bowel with a large amount of fecal contamination, laparotomy followed by repair and colostomy should be considered [33].

4. **Electro-thermal effect.** The sigmoid colon is especially vulnerable because of its close proximity to the uterus and ovaries. Colon injury caused by bipolar electrosurgery can be readily identified by viewing the area of blanch on the surface of the colon, as compared with monopolar electrosurgery which is more difficult to detect and evaluate [28]. Superficial thermal injuries to the bowel may be treated prophylactically with a laparoscopic-guided pursestring suture placed beyond the thermally affected tissue [56]. The spread of electro-thermal injuries is greater than the initial area of branching and can create a large area of necrosis; thus the depth of injury is difficult to assess even if they are noticed intraoperatively. The injury of a viscus or bile duct typical occurs only after several days have elapsed [31]. Thermal injury of the bowel necessitates segmental resection with a wide margin around the site of injury because thermal damage may extend for a considerable distance from the site of thermal contact (several centimetres) [33]. Excision of a generous segment up to 5 cm on each side of the margin of the injury site, to include this area of coagulation necrosis, is required to prevent subsequent reperforation. Currently, the best way to treat bowel injury during laparoscopic surgery is by traditional laparotomy. However, as laparoscopists become more experienced in laparoscopic surgery, laparoscopic suture repair will become another choice in the management [13]. The efficiency and accuracy of laparoscopic bowel suturing techniques have been proposed. In Reich's series, there are few indications for colostomy during the repair of bowel injuries noted during the course of a laparoscopic procedure [56].

5.2 Post-operative phase

1. **Being highly alert to postoperative warning signs.** During postoperative observation period, which may last 3 to 5 days, the surgical team should be highly alert to the early manifestations of peritonitis, especially for physicians who are on duty for coverage. Isolated small intestine injuries may not cause clear or rapid symptoms and abnormal laboratory values, while colon injury with or without combined ileal injuries, has grave outcomes. The degree of peritonitis depends on the amount of spillage and length of time between perforation and exploration. However, these warning signs may be insidious, and imply the importance of possible early intervention. For example, persistent excessive external fluid leak from the periumbilical area after laparoscopic surgery with no drainage from other incisional sides may suggest small-bowel injury. latrogenic, internal-external canalization between the small intestine and the skin masked clinical symptoms and signs of small-intestinal injury [63].

Abnormal laboratory and imaging tests are helpful in confirming the diagnosis, however, normal test result is not reassuring. Patients who do not void may have early manifestation of bowel injury. Lack of classic symptoms, signs, or changes in pertinent laboratory data did not rule out small-bowel perforation [63].

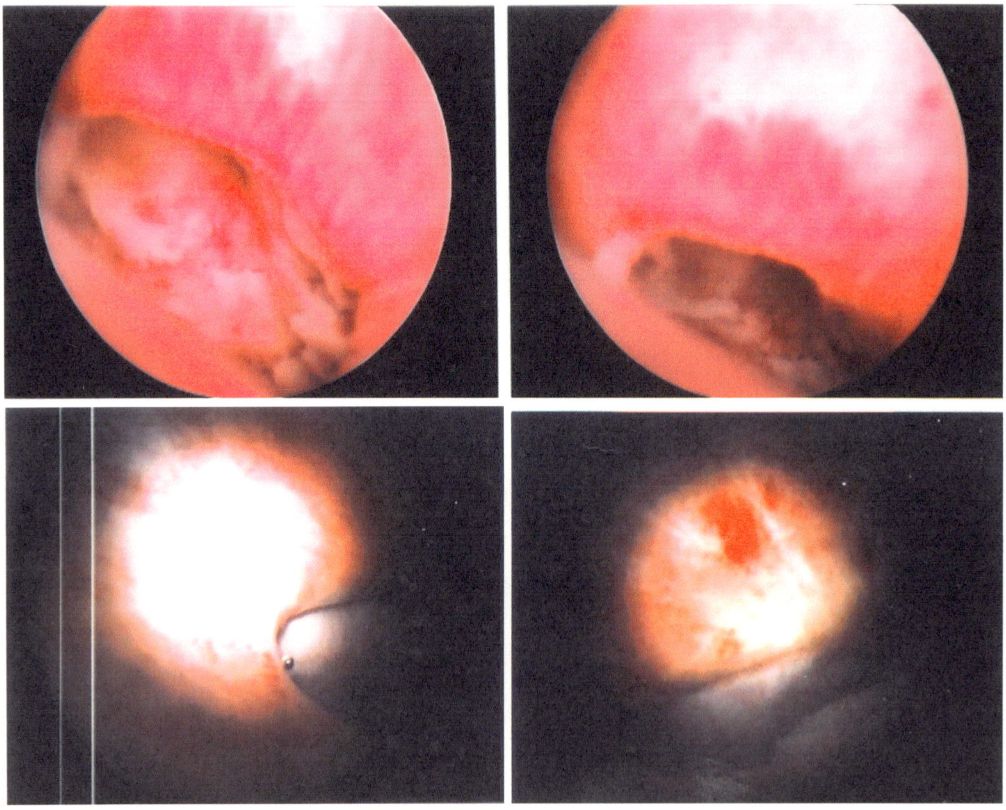

Fig. 7. Vesico-vaginal fistula happened with the delayed deterection of bladder injury.

2. **Patient education before discharge.** Bowel injury that is unrecognized at the time of surgery is one of the most dangerous complications of laparoscopic surgery. All

patients undergoing laparoscopy must be advised before discharge that they should feel progressively better, and that any worsening in their condition should prompt them to seek advice [26]. They may well make a reasonable initial recovery and be discharged home. Once at home, they may become unwell, develop pain and fever and start vomiting. On seeking medical help, it is essential that the attending staff have a very high degree of suspicion of bowel injury. In the case of postoperative peritonism or peritonitis, the early use of computed tomography scanning can be very useful in the diagnosis of bowel obstruction secondary to a port site hernia. Increasing abdominal pain after laparoscopic surgery demands an expedient evaluation, even if it requires a repeated laparoscopy with a negative finding [34]. The involvement of general surgeons and early recourse to exploratory surgery is essential to prevent a poor outcome [26].

3. **Delay detection of bladder injury** may result in vesico-vaginal fistula which demand repetitive repair if the first salvage procedure failed (Fig. 7) [15]. If a ureteric injury is suspected but not confirmed at the time of initial surgery, an intravenous pyelogram should be performed. Urological colleagues should be involved in the management of these complication [26]. Once ureteral injury was detected in a late post-operative period after the formation of ureteral fistula, ascites with urine content (urinoma) might complicate the situation. Laparotomy for end-to-end anastomosis is usually necessary in the cases with complete transection, ligation or electro-thermal injury-induced ischemic necrosis [15].

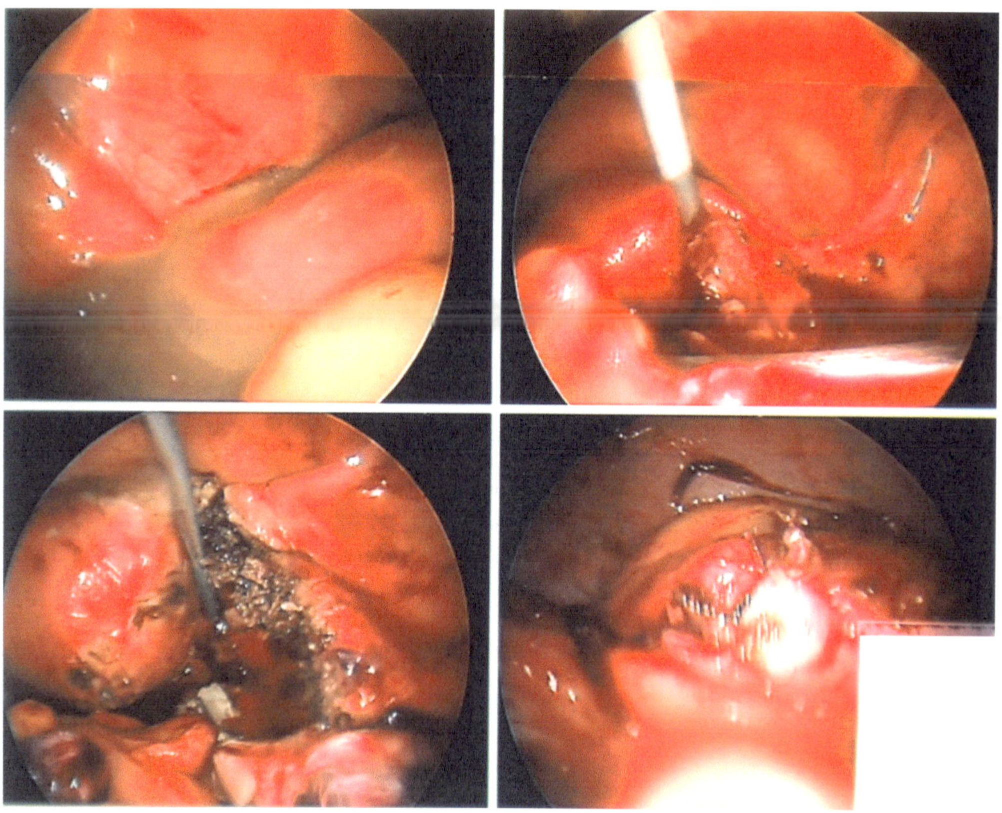

Fig. 8. Tubo-ovarian abscess is a risk factor associated with bowel injuries.

4. **Delay detection of bowel injury** may cause high morbidity and mortality. van der Voort *et al.* reported overall mortality rate associated with bowel injury complication 3.6% (16/ 450) The [17]. The clinical picture may be varied. The early manifestation may be non-specific, e.g. vomiting, abdominal pain, distension and malaise; which is followed by additional features, e.g. a localized peritoneal abscess or generalized peritonitis [33]. In this stage, fever, leukocytosis and even septic shock can occur. Bowel injury caused by direct trauma or electrothermal injury has different clinical courses and histo-pathologic findings [64]. Symptoms of bowel perforation after electrical injury usually arise 4 to 10 days after the procedures, whereas symptoms of traumatic perforation usually occur within 12 to 36 hours [56],[65],[34]. Most electro-thermal injuries, more common in large bowel, are unrecognized intraoperatively and lead to long-term sequelae. It may occur insidiously due to stray current, insulation failure or capacitive coupling, in addition to direct, active electrode injury [65]. As for the timing of detection, van der Voort *et al.* reported more than 10% unrecognized until the third post-operative day or later [17]. In Wu *et al.* series, some identifiable risk factors associated with bowel injuries were emergent, non-scheduled surgeries, tubo-ovarian abscess or uncertain preoperative diagnosis (Fig. 8) [15]. The original injury severity, e.g. multiple injuries, happened more commonly in managing tubo-ovarian abscess, especially combined with appendicitis. They had grave outcomes with prolonged hospitalizations and demanded multiple salvage procedures.

6. Conclusions

As complications are an inevitable reality of surgery, we need to be aware of the types of complications in a systematic way, train to respond in an appropriate way, and learn to communicate and deal with complications in laparoscopic surgery [8]. To achieve electrosurgical safety and to prevent potential electrosurgical injury, understanding the biophysics of electrosurgery, characteristics of their own equipment, desired tissue effects, types of injury, and the possible clinical manifestations are very important, as well as the mastering of laparoscopic surgical dexterity. Organizing a team-work including surgeons, perioperative nurses, biomedical engineers, and operation room personnel through team resource management. Intraoperative adjuvant protective maneuvers, early recognition and immediate implementation of salvage procedures will minimize the complications. Risk-aversive behaviors include paying particular attentions to placement of the first port, more liberal use of open laparoscopy or other adjuvant instrument, placement of all other ports under direct vision, elimination of intra-operative anatomy uncertainty, programmed inspection of the abdomen before withdrawing the laparoscope [31]. The dexterity improvement with hand-eye coordination and the knowledge of the mechanism of electrosurgical injury is important in recognizing and reducing potential electrosurgical complications [65]. Be highly alertness to postoperative warning signs including obvious signs of peritonitis or abdominal pain, and insidious ones. Patient education before discharge and detection of delay manifestation with salvage maneuver may minimize catastrophic disaster.

7. References

[1] Hoffman C P, Kennedy J, Borschel L, Burchette R, Kidd A: Laparoscopic hysterectomy: the Kaiser Permanente San Diego experience. *J Minim Invasive Gynecol* 2005;12:16-24.

[2] Medeiros L R, Rosa D D, Bozzetti M C, Fachel J M, Furness S, Garry R, et al.: Laparoscopy versus laparotomy for benign ovarian tumour. *Cochrane Database Syst Rev* 2009:CD004751.

[3] Nieboer T E, Johnson N, Lethaby A, Tavender E, Curr E, Garry R, et al.: Surgical approach to hysterectomy for benign gynaecological disease. *Cochrane Database Syst Rev* 2009:CD003677.

[4] Azziz R: Training, certification, and credentialing in gynecologic operative endoscopy. *Clin Obstet Gynecol* 1995;38:313-318.

[5] Peters J H, Ellison E C, Innes J T, Liss J L, Nichols K E, Lomano J M, et al.: Safety and efficacy of laparoscopic cholecystectomy. A prospective analysis of 100 initial patients. *Ann Surg* 1991;213:3-12.

[6] Magrina J F: Complications of laparoscopic surgery. *Clin Obstet Gynecol* 2002;45:469-480.

[7] Lam A, Kaufman Y, Khong S Y, Liew A, Ford S, Condous G: Dealing with complications in laparoscopy. *Best Pract Res Clin Obstet Gynaecol* 2009;23:631-646.

[8] Lam A, Khong S Y, Bignardi T: Principles and strategies for dealing with complications in laparoscopy. *Curr Opin Obstet Gynecol* 2010;22:315-319.

[9] Saidi M H, Vancaillie T G, White A J, Sadler R K, Akright B D, Farhart S A: Complications of major operative laparoscopy. A review of 452 cases. *J Reprod Med* 1996;41:471-476.

[10] Quasarano R T, Kashef M, Sherman S J, Hagglund K H: Complications of gynecologic laparoscopy. *J Am Assoc Gynecol Laparosc* 1999;6:317-321.

[11] Harkki-Siren P, Sjoberg J, Kurki T: Major complications of laparoscopy: a follow-up Finnish study. *Obstet Gynecol* 1999;94:94-98.

[12] Hulka J F, Levy B S, Parker W H, Phillips J M: Laparoscopic-assisted vaginal hysterectomy: American Association of Gynecologic Laparoscopists' 1995 membership survey. *J Am Assoc Gynecol Laparosc* 1997;4:167-171.

[13] Lee C L, Lai Y M, Soong Y K: Management of major complications in laparoscopically assisted vaginal hysterectomy. *J Formos Med Assoc* 1998;97:139-142.

[14] Wu M P, Lin Y S, Chou C Y: Major complications of operative gynecologic laparoscopy in southern Taiwan. *J Am Assoc Gynecol Laparosc* 2001;8:61-67.

[15] Tian Y F, Lin Y S, Lu C L, Chia C C, Huang K F, Shih T Y, et al.: Major complications of operative gynecologic laparoscopy in southern Taiwan: a follow-up study. *J Minim Invasive Gynecol* 2007;14:284-292.

[16] Brosens I, Gordon A, Campo R, Gordts S: Bowel injury in gynecologic laparoscopy. *J Am Assoc Gynecol Laparosc* 2003;10:9-13.

[17] van der Voort M, Heijnsdijk E A, Gouma D J: Bowel injury as a complication of laparoscopy. *Br J Surg* 2004;91:1253-1258.

[18] Advincula A P, Wang K: The evolutionary state of electrosurgery: where are we now? *Curr Opin Obstet Gynecol* 2008;20:353-358.

[19] Makai G, Isaacson K: Complications of gynecologic laparoscopy. *Clin Obstet Gynecol* 2009;52:401-411.

[20] Jones C M, Pierre K B, Nicoud I B, Stain S C, Melvin W V, 3rd: Electrosurgery. *Curr Surg* 2006;63:458-463.

[21] Wang K, Advincula A P: "Current thoughts" in electrosurgery. *Int J Gynaecol Obstet* 2007;97:245-250.

[22] Morris M L, Tucker R D, Baron T H, Song L M: Electrosurgery in gastrointestinal endoscopy: principles to practice. *Am J Gastroenterol* 2009;104:1563-1574.

[23] Lipscomb G H, Givens V M: Preventing electrosurgical energy-related injuries. *Obstet Gynecol Clin North Am* 2010;37:369-377.

[24] Frew J W: Performing surgery with a single electron: electrosurgery and quantum mechanics. *ANZ J Surg* 2009;79:680-682.

[25] Cooper M J, Fraser I: Training and accreditation in endoscopic surgery. *Curr Opin Obstet Gynecol* 1996;8:278-280.

[26] Jacobson T Z, Davis C J: Safe laparoscopy: is it possible? *Curr Opin Obstet Gynecol* 2004;16:283-288.

[27] Tucker R D, Voyles C R: Laparoscopic electrosurgical complications and their prevention. *Aorn J* 1995;62:51-53, 55, 58-59 passim; quiz 74-57.

[28] Nduka C C, Super P A, Monson J R, Darzi A W: Cause and prevention of electrosurgical injuries in laparoscopy. *J Am Coll Surg* 1994;179:161-170.

[29] Vilos G, Latendresse K, Gan B S: Electrophysical properties of electrosurgery and capacitive induced current. *Am J Surg* 2001;182:222-225.

[30] Ito M, Harada T, Yamauchi N, Tsudo T, Mizuta M, Terakawa N: Small bowel perforation from a thermal burn caused by contact with the end of a laparoscope during ovarian cystectomy. *J Obstet Gynaecol Res* 2006;32:434-436.

[31] Chandler J G, Voyles C R, Floore T L, Bartholomew L A: Litigious Consequences of Open and Laparoscopic Biliary Surgical Mishaps. *J Gastrointest Surg* 1997;1:138-145.

[32] Moak E: Electrosurgical unit safety. The role of the perioperative nurse. *Aorn J* 1991;53:744-746, 748-749, 752.

[33] Li T C, Saravelos H, Richmond M, Cooke I D: Complications of laparoscopic pelvic surgery: recognition, management and prevention. *Hum Reprod Update* 1997;3:505-515.

[34] Soderstrom R M: Bowel injury litigation after laparoscopy. *J Am Assoc Gynecol Laparosc* 1993;1:74-77.

[35] France D J, Leming-Lee S, Jackson T, Feistritzer N R, Higgins M S: An observational analysis of surgical team compliance with perioperative safety practices after crew resource management training. *Am J Surg* 2008;195:546-553.

[36] Granata M, Tsimpanakos I, Moeity F, Magos A: Are we underutilizing Palmer's point entry in gynecologic laparoscopy? *Fertil Steril*;94:2716-2719.

[37] Hasson H M: Window for open laparoscopy. *Am J Obstet Gynecol* 1980;137:869-870.

[38] Pelosi M A, 3rd, Pelosi M A: A simplified method of open laparoscopic entry and abdominal wall adhesiolysis. *J Am Assoc Gynecol Laparosc* 1995;3:91-98.

[39] Schoonderwoerd L, Swank D J: The role of optical access trocars in laparoscopic surgery. *Surg Technol Int* 2005;14:61-67.

[40] Berch B R, Torquati A, Lutfi R E, Richards W O: Experience with the optical access trocar for safe and rapid entry in the performance of laparoscopic gastric bypass. *Surg Endosc* 2006;20:1238-1241.

[41] Turner D J: A new, radially expanding access system for laparoscopic procedures versus conventional cannulas. *J Am Assoc Gynecol Laparosc* 1996;3:609-615.

[42] Ahmad G, Duffy J M, Phillips K, Watson A: Laparoscopic entry techniques. *Cochrane Database Syst Rev* 2008:CD006583.

[43] Tarnay C M, Glass K B, Munro M G: Entry force and intra-abdominal pressure associated with six laparoscopic trocar-cannula systems: a randomized comparison. *Obstet Gynecol* 1999;94:83-88.
[44] Nezhat C H, Nezhat F, Brill A I, Nezhat C: Normal variations of abdominal and pelvic anatomy evaluated at laparoscopy. *Obstet Gynecol* 1999;94:238-242.
[45] Voyles C R, Tucker R D: Education and engineering solutions for potential problems with laparoscopic monopolar electrosurgery. *Am J Surg* 1992;164:57-62.
[46] Bradshaw A D, Advincula A P: Optimizing patient positioning and understanding radiofrequency energy in gynecologic surgery. *Clin Obstet Gynecol*;53:511-520.
[47] Mayooran Z, Pearce S, Tsaltas J, Rombauts L, Brown T I, Lawrence A S, et al.: Ignorance of electrosurgery among obstetricians and gynaecologists. *Bjog* 2004;111:1413-1418.
[48] Harold K L, Pollinger H, Matthews B D, Kercher K W, Sing R F, Heniford B T: Comparison of ultrasonic energy, bipolar thermal energy, and vascular clips for the hemostasis of small-, medium-, and large-sized arteries. *Surg Endosc* 2003;17:1228-1230.
[49] Carbonell A M, Joels C S, Kercher K W, Matthews B D, Sing R F, Heniford B T: A comparison of laparoscopic bipolar vessel sealing devices in the hemostasis of small-, medium-, and large-sized arteries. *J Laparoendosc Adv Surg Tech A* 2003;13:377-380.
[50] Richter S, Kollmar O, Schilling M K, Pistorius G A, Menger M D: Efficacy and quality of vessel sealing: comparison of a reusable with a disposable device and effects of clamp surface geometry and structure. *Surg Endosc* 2006;20:890-894.
[51] Ott D: Smoke production and smoke reduction in endoscopic surgery: preliminary report. *Endosc Surg Allied Technol* 1993;1:230-232.
[52] Wu M P, Lin C C, Tian Y F, Huang K F, Chiu A W: The feasibility of an internal bladder retractor in facilitating bladder dissection during laparoscopic-assisted vaginal hysterectomy. *J Am Assoc Gynecol Laparosc* 2004;11:283-284.
[53] Lin Y S, Chou C Y: A modified procedure of laparoscopic hysterectomy: preligating the uterine arteries with polydioxanone clips. *J Gynecol Surg* 1996;12:173-176.
[54] Chang W C, Torng P L, Huang S C, Sheu B C, Hsu W C, Chen R J, et al.: Laparoscopic-assisted vaginal hysterectomy with uterine artery ligation through retrograde umbilical ligament tracking. *J Minim Invasive Gynecol* 2005;12:336-342.
[55] Gomel V, James C: Intraoperative management of ureteral injury during operative laparoscopy. *Fertil Steril* 1991;55:416-419.
[56] Reich H: Laparoscopic bowel injury. *Surg Laparosc Endosc* 1992;2:74-78.
[57] Saidi M H, Sadler R K, Vancaillie T G, Akright B D, Farhart S A, White A J: Diagnosis and management of serious urinary complications after major operative laparoscopy. *Obstet Gynecol* 1996;87:272-276.
[58] Deziel D J, Millikan K W, Economou S G, Doolas A, Ko S T, Airan M C: Complications of laparoscopic cholecystectomy: a national survey of 4,292 hospitals and an analysis of 77,604 cases. *Am J Surg* 1993;165:9-14.
[59] Birns M T: Inadvertent instrumental perforation of the colon during laparoscopy: nonsurgical repair. *Gastrointest Endosc* 1989;35:54-56.
[60] Curran T J, Borzotta A P: Complications of primary repair of colon injury: literature review of 2,964 cases. *Am J Surg* 1999;177:42-47.

[61] Reich H, McGlynn F, Budin R: Laparoscopic repair of full-thickness bowel injury. *J Laparoendosc Surg* 1991;1:119-122.

[62] Redwine D B, Koning M, Sharpe D R: Laparoscopically assisted transvaginal segmental resection of the rectosigmoid colon for endometriosis. *Fertil Steril* 1996;65:193-197.

[63] Ostrzenski A: Laparoscopic intestinal injury: a review and case presentation. *J Natl Med Assoc* 2001;93:440-443.

[64] Levy B S, Soderstrom R M, Dail D H: Bowel injuries during laparoscopy. Gross anatomy and histology. *J Reprod Med* 1985;30:168-172.

[65] Wu M P, Ou C S, Chen S L, Yen E Y, Rowbotham R: Complications and recommended practices for electrosurgery in laparoscopy. *Am J Surg* 2000;179:67-73.

Part 5

Endoscopic Entry Techniques

6

Laparoscopic Access Techniques

Mieszko Norbert Opilka, Zbigniew Lorenc and Jacek Starzewski
Higher Medical School in Sosnowiec, Silesian Medical University in Katowice, Saint's Barbara Memorial Main District Hospital no 5 in Sosnowiec
Poland

1. Introduction

The introduction of the first trocar, often following creation of the pneumoperitoneum is considered as crucial, and the most dangerous step of a laparoscopic procedure. Throughout the years individual methods of laparoscopic entry were described. The first person to create the pneumoperitoneum was German surgeon Georg Kelling (1866-1945). He performed this procedure on dogs. Among the methods actually used, arguably the most popular method of the closed laparoscopic entry probably was introduced in 1947 by Raol Palmer (1904-1945) French gynaecologist, who was also the inventor of an insuflator, which was adapted from a colposcopy pressure measuring device. He was followed by Kurt Semm (1927-2003) German gynaecologist, who invented also an automated electronic insuflation device. They both used in this technique the needle formerly developed in 1938 by a Hungarian, Janos Veres[1] (1903-1979) which had been primarly used for the creation of a pneumothorax. The last two, but not least to mention are Harrith M. Hasson, an American who described the open access laparoscopy in 1970, arguably considered as the safer than the classic closed (blind) method, and JR Dingfelder, who developed the direct laparoscopic trocar insertion technique in 1978.

2. Pneumoperitoneum techniques

There are numerous techniques of the intraperitoneal laparoscopic entry which can be found in various publications. However there are two main streams to be distinguished: the most popular methods with the creation of the pneumoperitoneum, and these performed without it. Some other techniques need to be mentioned, used mainly for retroperitoneal, or extraperitoneal access, however these should be considered as a part of the first mentioned group, and are more specific for disciplines other than surgery (urology).

2.1 Pneumoperitoneum

Pneumoperitoneum is a condition, when the whole intraperitoneal space is filled with gas (most often carbon dioxide). That causes an organ separation, and the space obtained this way is one of the crucial conditions for an introduction of necessary instruments, camera and the making of the intra-abdominal manoeuvres possible.

---

[1] Veres has been using his name with a double and single s, however his birth certificate states Veres.

2.1.1 Gases used

Actually the most popular gas used for laparoscopy is carbon dioxide. Other gases that are used for insuflation are nitrous oxide, argonium, helium, xenon, and also room air. It appears that there are significant differences between these, not only in physical matter. Many reports show the different effect on tumor biology during the laparoscopic procedure, and the helium, and especially the xenon seem to decrease tumor volume. The helium and the argonium are also found to be safer for the cardio-circulatory system.

2.1.2 Insuflator

Insuflator (laparoflator) is a device used for introduction of the gas under specified volume and pressure into peritoneal cavity. First, old devices were set manually, nowadays mainly automatic electronically controlled insuflators are used. These allow to set a precise flow of the introduced gas (in l/min), and at a constant pressure (12-14 mmHg). Some of the sets are equipped with bacteriological filters, and an endothermic system (to maintain adequate temperature of insufflated gas). In some cases a controlled desuflation is also used to remove a surgical smoke.

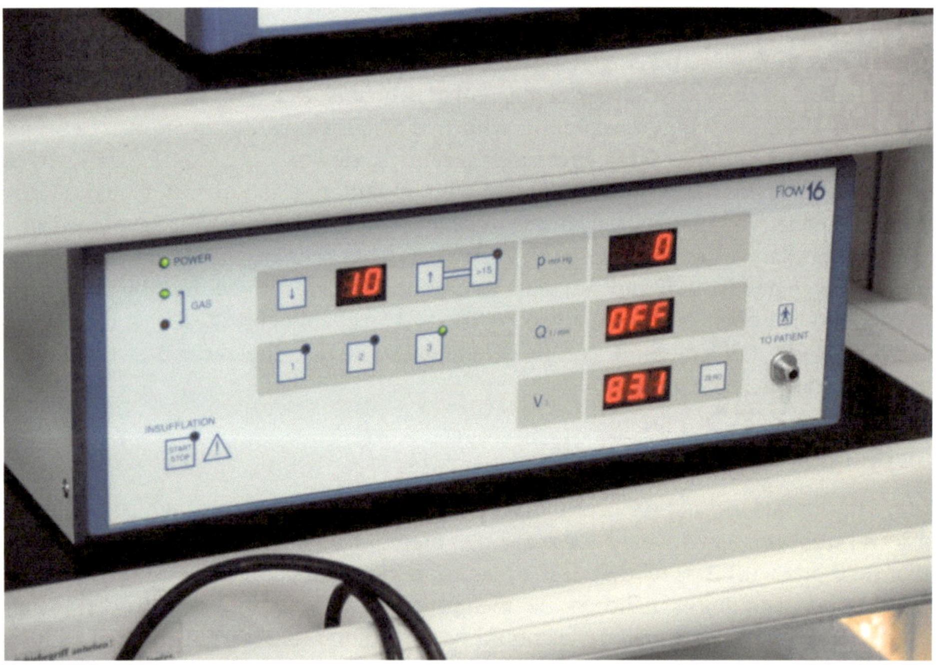

Fig. 1. Fully automated electronic insuflator at work.

2.1.3 Physiological consequences

Pneumoperitoneum is a specific situation, distinctly differentiating laparoscopy and open surgery. Recognition of physiological consequences of laparoscopy, as well as the pneumoperitoneum is crucial for safety of the techniques. Most of the consequences come from the use of the gas for the insufflation, especially the most popular carbon dioxide. Introduced gas (if endothermic system is not in use) causes a significant body temperature lost, it may also be the potential source of infection. Obviously it is not a single impact on the human organism. The peritoneum has the well known ability to absorb gases, particularly the carbon dioxide which must be subsequently exhaled. Therefore a respiratory acidosis, as well as a sympathetic stimulation, and an arrhythmia may occur. In the high pressure pneumoperitoneum (significantly above 12 mmHg) the risk of decrease of the heart stroke volume, and a flow in the inferior vena cava, as well as in the mesenteric vein exists, therefore the risk of a portal hypertension occur. The impaired blood flow concerns may be present also in the veins of the lower limbs, increasing the risk of a deep venous thrombosis and pulmonary embolism. It is followed by an increase in the intracranial pressure with the risk of a low cerebral blood flow These conditions are potentiated also by the Trendelenburg position, typically used in laparoscopy. Nevertheless many authors are using high pressure entries (up to 30mmHg) advocating that these minimize the risk of injuries, and do not affect significantly a cardiopulmonary functions in healthy patients.

2.1.4 Complications

One of the main advantages of laparoscopic surgery, when compared with open surgery is the lesser complication rate. Nevertheless, what is obvious, the minor, severe or even fatal complications may also occur. Serious ones such as a gas embolus (0,001%), the major vascular injury (0,003-1,33%), or visceral injury (0,04-4%) have been described in various publications, and are rather rare. Minor (0,1-0,5%) complications are the port site infection, subcutaneous emphysema, or bleeding from the epigastric vessels. Management depends on the type of the complication. Major vascular injury as the laceration of the abdominal aorta, or illiac vessels (caused mainly by a poor technique, but also too low pressure of a pneumoperitoneum) is an indication for an urgent laparotomy. Minor complications can be easily controlled, as in a case of the epigastric vessels injury with a Foley catether.

2.2 Closed laparoscopic access

Arguably is the most popular technique used for a laparoscopic entry, especially popular with gynaecologists. The closed method is also called a blind method, because of the first trocar which is pushed through the abdominal wall without the sight control. Prior to this step a pneumoperitoneum with the use of the Veres needle is made to avoid complications such as organs or main vessels injuries.

2.2.1 Instrumentarium

The Veres needle is undoubtedly the most characteristic instrument for a closed laparoscopic entry. Disposable or not disposable, they are available in many sizes, also equipped with the movable blunt tip to avoid incidental injuries. The Veres needle is connected through the isolated cord, often equipped with bacterial filters to an insuflator. It is possible to close the gas flow with the valve placed on the stalk of the needle. There are also other more sophisticated Veres needle modifications, like the units equipped with pressure sensor, or fiberoptic minilaparoscope. The first trocar which, in this method, is pushed through the abdominal wall into the peritoneal cavity, should also be equipped with the blunt tip, automatically popping out while reaching the peritoneal cavity (or an analogical protective tube around the trocar blade). It must be also equipped with a gas valve which allows passing the gas inside. The introduction of the first trocar is the last step of the closed laparoscopic entry procedure.

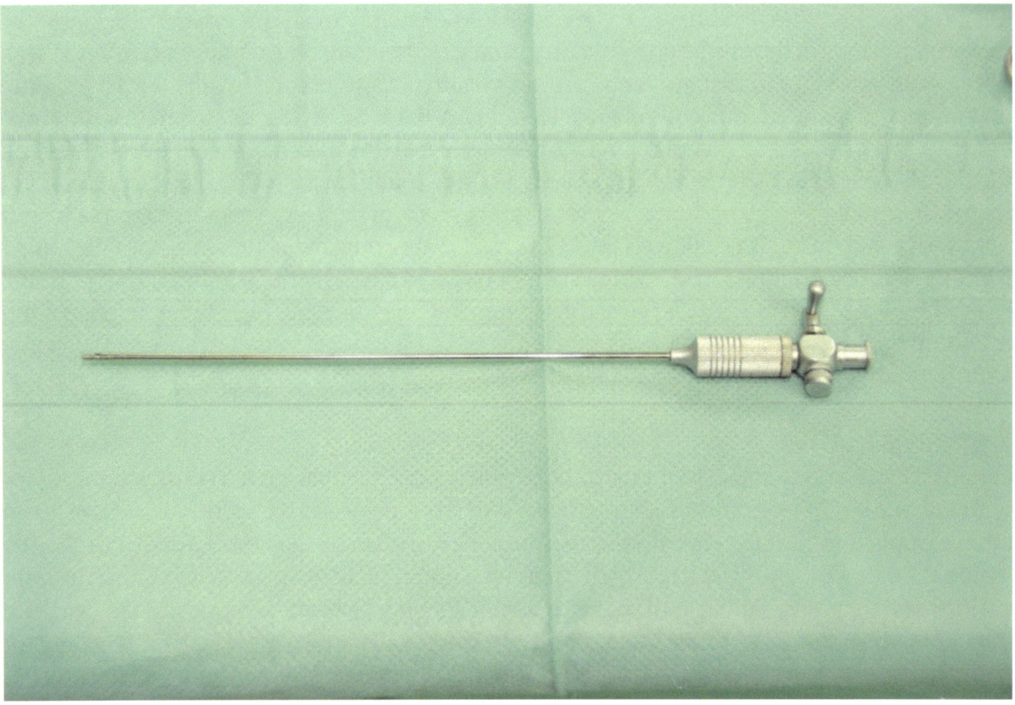

Fig. 2. Nondisposable Veres needle with blunt tip.

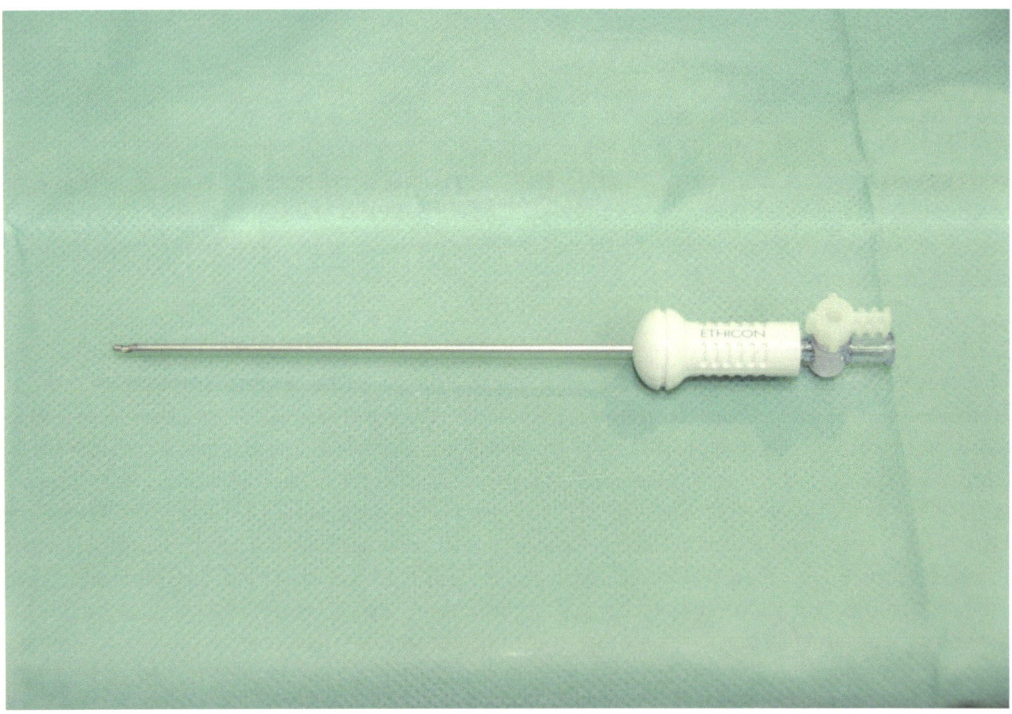

Fig. 3. Disposable Veres needle with blunt tip.

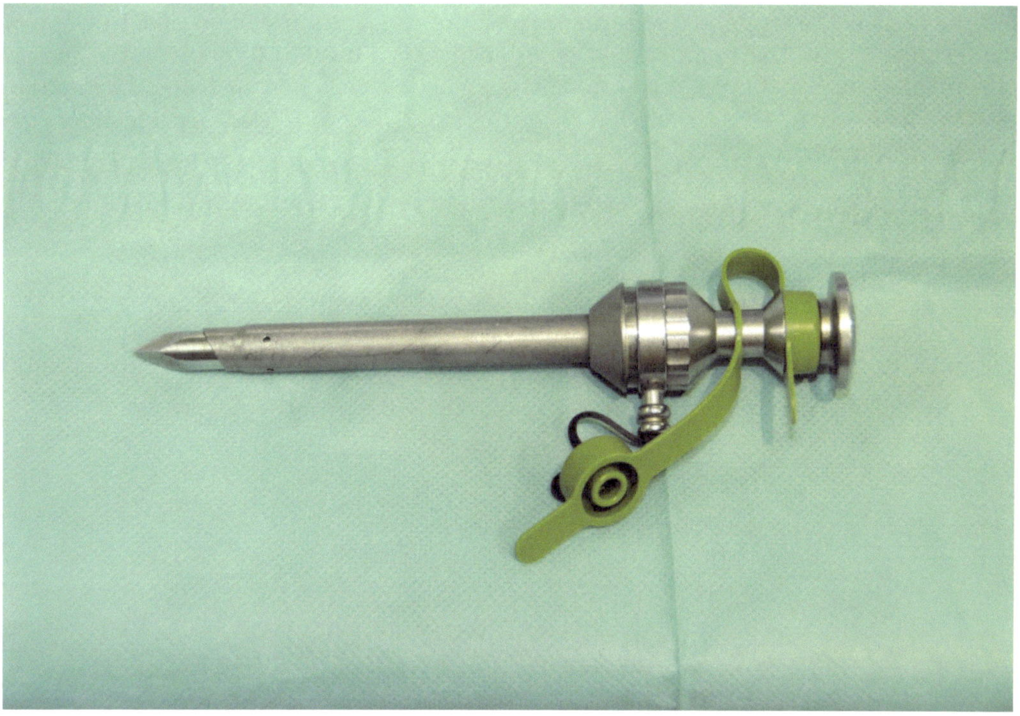

Fig. 4. Classic nondisposable trocar.

2.2.2 Key steps

In the first step of this technique a small (up to 2 cm) incision, above, under, or in the lateral (most often left side) of the umbilicus is made.

Many authors recommend then to lift the anterior abdominal wall (using Mikulicz forceps or Backhaus clamp), or stabilize it before the Veres needle is inserted. It is considered that only three attempts for successful pneumoperitoneum estabilishment are acceptable, fourth attempt should be made in an alternative site. One of these sites is the Palmer's point localized about 3 cm below the left costal margin in the midclavicular line. This is the site especially recommended in extremely obese and thin patients, and always requires prior stomach suction by a nasogastric tube. Contraindications for using this site are hepatosplenomegaly, portal hypertension, and other pathologies in this region. Other less popular alternative sites are anterior and posterior vaginal fornix, and IX-X intercostal space.

It is considered that the Veres needle should be inserted in angle from 45° in non-obese to 90° in obese patients. There are various methods like hanging drop of saline test, the "hiss" sound test, aspiration and syringe test, that are believed to prove correct localization of the needle, however in view of recent findings these do not have any support in evidence.

As said before, the last step of the blind laparoscopic entry is the introduction of the first trocar, the manoeuvre especially critical in an aspect of potential major vessels, or organ injuries. It is strongly recommended to elevate the anterior abdominal wall with the hand, or Backhaus clamp during the trocar insertion, which helps to avoid major complications. The insertion should be made just after the removal of the Veres needle to avoid escape of the insufflated gas. The trocar should be gripped for its handle 90° angle to the surface of abdominal wall, and introduced carefully with the rotary motion. Just after the insertion of the first trocar, the insufflation cord should be connected to maintain the pneumoperitoneum.

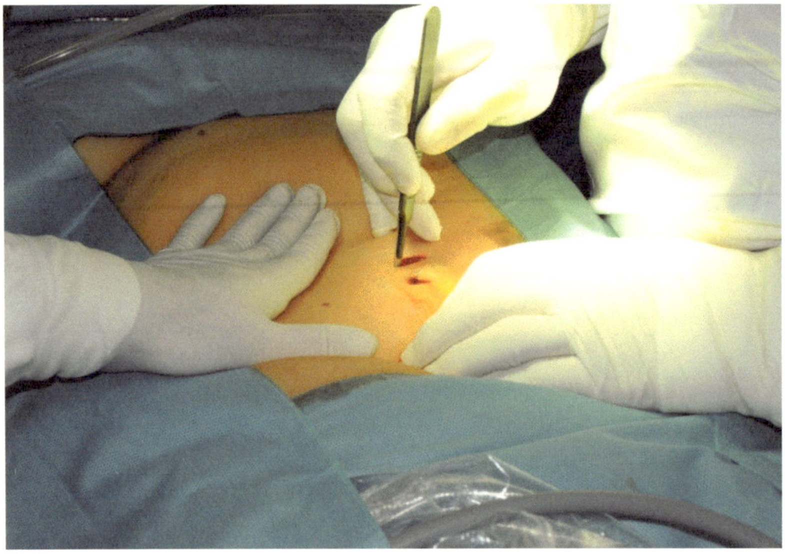

Fig. 5. Skin incision in a closed technique.

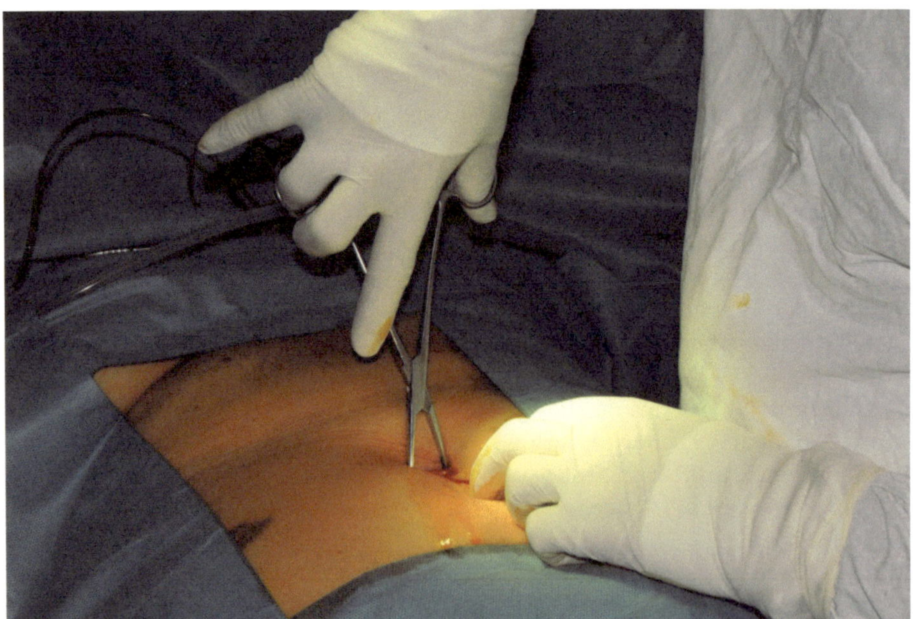

Fig. 6. Dissection of the anterior abdominal cavity wall in a closed technique.

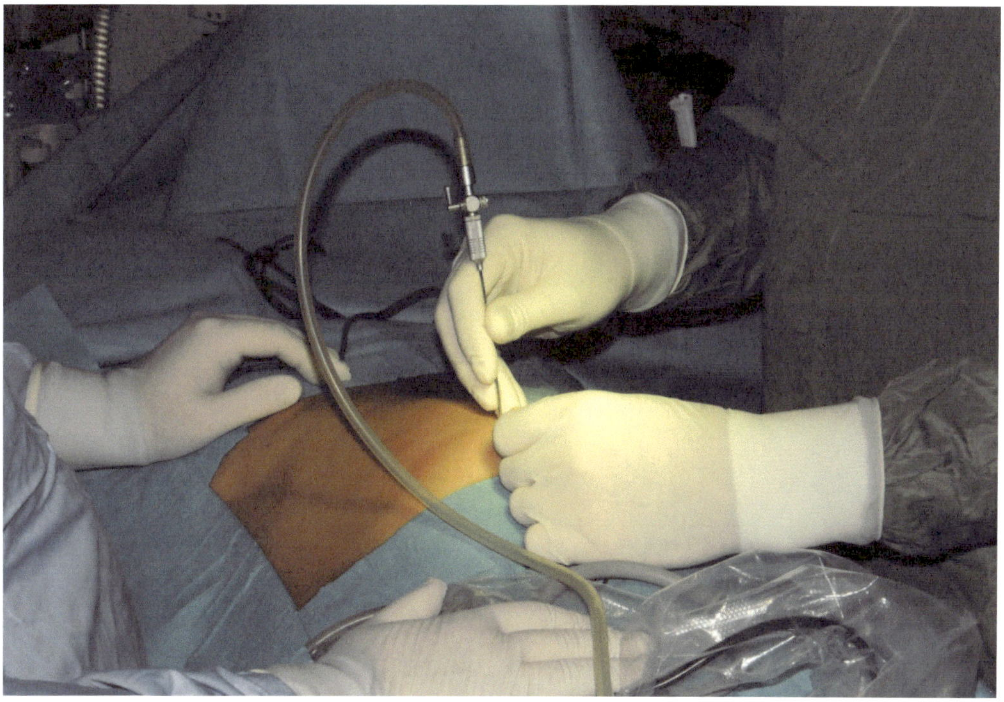

Fig. 7. Veres needle insertion.

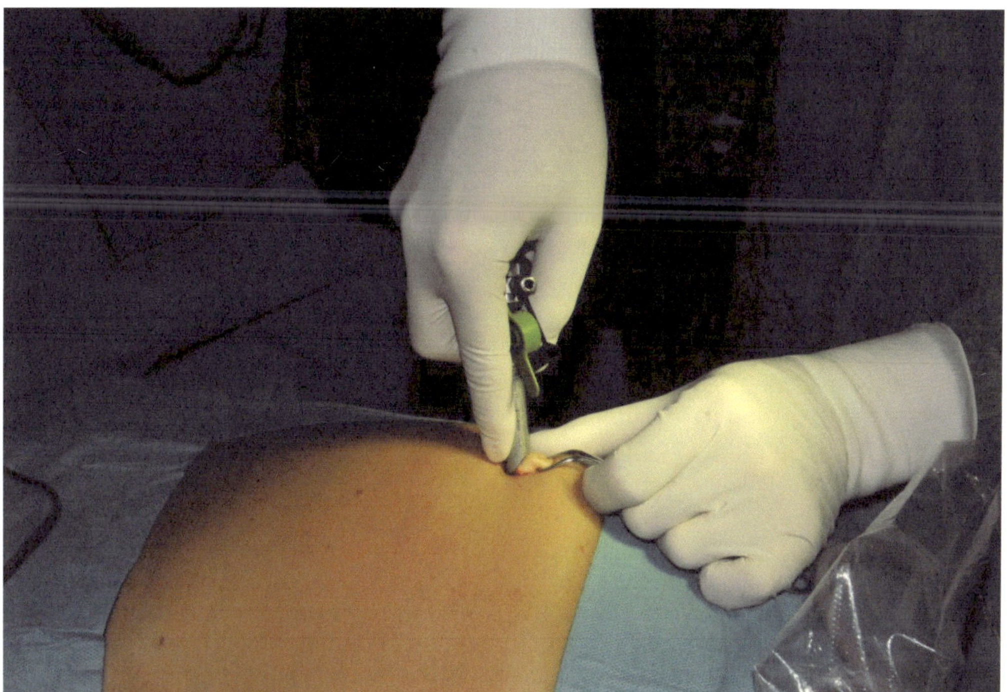

Fig. 8. Blind first trocar insertion in a closed technique.

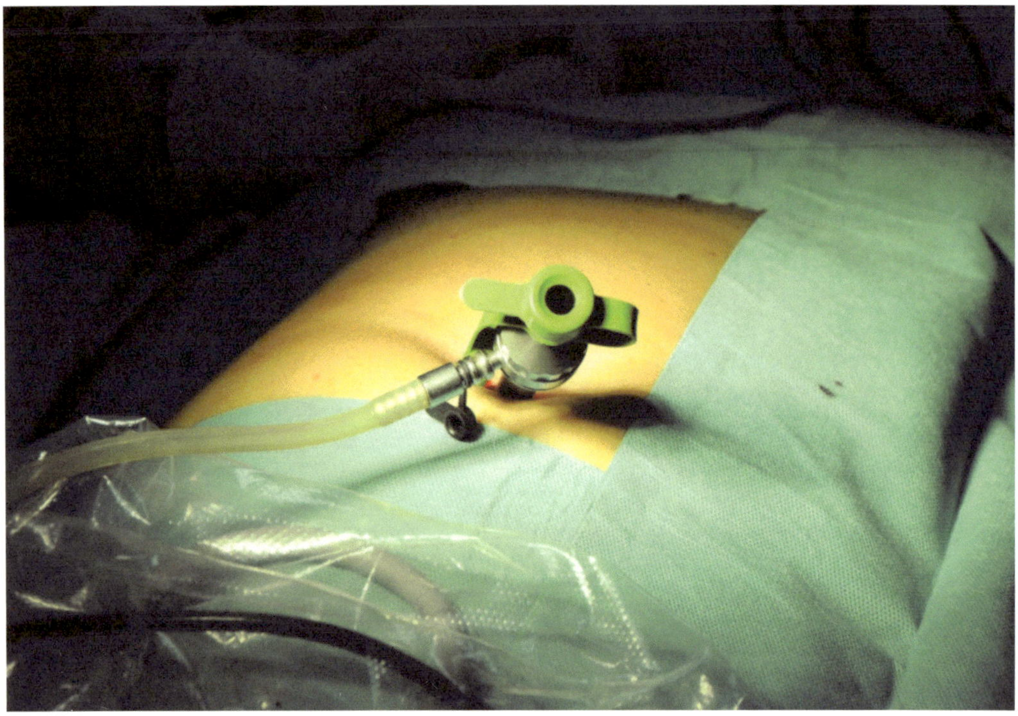

Fig. 9. First trocar in its place.

2.3 Open laparoscopic access

Open laparoscopic access was developed by HM. Hasson as the alternative for the closed laparoscopic entry. The notable difference between techniques is, that the first trocar is inserted before the pneumoperitoneum is estabilished, and with a prior dissection of the anterior abdominal cavity wall, with an incision of the fascia and the peritoneum under the control of the sight.

2.3.1 Instrumentarium

The most specific part of the instrumentarium used in open laparoscopic entry is Hasson trocar. It consists of a canula and a blunt obturator, which helps to avoid injuries during an insertion, and a specific sealing cone with tabs to fix the sutures. Alternativelly a standard 10 mm trocar, without its blade may be used, however adequate sealing sutures must be used. The insufflation equipment remains the same as in the closed method.

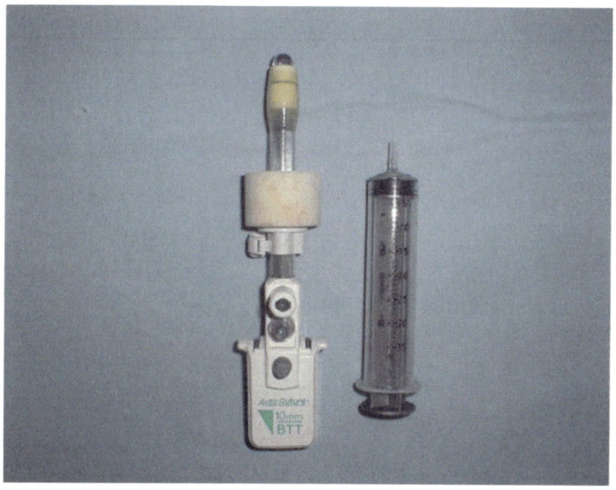

Fig. 10. Modificated Hasson-like trocar.

2.3.2 Key steps

As described before, the first step in the open laparoscopic entry is the dissection of the anterior abdominal cavity wall. The skin incision is rather longer than in a closed laparoscopic entry, so it has to fit the wider Hasson trocar, it is localized typically as in closed technique. After the incision of subcutaneous tissue, the fascia (up to 5mm) and the peritoneum, pursestring sutures are placed, and after the exposition of the prepared hole, and optional finger control of the space, the Hasson trocar is placed into the peritoneal cavity.

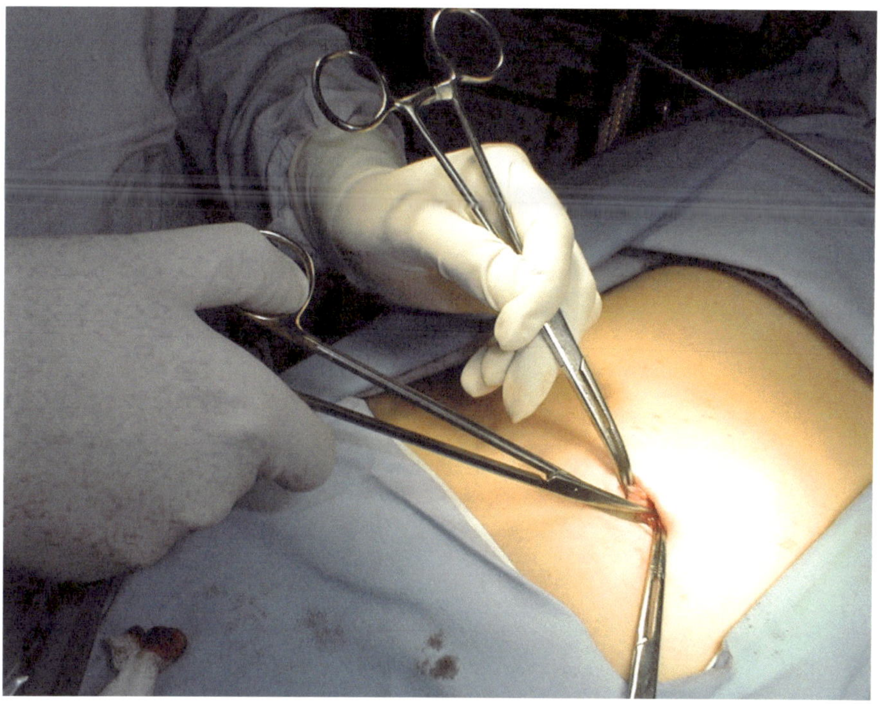

Fig. 11. Dissection of the anterior abdominal cavity wall in an open technique.

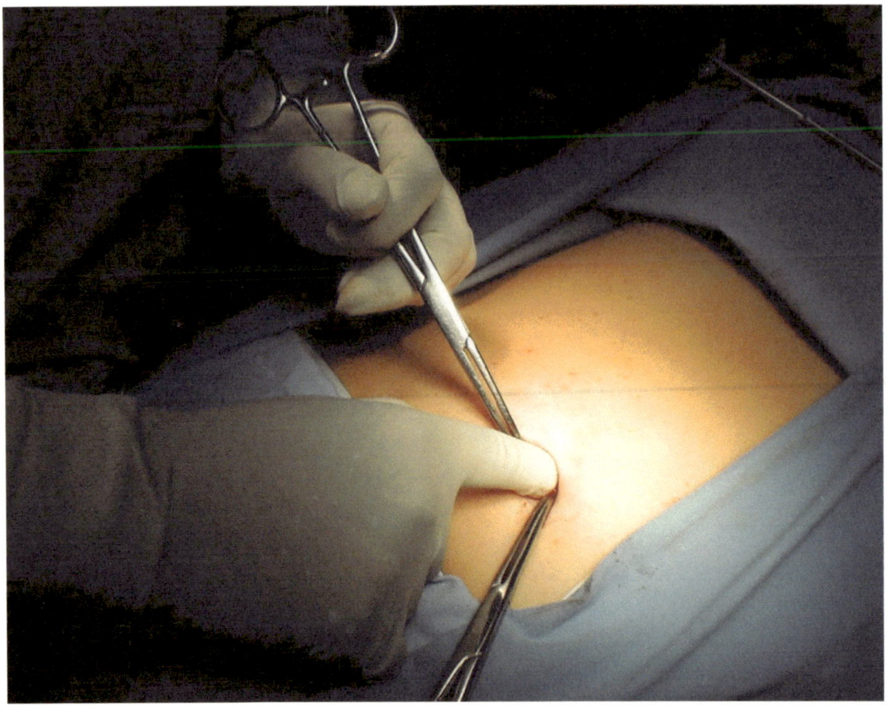

Fig. 12. Finger control of the place for trocar insertion inside the abdominal cavity.

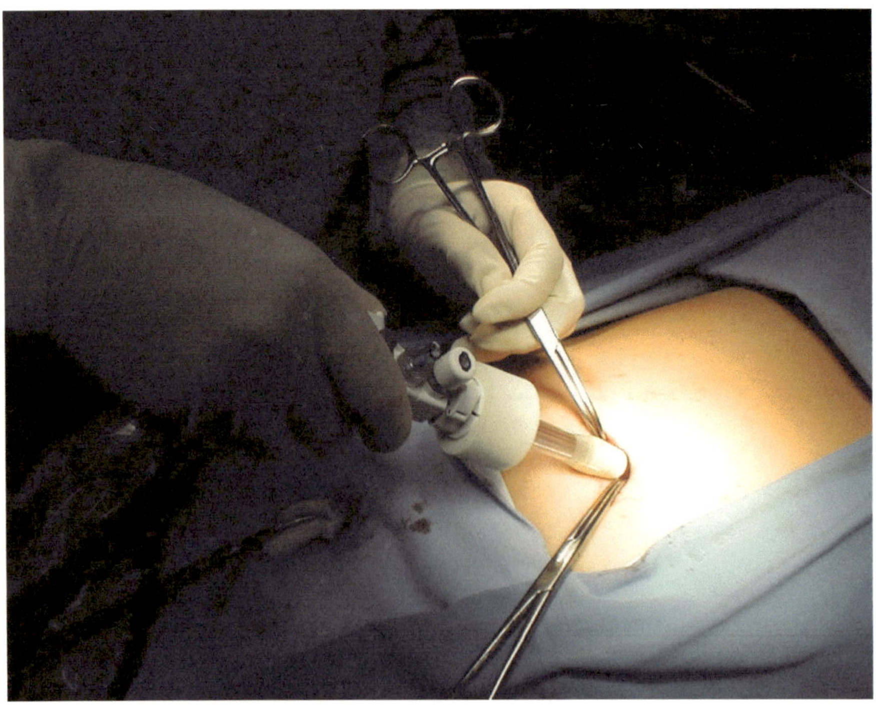

Fig. 13. Hasson-like trocar insertion.

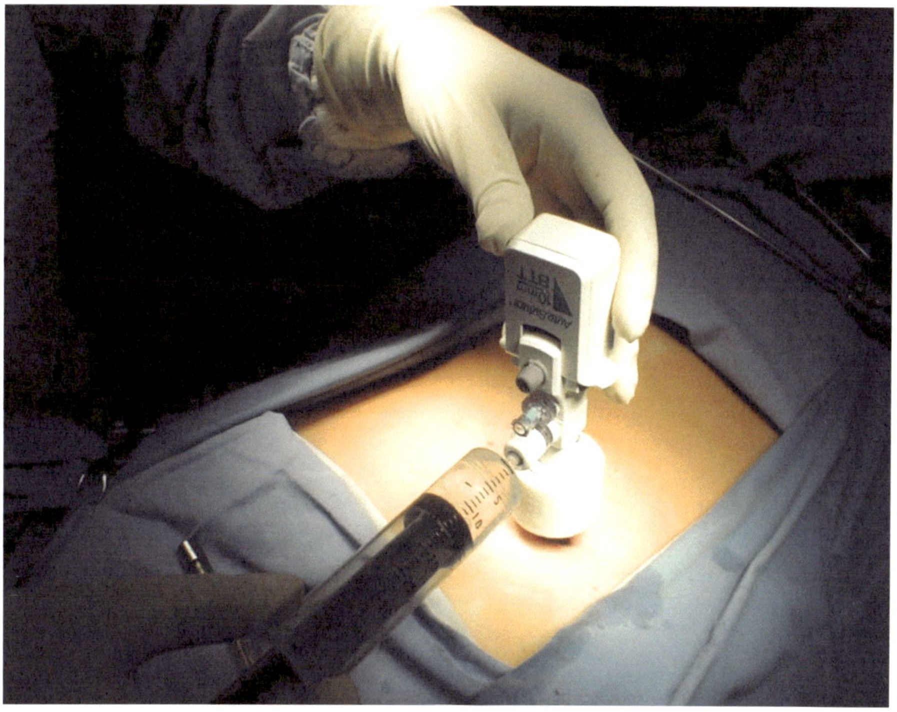

Fig. 14. Trocar cuff insufflation.

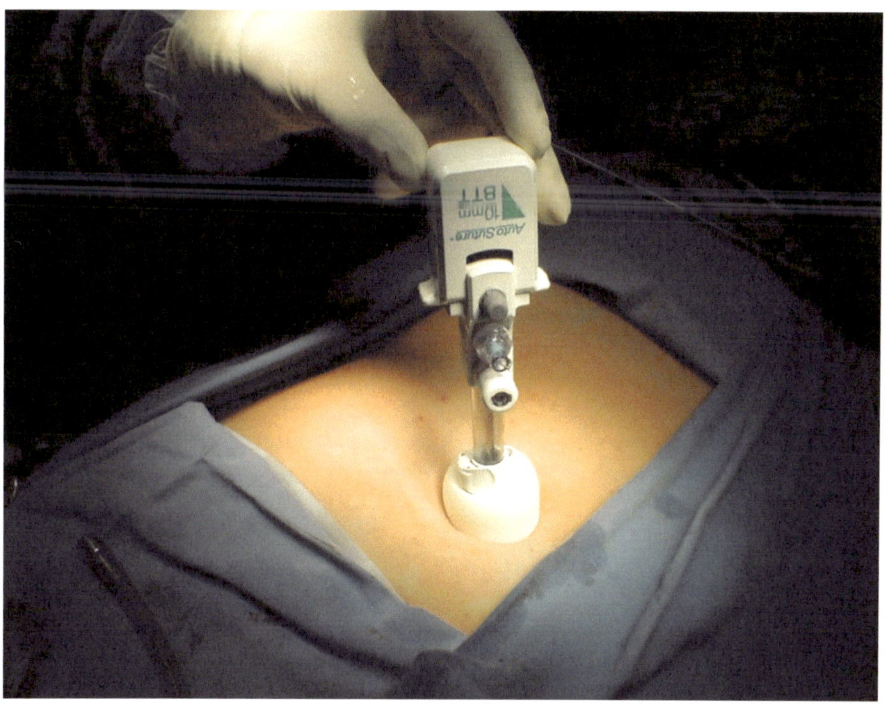

Fig. 15. Trocar in its place.

2.4 Indirect laparoscopic access (optic trocar technique)

The intermediate method between the open and the closed laparoscopic access, which allows to avoid the need of the blind Veres needle and trocar traversion, and at the same time does not require an anterior abdominal wall dissection. However, it must be mentioned, that in this case a sophisticated instrumentarium (an optical trocar) is needed.

2.4.1 Instrumentarium

There are many various optical access trocar systems available nowadays. The complete system consists most often of three main parts: standard 10 mm port, blunt trocar with optical lens, and the standard optic with 0° angle. The most popular systems are Optiview, Johnson&Johnson, Ethicon Endo-Surgery, and Visiport, Autosuture. The first one is equipped with a conical clear tip which allows for a traversion through abdominal wall by dilating, the second with a cutting blade is able to penetrate through the layers for the same reason. In both cases the whole procedure is controlled on the screen of the camera. Previously other solutions were also proposed, the example would be the Trocarless Rotational Access Cannula (TRAC). It consisted also of a trocarless canula in 5 or 10 mm diameter, where also a standard 0° optic may be inserted. The canula had the screw-like threads for its whole length, therefore can be countersinked through the abdominal cavity wall also under the vision control.

2.4.2 Key steps

In the first step, a standard (up to 2 cm) incision is made, usually under the umbilicus, and the optical trocar is advanced into a wound. All of the traversed layers are seen on the screen, subsequently these are: skin and subcutaneous tissue, anterior and posterior fascia of the abdominal rectus muscle (also seen), transversalis fascia, and at last peritoneum. Insufflation is started only when the peritoneum is punctured. The other steps follows as in the open and closed laparoscopic entries.

2.5 Direct trocar insertion

Direct trocar insertion seemed to be far more dangerous than other methods of a laparoscopic entry, but in reality it is considered as a relatively safe alternative for a closed laparoscopic access, when performed properly. The procedure also starts with a skin incision, most often below the umbilicus, the abdominal wall is lifted with a hand of an operator, or with Backhaus clamps, and the trocar is inserted in a pelvic direction. The crucial point of this method is the sharpness quality of a trocar, therefore mainly good quality disposable trocars are in use. In the last step, the blade of a trocar is removed, and the optics of the camera is passed through to assess the localization of introduced canulas. This method allows to avoid most of the complications related to the insuflation procedure like a pneumoembolism, more common in Veress needle insertion, being much faster method at once.

2.6 Low pressure pneumoperitoneum

It is controversial to define the concept of a low pressure pneumoperitoneum. It may be described as the pressure of the gas insufflated lower than used usually. The conception is to decrease the risk of complications of the pneumoperitoneum, when a higher pressure is not necessary due to the anatomical conditions. Obviously, rather smaller procedures can be performed in these circumstances, for example jejunostomy, sigmoideostomy, and peritoneal dialysis catethers manoeuvres.

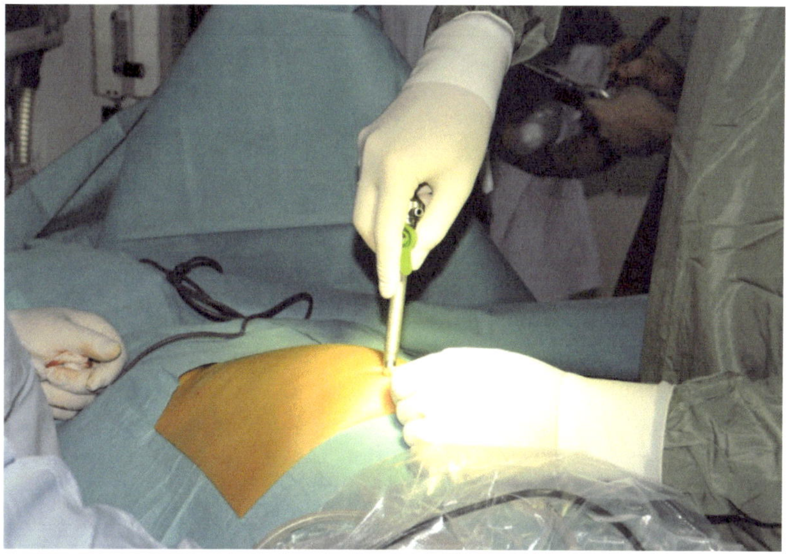

Fig. 16. Direct trocar insertion.

2.7 Pneumoperitoneum techniques summary

It is absolutely not possible to point out the best method of the laparoscopic entry. Hasson's technique, developed to avoid major complications, helped indeed to lower the risk of major vessels injuries, however did not alter (or even increased) the incidence of intestine perforations. The reason could be that it is more often used in patients after prior surgery with peritoneal adhesions. Additionally, closed laparoscopic entry is arguably most often used among the surgeons, especially gynaecologists, who point at its superiority as a faster technique. This also cannot be advocated, because with the correct technique used, open access is comparable, or even faster then the one with use of Veres needle. The open technique is also recommended for pregnant women from third semester. Unsurprisingly, also the optical trocar system is not a complications free method, as the major complications were also described. Despite this, the costs of these more sophisticated techniques can be an essential barrier, therefore these devices are often used as second-line techniques for the creation of the pneumoperitoneum.

3. Non pneumoperitoneum (low pressure pneumoperitoneum) techniques

Laparoscopic pneumoperitoneum techniques appear as minimally invasive with relatively low risk of complications, however there are still various clinical situations, when these become too great danger for the patients. Primarily it concerns older ones with significant cardiopulmonary dysfunctions, when the pneumoperitoneum characteristic with its physiological consequences may cause a life threatening risk for the patients. That has resulted in developing techniques of the laparoscopic entry without the necessity for the pneumoperitoneum creation.

3.1 Techniques used

Following techniques may be performed with an initial low pressure pneumoperitoneum in the first step, or without the need of the pneumoperitoneum creation at all. Despite of the method used, the next steps of the laparoscopic procedure are performed without the need of an insuflation, or only with a low pressure gas flow. These also appear to be useful in extremely obese patients, to limit the utilization of gases for pneumoperitoneum, however in all of the cases the proper relaxation is necessary. The following suspension techniques are described mainly for use in a hepatobiliary laparoscopic surgery.

3.1.2 Cutaneous suture suspension

In the first step of this technique the low pressure pneumoperitoneum is performed (however it is not obligatory), then the strong sutures are placed in a right subcostal region in midclavicular and middle line of the patient's body, through all the layers of the abdominal cavity wall. This step is performed under the eye-control, through the introduced previously optics. The sutures are fastened to the frame of the operation table. In the other type of the cutaneus sutrure suspension, the first suture is placed, after a minilaparotomy (like in an open access laparoscopy) most often under the umbilicus. Often additional sutures are placed in the right subcostal region, like in the first type of this method, enabling easier maneuveration. The sutures are subsequently attached to the operation table frame. These methods of laparoscopic entry enable the operation with an use of a low pressure pneumoperitoneum, or without it.

3.1.3 Kirschner wire suspension

This method is analogical to other suspension methods described above, however instead of the sutures, Kirschner wire is in use. In the first step low pressure pneumoperitoneum is achieved and the bent wire is inserted subfascially in the right subcostal region also between right midclavicular and midline. Afterwards, the wire is attached to the table frame. Then the operation without the pnuemoperitoneum, or with low pressure insufflations may be performed.

3.1.4 Laparolift technique

Laparolift (Autosuture) device consists of a hydropneumatic elevator, and specific interchangeable body hooks in V or C shape. It enables to achieve laparoscopic entry completely without the creation of a pneumoperitoneum, with relatively low invasiveness (however incomparably greater than in other methods of laparoscopic entry described above). The hooks are introduced to the abdominal cavity through the minilaparotomy folded, and subsequently assembled inside, then the anterior abdominal wall is being elevated, and the hook is attached to the hydropneumatic elevator. The similar method to the one described above is the one with an use of the tire shape balloon instead of laparolift hooks (device like Origin Airlift), it is arguably considered as the safer method. These two methods may be used in the most of the laparoscopic operations.

3.2 Non –pneumoperitoneum (low pressure pneumoperitoneum) techniques summary

The methods of non-pneumoperitoneum techniques are certainly less popular than the open and closed laparoscopic entries. Most of the problems related to the creation of the pneumoperitoneum may be omitted by discerning anaesthesiology, what with limited equipment, makes suspension methods useful only in a very selected group of patients.

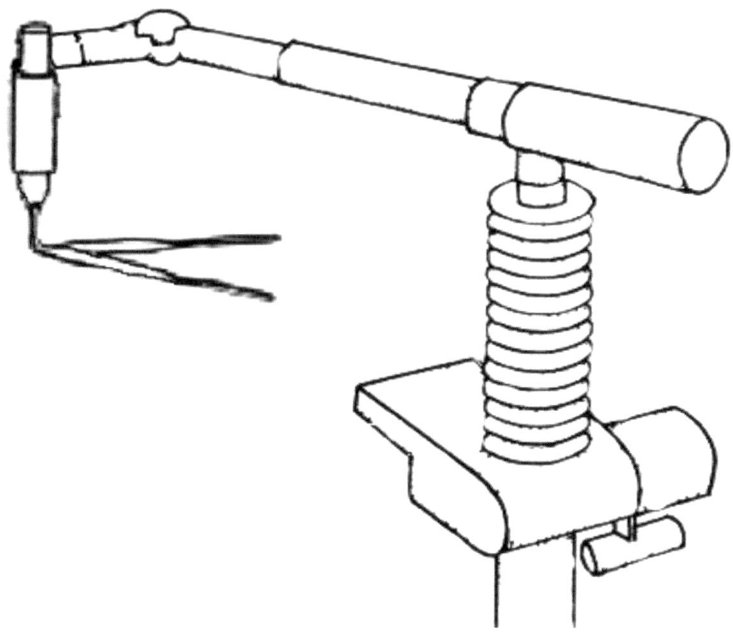

Fig. 17. Laparolift device.

4. The wind of change. Single port and NOTES laparoscopy

It appears obvious, that the future belongs to these even less invasive procedures. Both NOTES and single port laparoscopy, without exception also demand the laparoscopic entry. These are mainly based on the access methods with use of a pneumoperitoneum, like in the single port laparoscopic surgery, where the paraumbilical minilaparotomy is performed, to insert larger port. Also in NOTES, the need for creation of a pneumoperitoneum is achieved through the closed entry like access, with an use of a needle introduced to the abdominal cavity through the vaginal fornix. It must be however said that there are also some other methods assigned to the NOTES surgery, with the use of other access procedures, like the flexible endoscope introduced to the abdominal cavity through a cut in a stomach wall, and the pneumoperitoneum achieved this way.

5. References

Agresta F. et al. (2004). Direct trocar insertion vs needle in nonobese patients undergoing laparoscopic procedures. *Surg Endosc* Vol. 18: pp. 1778-1781. ISSN 1432-2218.

Ahmad G. et al. (2008). Laparoscopic Entry Techniques (Review). *Cochrane Database Syst. Rev.* Apr 16(2): CD006583.

Antoniou SA., Pointner R., Granderath FA. (2011). Single-incision laparoscopic cholecystectomy: a systematic review. *Surg Endosc* Vol 25: pp. 367-377.

Berch RB. et al. (2006). Experience with the optical access trocar for safe and rapid entry in the performance of laparoscopic gastric bypass. *Surg Endosc* Vol 20: pp. 1238-1241.

Catarci M. et al. (2001). Major and minor injuries during the creation of pneumoperitoneum. A multicenter study on 12,919 cases. *Surg Endosc* Vol 15: pp. 566-569.

Channa GA., Siddiqui AJ., Zafar SN. Open versus closed method of establishing pneumoperitoneum for laparoscopic cholecystectomy. J Coll Physicians Surg Pak Vol 19 No 9: pp. 557-560.

Collinet P. et al. (2010). Risks associated with laparoscopic entry. *J Gynecol Obstet Biol Reprod* Vol 39 No 8 suppl 2: p. 123-135.

Daehn S. et al. (2005). Influence of different gases used for laparoscopy (helium, carbon dioxide, room air, and xenon) on tumor volume, histomorphology, and leukocyte-tumor-endothelium interaction in intravital microscopy. *Surg Endosc* Vol. 19: pp. 65-70.

Kostewicz W. (2002). Operacje laparoskopowe w warunkach odmy niskociśnieniowej lub bez wytwarzania odmy otrzewnowej, In : *Chirurgia Laparoskopowa*, Kostewicz W., pp. 117-121, PZWL, ISBN 83-200-2440-4, Warszawa, Poland.

Laffularde T., Van Hee R., Gys T. (1999). A safe and simple method for routine open access in laparoscopic procedures. *Surg Endosc* Vol 13: pp. 769-772.

Langwieler TE., Nimmesgern T., Back M. (2009) Single-port access in laparoscopic cholecystectomy. *Surg Endosc* Vol 23: pp. 1138-1141.

Leszczyszyn J. (2002). Wytwarzanie odmy otrzewnowej, In : *Chirurgia Laparoskopowa,* Kostewicz W., pp. 89-96, PZWL, ISBN 83-200-2440-4, Warszawa, Poland.

Liu HF., Chen X., Liu Y. (2009). A multi-center study of a modified open trocar first puncture approach in 17 350 patients for laparoscopic entry. Chin Med J Vol 122 No 22: pp. 2733-2736.

Moberg AC.,Montgomery A. (2005). Primary access-related complications with laparoscopy. *Surg Endosc* Vol 19: pp. 1196-1199.

Opilka MN., et al. (2009). Open versus closed laparoscopy entry – which are evidences? Hepatogastroenterology Vol 56 No 89: pp. 75-79.

Perreta S. et al. (2009). Adrenalectomy using natural orifice translumenal endoscopic surgery (NOTES): A transvaginal retroperitoneal approach. Surg Endosc Vol 23: p.1390.

Rosen DM. et al. (1998). Methods of creating pneumoperitoneum: a review of techniques and complications. *Obstet Gynecol Surv* Vol 53 No 3: pp. 167-174.

Sharp HT. et al. (2002). Complications associated with optical-access laparoscopic trocars. Obstet Gynecol Vol 99 No 4: pp. 553-555.

String A. et al. (2001). Use of the optical access trocar for safe and rapid entry in various laparoscopic procedures. *Surg Endosc* Vol 15: pp. 570-573.

Tagaya N., Kubota K. (2009). NOTES: approach to the liver and spleen. *J Hepatobiliary Pancreat Surg* Vol 16: pp. 283-287.

Targarona EM. et al. (2011). Single-port splenectomy: Current update and controversies. *J Min Access Surg* Vol 7 No 1: pp. 61-64.

Ternamian AM. (1997). Laparoscopy without trocars. *Surg Endosc* Vol 11: pp. 815-818.

Tinelli A. et al. (2010). Abdominal access in gynecological laparoscopy: a comparision between direct optical and blind closed access by Veress needle. Eur J Obstet Gynecol Reprod Biol Vol 148 No 2: pp.191-194.

Tinelli A. et al. (2011). Laparoscopy entry in patients with previous abdominal and pelvic surgery. *Surg Innov* Vol 18 Epub ahead of print.

Vilos GA. et al. (2007). Laparoscopic entry: a review of techniques, technologies, and complications. *J Obstet Gynaecol Can* Vol 29 No 5: 433-465.

Zakherah MS. (2010). Direct trocar versus needle entry for laparoscopy: a randomized clinical trial. *Gynecol Obstet Invest* Vol 69 No 4: pp. 260-263.

7

Single-Port Access Laparoscopic Surgery in Gynecology: Technical Tips

Jiheum Paek[1] and Sang Wun Kim[2]
[1]*Department of Obstetrics and Gynecology, Ajou University School of Medicine, Suwon,*
[2]*Division of Gynecologic Oncology, Department of Obstetrics and Gynecology, Yonsei University College of Medicine, Seoul, Korea*

1. Introduction

Numerous studies have reported various laparoscopic techniques since the idea of "minimal invasive access surgery" was introduced in the early 1990s (1). One of them is the transumbilical endoscopic surgery (TUES). TUES is a single-port access (SPA) surgery approach to the umbilicus, an embryologic natural orifice (2). Other names of this technique include SPA surgery, scarless surgery, single-port laparoscopy (3), one-port umbilical surgery, natural orifice transumbilical surgery (4), laparoendoscopic single-site surgery (LESS) (5), and embryonic natural orifice transumbilical endoscopic surgery (6). Recently, with improvements in surgical expertise with optimal instrumentation, the interests of minimally invasive surgery have increased. As a result, many surgeons have tried to reduce the number and size of ports in laparoscopic surgery for reducing morbidity and better cosmetic outcome.

It has been reported that SPA surgery has less postoperative pain compared to conventional laparoscopy in the gynecologic field (7). In addition, SPA surgery is expected to offer better cosmetic results and to reduce operative complications related to the trocar insertion as it involves less inserted trocars (8). However, SPA surgery has systemic limitations, including crashes between instruments or between instruments and endoscope, a limited number of instruments, an unstable camera platform, and the limited mobility of straight laparoscopic instruments because surgical instruments work through only one port. These technical problems cause lower accuracy of the operation and longer operation time compared to conventional laparoscopy. To overcome the technical difficulties, newly developed instruments, including an angled laparoscope or instrument have been introduced. However, there are limitations for popular use of SPA surgery, including high cost. Therefore, we suggest useful surgical techniques for SPA surgery using conventional laparoscopic instruments.

2. Port placement

Several commercial port systems have been introduced for SPA laparoscopy. We introduce a home-made single-port system using wound retractor and surgical gloves (Fig. 1). After making a 1.2~1.5-cm vertical intra-umbilical skin incision (Fig. 2), the Alexis® wound retractor (Applied Medical, CA, USA) is inserted into the peritoneal cavity through the umbilicus (Fig. 3). Because it is often difficult to remove the wound retractor after surgery, a 1-0 Black Silk is tied at the inner ring of the wound retractor (Fig. 4). An operator has only to pull on the thread that is positioned out of the skin. A 7½ surgical glove is fixed to the outer ring of the wound retractor. After making small incisions in the finger tip portions of the glove, two 5-mm trocars and one 11-mm trocar are inserted. A rigid 30-degree, 5-mm, endoscope 45 cm long is used (Fig. 5A).

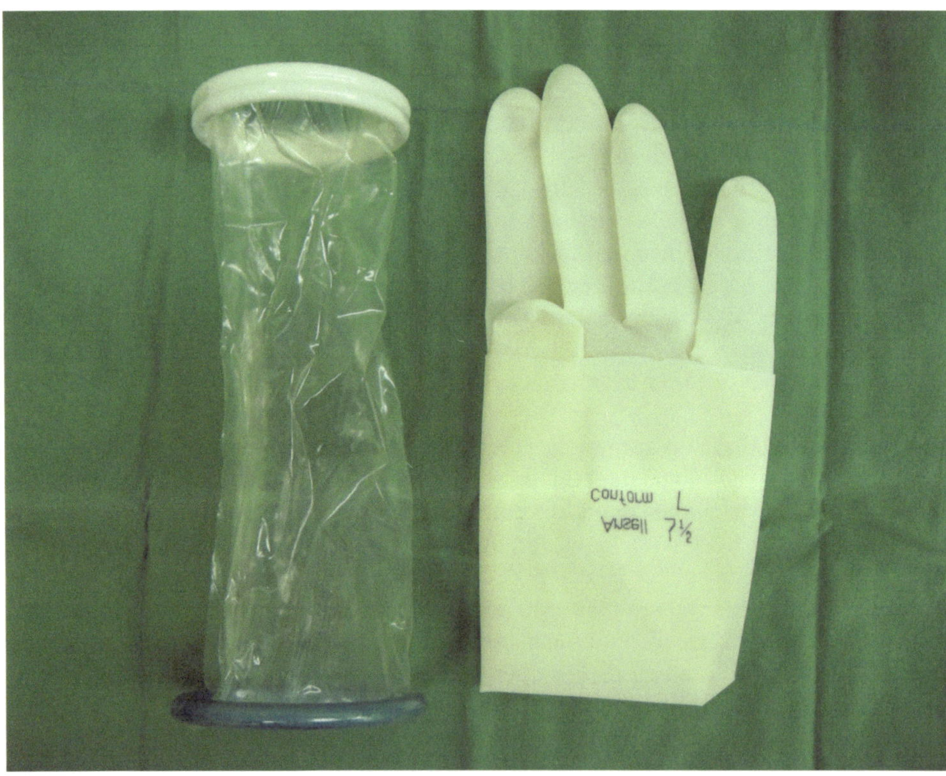

Fig. 1. A homemade single-port system using the Alexis® wound retractor (Applied Medical, CA, USA) and a 7½ surgical glove.

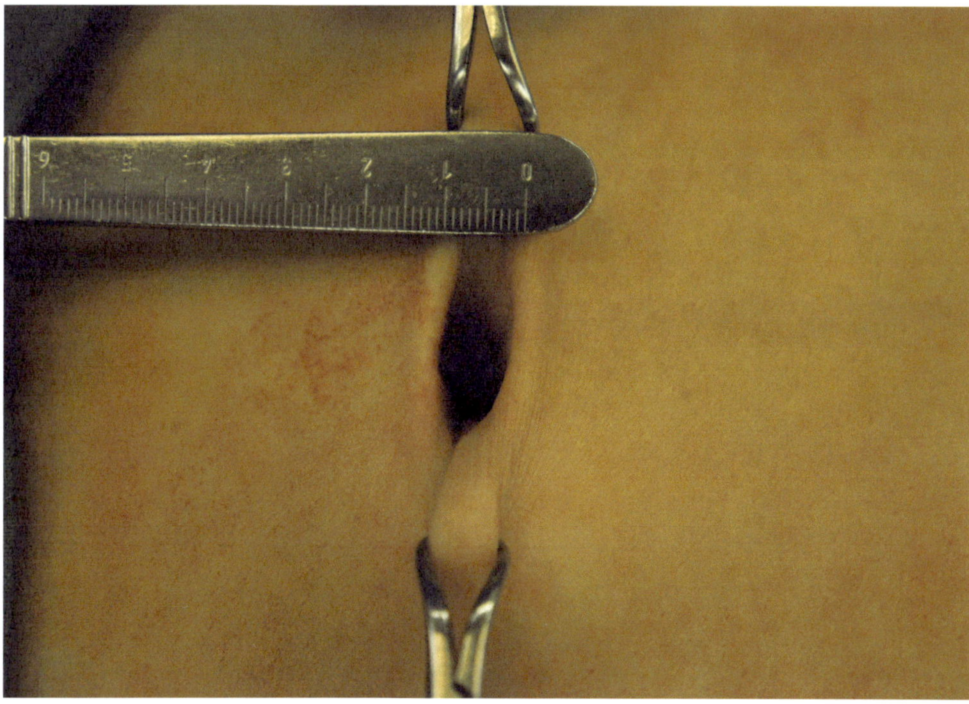

Fig. 2. A 1.5-cm vertical intra-umbilical skin incision.

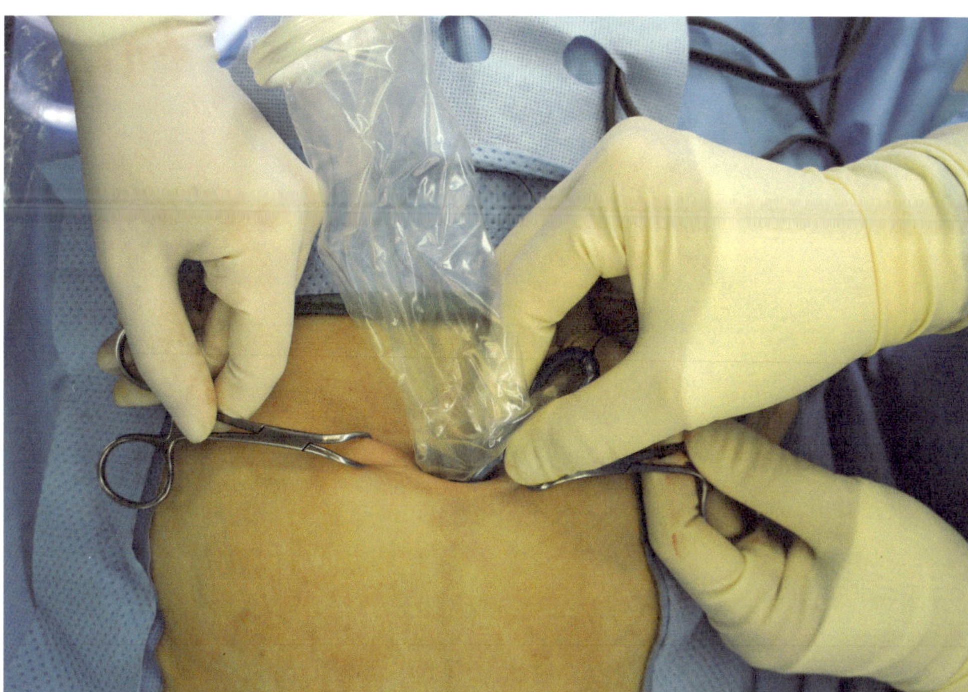

Fig. 3. Insertion of wound retractor into the peritoneal cavity through the umbilicus.

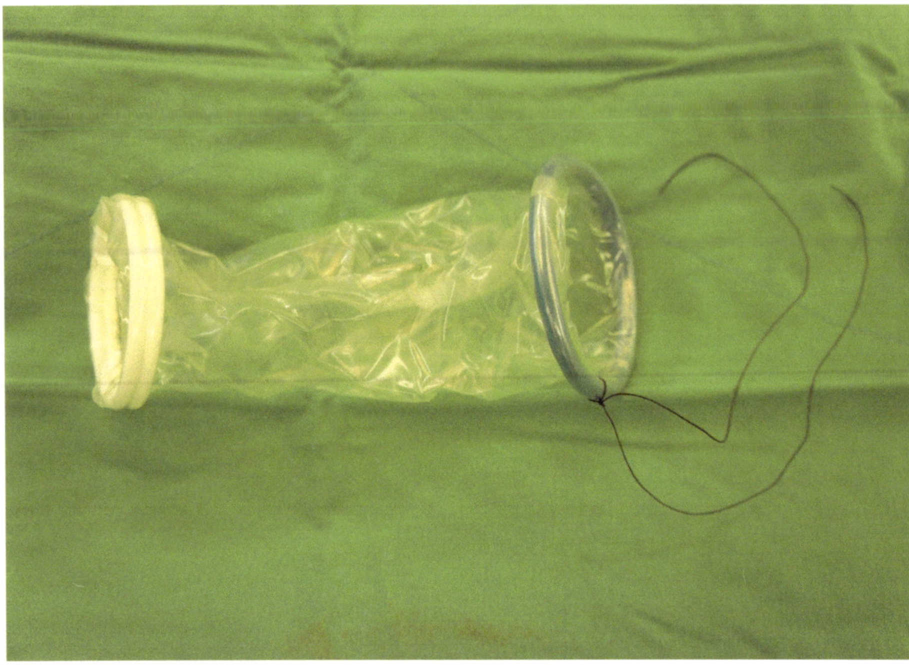

Fig. 4. A 1-0 Black Silk is tied at the inner ring of the wound retractor to remove the wound retractor after surgery.

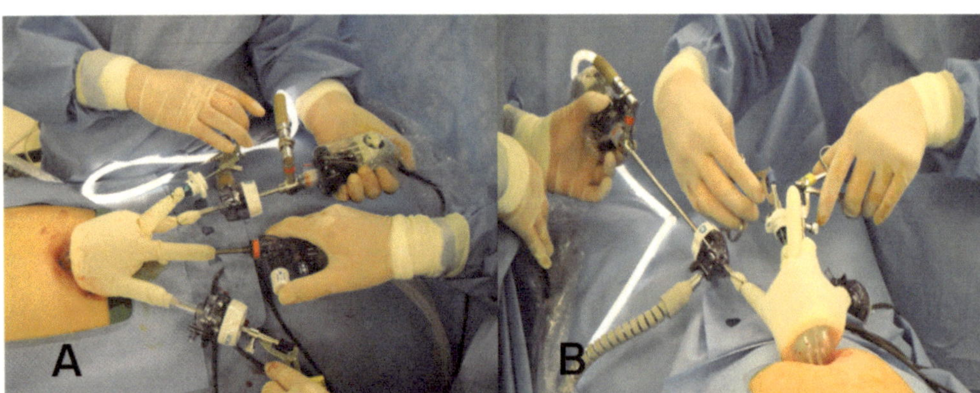

Fig. 5. (A, B) Two 5-mm trocars and one 11-mm trocar are inserted. A rigid 30-degree, 5-mm, endoscope 45 cm long is used. Using a 5-mm trocar-threaded cannula and seal (Applied medical, CA, USA) and 3-mm hole on the tip of the surgical glove without a trocar.

3. Surgical applications

Total laparoscopic hysterectomy (TLH)

Hysterectomy is the most common surgery in gynecologic field. Recently, it has been reported that hysterectomy using the SPA system was feasible (7, 9-14). For an analysis of SPA hysterectomy other than small case series, Park et al evaluated a total of 105 cases of

SPA laparoscopy-assisted vaginal hysterectomy (15). In this analysis, 4 of 105 patients needed additional port and one case was converted to a laparotomy. The operating time was 120 min and the complication rate was 4%. In addition, the authors analyzed the learning curve of 100 consecutive patients underwent SPA-TLH. There was no conversion to conventional laparoscopy or laparotomy. The median time until the removal of a specimen (T_R) was 45 min and the median time for closure of the vaginal cuff (T_C) was 18 min. The median total operating time from skin opening to closure (T_O) was 80 min. T_R, T_C, T_O, and decreased significantly over the study period. The T_C decreased significantly from the first 20 cases to the next 20 ($p = 0.028$) and the T_O from the second 20 cases to the next 20 ($p = 0.029$). Compared to multiple-port access TLH, SPA-TLH seems to be feasible without increased complication rates and is expected to have an improved cosmesis with the surgical incision hidden in the umbilicus.

Laparoscopic adnexal surgery

It is important issue for most of woman to have less surgical scar regardless of age. Moreover, age of woman who undergo an adnexal surgery is younger compared to other gynecologic surgery. In addition, the specimen can be easily removed through a laparoscopic bag inserted through an umbilical trocar. When surgical gloves and wound retractor are used for an umbilical port, 1.5 cm incision in the umbilicus is more useful to remove the specimen compared to conventional laparoscopy or commercial single port system. However, it is not always easy to perform an SPA adnexal surgery in severe endometriosis or huge ovarian tumor. Therefore, the SPA adnexal surgery often needs to have surgical techniques and experiences.

Others

Escobar et al reported a retrospective, multi-institutional analysis of BRCA carriers and women at high risk for breast/ovarian cancer who underwent LESS risk-reducing salpingo-oophorectomy with and without hysterectomy. A total of 58 patients were evaluated surgical proficiency was possible after 10–15 cases in this study (16). Additionally, for gynecologic cancer operation, lymph node dissection with single-port has been introduced (17).

4. Technical tips with conventional instruments

The authors have performed more than 400 SPA laparoscopy surgeries in the gynecologic field. Based on our abundant experiences, we have introduced surgical tips to overcome technical difficulties in SPA surgery (18). A collision between the camera and surgical instruments is one of problems with which the operator is faced in SPA surgery. With a 0-degree endoscope, the endoscope and the surgical instrument are positioned in parallel to each other, which limits the field of vision and makes it difficult to avoid collision between the endoscope and the surgical instruments. The use of a 30-degree endoscope provides the operator a wider vision. In this situation, the endoscope is not in parallel with the surgical instruments and can keep a distance from the instruments without a change of the visual field. By changing the angle of the endoscope via the endoscope-holder, the operator can accurately see the structure that he intends to operate on, and can avoid instrumental collision as well. Moreover, the operator can see the field that is invisible when using a 0-degree endoscope. The collision between the light cable and the operator's hands often occurs because the angle between the light cable and the endoscope is generally 90°. Such a collision can be avoided by using a 90-degree light cable adaptor. Generally, the length of a commonly used endoscope is 30 cm. However, the 45-cm endoscope that enables the head of the camera and the light cable to be positioned 15 cm behind of the operator's hands can effectively prevent the collision between the camera and the operator's hands (Fig. 5B).

A collision between trocars is caused by the head portion of the trocar which is greater in size compared with a diameter of the trocar. Such a collision can be avoided by using a trocar with a smaller-sized head portion, such as a 5-mm trocar-threaded cannula and seal (Applied medical, CA, USA). In addition, to avoid the collision between the trocars, we make an approximately 3-mm hole on the tip of the surgical glove that forms a part of the SPA system without using a trocar. Then, a singular instrument is inserted through the holes of the glove (Fig. 5B).

In some circumstances, it may require one additional instrument for grasping tissue or traction. Particularly, there are many cases that one grasper is not sufficient for surgical procedures, such as dissection of an ovarian tumor, coagulation after dissection, and dissection of pelvic adhesion. The surgical glove may allow simultaneously insertion of up to 5 surgical instruments, which means a maximum of 4 surgical instruments other than the endoscope. The 2-mm grasper (Christian Diener Gmbh. & CO. K.G., Germany) can be used without increasing the length of the umbilical incision, and this instrument is flexible so that adding it does not cause a crash with other surgical instruments (Fig. 6).

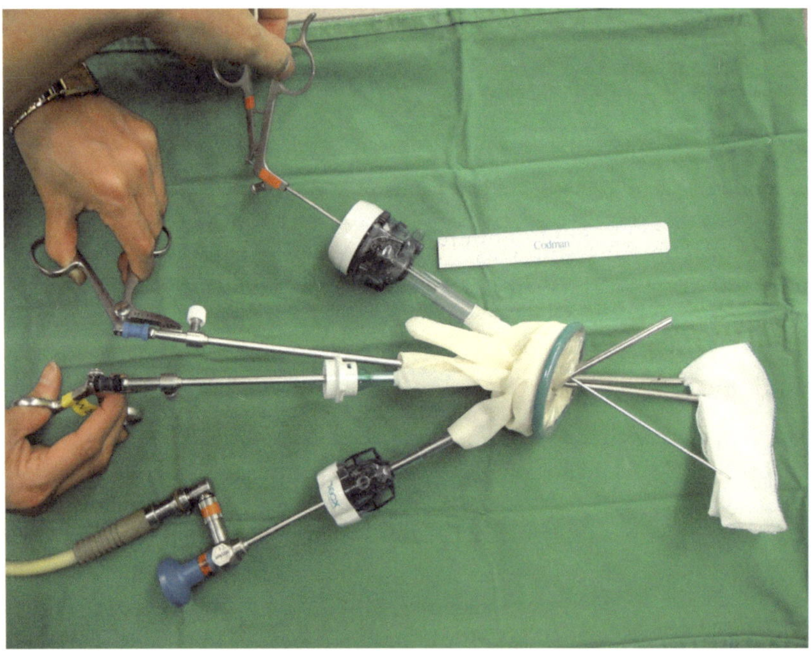

Fig. 6. An additional 2-mm instrument can be used to perform traction of tissue.

Suturing and tying can be the most difficult procedure in surgical techniques for SPA surgery. In gynecologic surgery, suturing and tying are mostly performed to close the vaginal cuff after a hysterectomy or to repair the uterine wall after a myomectomy or parenchyma of ovary after cystectomy. Because these operations are parts of the most common surgeries in gynecology and the incidence of using the SPA system continues to rise, it is necessary to find the most effective and accurate method of suturing and tying which is specifically suitable for these surgeries. Among conventional instruments, a needle holder which has a curved end seems to be the most adequate instrument for SPA laparoscopic surgery. The curved end of the needle holder allows the operator to have an optimal angle between the needle and tissue of the vaginal cuff. Besides, the handle is so simple that the operator can easily control it without much collision with other instruments. The suture could be knotted extracorporeally or intracorporeally. For extracorporeal tying, 90-cm long sutures and the Clarke-Reich knot pusher (Cook Medical, IN, USA) are needed. Because there are technical difficulties to perform an intracorporeal tying, reducing the number of intracorporeal tying could be helpful. The first intracorporeal tying could be omitted by making a slipknot on the tip of a suture before inserting the suture in the abdominal cavity (Fig. 7).

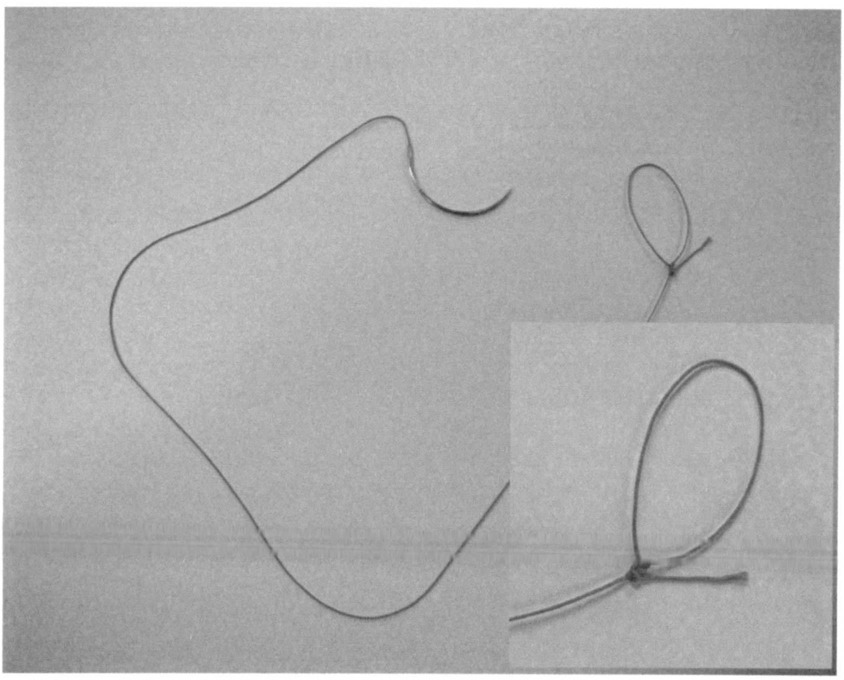

Fig. 7. The first intracorporeal tying can be omitted by making a slipknot on the tip of a suture

5. Conclusion

As the technical difficulties are overcome, SPA laparoscopic surgery will be a more and more widespread procedure in gynecology with only minimal skin incision.

6. References

[1] Podolsky ER, Rottman SJ, Poblete H, King SA, Curcillo PG. Single port access (SPA) cholecystectomy: a completely transumbilical approach. Journal of laparoendoscopic & advanced surgical techniques. 2009;19(2):219-22.

[2] Remzi FH, Kirat HT, Kaouk JH, Geisler DP. Single-port laparoscopy in colorectal surgery. Colorectal disease. 2008;10(8):823-6.
[3] Cuesta MA, Berends F, Veenhof AA. The "invisible cholecystectomy": A transumbilical laparoscopic operation without a scar. Surgical Endoscopy. 2008;22(5):1211-3.
[4] Nguyen NT, Reavis KM, Hinojosa MW, Smith BR, Wilson SE. Laparoscopic transumbilical cholecystectomy without visible abdominal scars. Journal of gastrointestinal surgery. 2009;13(6):1125-8.
[5] Fader AN, Escobar PF. Laparoendoscopic single-site surgery (LESS) in gynecologic oncology: technique and initial report. Gynecologic Oncology. 2009;114(2):157-61.
[6] Canes D, Desai M, Aron M, Haber G, Goel RK, Stein RJ, et al. Transumbilical single-port surgery: evolution and current status. European urology. 2008;54(5):1020-9.
[7] Yim GW, Jung YW, Paek J, Lee SH, Kwon HY, Nam EJ, et al. Transumbilical single-port access versus conventional total laparoscopic hysterectomy: surgical outcomes. American journal of obstetrics and gynecology. 2010;203(1):26.e1-.e6.
[8] Desai M, Rao P, Aron M, Pascal-Haber G, Desai MR, Mishra S, et al. Scarless single port transumbilical nephrectomy and pyeloplasty: first clinical report. BJU international. 2008;101(1):83-8.
[9] Jung YW, Kim YT, Lee DW, Hwang YI, Nam EJ, Kim JH, et al. The feasibility of scarless single-port transumbilical total laparoscopic hysterectomy: initial clinical experience. Surg Endosc2009.
[10] Lee YY, Kim TJ, Kim CJ, Kang H, Choi CH, Lee JW, et al. Single-port access laparoscopic-assisted vaginal hysterectomy: a novel method with a wound retractor and a glove. J Minim Invasive Gynecol. 2009 Jul-Aug;16(4):450-3.
[11] Kim TJ, Lee YY, Cha HH, Kim CJ, Choi CH, Lee JW, et al. Single-port-access laparoscopic-assisted vaginal hysterectomy versus conventional laparoscopic-assisted vaginal hysterectomy: a comparison of perioperative outcomes. Surg Endosc. 2010 Sep;24(9):2248-52.
[12] Song T, Kim TJ, Kim MK, Park H, Kim JS, Lee YY, et al. Single port access laparoscopic-assisted vaginal hysterectomy for large uterus weighing exceeding 500 grams: technique and initial report. J Minim Invasive Gynecol. 2010 Jul-Aug;17(4):456-60.
[13] Yoon G, Kim TJ, Lee YY, Kim CJ, Choi CH, Lee JW, et al. Single-port access subtotal hysterectomy with transcervical morcellation: a pilot study. J Minim Invasive Gynecol. 2010 Jan-Feb;17(1):78-81.
[14] Jung YW, Lee M, Yim GW, Lee SH, Paek JH, Kwon HY, et al. A randomized prospective study of single-port and four-port approaches for hysterectomy in terms of postoperative pain. Surg Endosc. 2011 Feb 7.
[15] Park HS, Kim TJ, Song T, Kim MK, Lee YY, Choi CH, et al. Single-port access (SPA) laparoscopic surgery in gynecology: a surgeon's experience with an initial 200 cases. Eur J Obstet Gynecol Reprod Biol. 2011 Jan;154(1):81-4.
[16] Escobar PF, Starks DC, Fader AN, Barber M, Rojas-Espalliat L. Single-port risk-reducing salpingo-oophorectomy with and without hysterectomy: surgical outcomes and learning curve analysis. Gynecol Oncol. 2010 Oct;119(1):43-7.
[17] Hahn HS, Kim YW. Single-port laparoscopic pelvic lymph node dissection with modified radical vaginal hysterectomy in cervical cancer. Int J Gynecol Cancer. 2010 Nov;20(8):1429-32.
[18] Paek J, Nam EJ, Kim YT, Kim SW. Overcoming technical difficulties with single-port access laparoscopic surgery in gynecology: using conventional laparoscopic instruments. J Laparoendosc Adv Surg Tech A. 2011 Mar;21(2):137-41.

8

Transvaginal Natural Orifice Transluminal Endoscopic Surgery (Notes): Surgical Technique and Results

William Kondo et al.*
[1]Hospital da Cruz Vermelha, Curitiba, Paraná,
[2]Centro Médico-Hospitalar Sugisawa, Curitiba, Paraná,
[3]University Hospital Teresopolis HCTCO-FESO, Rio de Janeiro,
[4]CHU Estaing, Clermont-Ferrand,
[1,2,3]Brazil
[4]France

1. Introduction

In recent decades, surgical specialties have experienced numerous changes and developments, and minimally invasive surgical techniques have been adopted to reduce patient morbidity (Branco et al., 2008a). Laparoscopy has a well-established role in the modern era of surgery. Despite the difficulties in terms of learning curve early in the clinical implementation of this method, almost all surgical specialties have adopted the minimally invasive surgical approach as the gold standard. This results in less postoperative pain, shorter hospital stay, faster recovery and better aesthetic results (Jin et al., 2009; Keus et al., 2010; Kondo et al., 2006).

Recently, a new minimally invasive surgical approach has been increasingly described in the literature as NOTES (Natural Orifice Transluminal Endoscopic Surgery). This is an access to the abdominal cavity without any incisions in the abdominal wall (scarless surgery), and the natural orifices serve as the gateway to the peritoneal cavity. Thus, an endoscope is inserted into the abdominal cavity through the stomach, vagina, bladder or colon (de la Fuente et al., 2007). The first report of this surgical technique was described by Gettman et al. (2002), at The University of Texas in 2002, which demonstrated that transvaginal nephrectomy in an experimental animal model was feasible. Two years later, Kalloo et al. (2004) performed transgastric liver biopsies at the Johns Hopkins University. After these initial reports, several researchers have demonstrated the safety of the transgastric access to perform tubal ligation (Jagannath et al., 2005), cholecystectomy (Park et al., 2005), gastrojejunostomy (Kantsevoy et al., 2005), subtotal hysterectomy with oophorectomy (Wagh et al, 2005; Wagh et al, 2006), splenectomy (Kantsevoy et al., 2006), gastric bypass (Kantsevoy et al., 2007), nephrectomy (Lima et al., 2007) and pancreatectomy (Matthes et al., 2007), all based on experimental studies in the porcine model.

Since 2007, reports of cholecystectomy (Branco Filho et al., 2007; Marescaux et al., 2007; Zorrón et al., 2007), nephrectomy (Branco et al., 2008b) and tubal ligation (Kondo et al., 2009)

---

*Anibal Wood Branco, Alcides José Branco Filho, Rafael William Noda, Monica Tessmann Zomer, Lorne Charles, Nicolas Bourdel and Ricardo Zorron.

using transvaginal NOTES in humans appeared in the literature. In this chapter we will discuss Natural Orifice Transluminal Endoscopic Surgery with the vagina as the point of entry into the abdominal cavity.

2. Overview of the previous studies

2.1 Transvaginal endoscopic access in animal models

The transvaginal endoscopic approach has been tested in animal models in General Surgery, Urology and Gynecology.

2.1.1 General surgery

Several procedures in the field of General Surgery have been performed in animal models by transvaginal endoscopic approach. Cholecystectomy is the simplest procedure for training and it can be performed by the hybrid technique (transvaginal access associated with transabdominal laparoscopic punctures) (Bessler et al., 2008; Horváth et al., 2009) or by the purely vaginal approach (Sánchez-Margallo et al., 2009). The use of the hybrid technique facilitates the procedure and is recommended at the beginning of training in NOTES.

The repair of abdominal wall hernias using the endoscopic transvaginal approach has also been studied by some authors (Lomanto et al., 2009b; Powell et al., 2010). Lomanto et al. (2009b) performed 5 abdominal wall hernia repairs using a transvaginal approach. The procedures were performed using a double-channel endoscope under general endotracheal anesthesia. A mesh was placed and fixed to the abdominal wall using laparoscopic and endoscopic standard equipment. The animals survived for 2 weeks and were subsequently euthanized. At the autopsy all meshes were in place and mild adhesions were recorded in one animal with a small subcutaneous abscess. In a study by Powell et al. (2010), transvaginal placement of a large synthetic mesh to repair the hernia was feasible in seven porcine animal models with a mean operative time of 133 minutes. No gross contamination was seen at autopsy. However, five animals had positive mesh cultures; 7 had positive cultures from the rectouterine space in enrichment broth or by direct culture. They concluded that future studies need to be conducted to develop better techniques and determine the significance of mesh contamination.

Even more complex surgical procedures such as partial gastrectomy (Nakajima et al., 2008) and distal pancreatectomy (Allemann et al., 2009) have been successfully performed using the endoscopic transvaginal access in animal model.

Lomanto et al (2009a) assessed the safety of transluminal surgery by investigating the intraperitoneal bacterial load and contamination during transgastric and transvaginal surgeries. Twelve female pigs underwent transgastric (n = 7; tubal ligation and oophorectomy) and transvaginal procedures (n = 5; cholecystectomy), and all animals were sacrificed after 2 weeks. In the transgastric group, six animals completed the surgical procedures and survived. Three pigs demonstrated signs of postoperative adhesions and abscesses with peritonitis and *Escherichia coli* was isolated at autopsy. In the transvaginal group, cholecystectomy was performed without any technical problems in the animals. No signs of postoperative sepsis or bacterial growth were observed in the microbiologic samples. The authors concluded that the transvaginal approach seemed to be safer and produced less contamination and intra-abdominal sepsis, compared to the transgastric route.

2.1.2 Urology

The first report of transvaginal NOTES in Urology was in 2002 by Gettman et al. They performed six transvaginal laparoscopic nephrectomies in female pigs. In one renal unit, the laparoscopic nephrectomy was completed entirely by way of the vagina. In five renal units, a single, 5-mm transbdominal laparoscope was required to facilitate visualization. In one case an uncontrollable vascular injury occurred during placement of the Endo-GIA stapler, resulting in exsanguination. After this initial report, other authors published their experience on transvaginal NOTES nephrectomy with success (Aminsharifi et al., 2009; Clayman et al., 2007; Haber et al., 2009; Isariyawongse et al., 2008), using the hybrid or pure technique. Also, Raman et al. (2009) demonstrated that the use of magnetically anchored instrumentation can improve shortcomings of previously reported NOTES nephrectomies in that triangulation, instrument fidelity, and visualization are preserved while hilar ligation is performed using a conventional stapler without need for additional transabdominal trocars. The exploration of the retroperitoneum's via NOTES using transvaginal access in a porcine model was evaluated by Zacharopoulou et al (2009). An excellent view of the retroperitoneal space and structures, such as the vascular and lymphatic tissues, the kidney, the adrenal gland, and the ureter, was obtained.

2.1.3 Gynecology

Transvaginal endoscopic retroperitoneal lymphadenectomy in a pig model was first demonstrated by Nassif et al. (2009). They performed three pelvic lymphadenectomies and three retroperitoneal lymphadenectomies (inter-aortocaval, lateral-aortic and lateral caval) successfully. The group of Clermont-Ferrand (CHU Estaing) (Bourdel et al., 2009) also evaluated this access in the performance of retroperitoneal sentinel lymph node resection in 10 pigs. After injection of methylene blue in the paracervical region (Figures 1A and 1B), the endoscope was inserted through a colpotomy incision on the right side. The internal iliac vessels were visualized, followed by identification of the bilateral external iliac vessels, aorta and vena cava (Figures 1C to 1E). The blue stained sentinel nodes were dissected bluntly and removed (Figures 1F to 1I). The mean operative time was 56 minutes and the average number of lymph nodes removed per animal was 1.75. After transvaginal NOTES lymphadenectomy, a laparoscopic procedure was performed and the removal of 19 of 20 sentinel nodes was confirmed. No major complication occurred in 10 animals. Of the 19 sentinel nodes, 11 were located on the left side and 8 on the right side. Fifteen lymph nodes were obtained from the iliac vessels or the region of the promontory and four from the pre-aortic or lateral aortic regions.

2.2 Transvaginal endoscopic access in human cadavers

2.2.1 General surgery

Sugimoto et al. (2009) performed one case of transvaginal NOTES cholecystectomy in a human female cadaver. The surgical time was 87 minutes and there was no major complication.

Some cases of transvaginal NOTES gastric bypass in human cadavers have been reported in the literature (Hagen et al., 2008; Madan et al., 2008). Nevertheless, several factors made this technique very challenging and time-consuming. A lack of proper instrumentation resulting in insufficient tissue traction, countertraction, and instrument manipulation complicated several steps during the procedure. A combination of flexible with rigid endoscopic techniques offers specific advantages for aspects of this type of surgery. Changes in instrument design are required to improve ergonomics in more complex endosurgical procedures (Hagen et al., 2008).

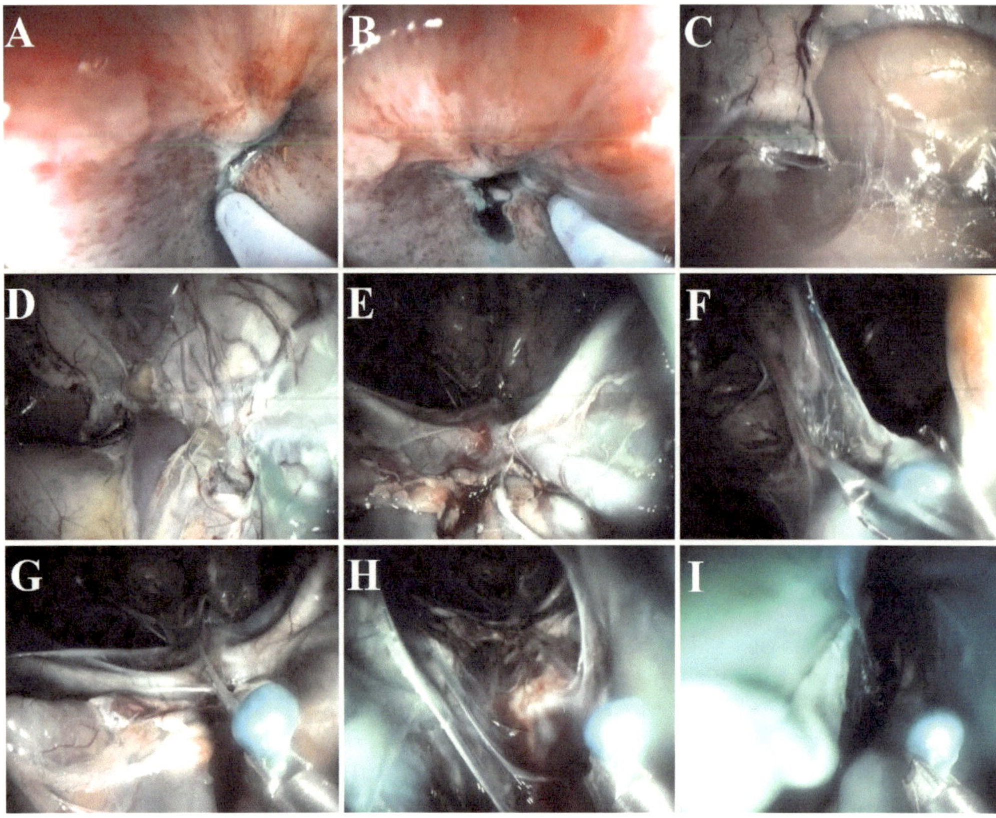

Fig. 1. Sentinel lymph node biopsy by retroperitoneal transvaginal NOTES in an animal model. (A and B) Injection of methylene blue in the paracervical region. (C) Visualization of the left kidney. (D) Identification of the right kidney and inferior vena cava. (E) Bifurcation of the iliac vessels. (F, G, H and I) Removal of the blue-stained sentinel lymph node in the region of the iliac vessels.

2.2.2 Urology

Allemann et al. (2010) described their experience with the pure transvaginal access for exploration of the retroperitoneum in cadavers to simulate the procedure of nephrectomy, adrenalectomy and pancreatectomy. The experiments were conducted in three fresh human cadavers, warmed at room temperature for 12 hours. The colpotomy was performed on the posterior wall of the vagina approximately 3 cm proximal to the posterior fornix. A posterior and left lateral tunnel was created under direct vision, using open surgical and laparoscopic instruments. Upon entry into the pararectal space, a 12mm dual channel endoscope was introduced and the carbon dioxide insufflation was achieved through one of the channels. The anatomic landmarks identified were the obturator nerve and artery entering the canal of Alcock, the sacral nerves, the median rectal artery, external iliac vessels, the inferior epigastric artery and the left lower pole of the kidney. The access was performed correctly up to the level of the iliac vessels in three cadavers. In the first case, the frozen tissue prevented the complete dissection up to the kidney. In the other two cadavers, the inferior pole of the kidney was clearly visualized. The mean surgical access time was 52 minutes.

Perreta et al. (2009b) confirmed the feasibility of the transvaginal retroperitoneal access for nephrectomy in two cadavers but a complete dissection of the kidney was not possible because of the rigor of the surrounding tissues. This access was also effectively reproduced in a cadaver model for adrenalectomy by the same authors (Perretta et al., 2009a).
Aron et al. (2009) tried a novel port called QuadPort (Advanced Surgical Concepts, Wicklow, Ireland) to perform transvaginal nephrectomy using standard and articulating laparoscopic instruments in four fresh female cadavers. One procedure was aborted due to dense pelvic adhesions from previous pelvic surgery. In the first 2 cadavers the assistance from an umbilical port was required to divide the attachments between the upper renal pole and the diaphragm. In the third case the dissection was completely performed by transvaginal means using a flexible gastroscope.

2.2.3 Gynecology

The gynecology group of Clermont-Ferrand (CHU Estaing) also performed the endoscopic approach for transvaginal retroperitoneal evaluation in cadavers, but the results were not published. The same surgical steps described above by Allemann et al. (2010) were performed in two cadavers with a mean operative time of 60 minutes (Figures 2A and 2B).

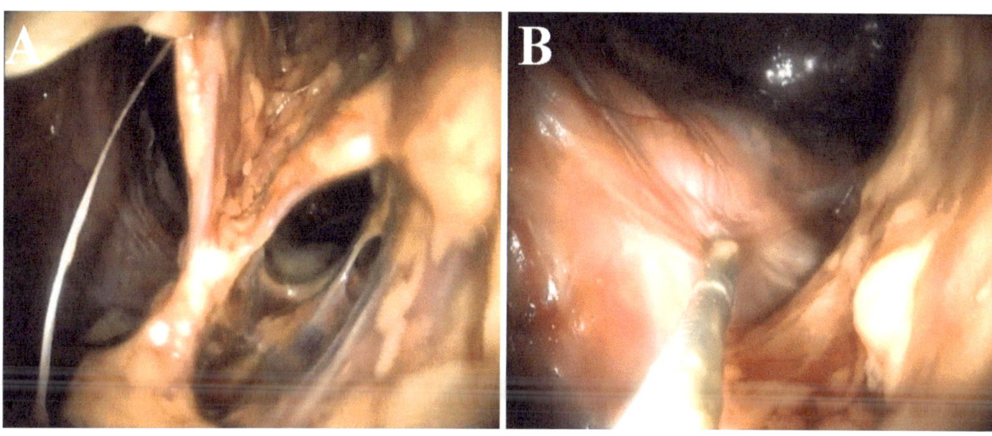

Fig. 2. (A) Retroperitoneal dissection prior to the sacral bone. (B) Identification of the promontory and the bifurcation of the iliac vessels.

2.3 Transvaginal endoscopic access in humans

2.3.1 Use of the rigid endoscope

The vaginal access has been used to visualize pelvic and intra-abdominal organs since the early 1900s, when it was called culdoscopy. On April 19, 1901, the Russian surgeon Dr. Dmitri von Ott first described the ventroscopy through colpotomy in Trendelenburg position at the Meeting of the Society of Gynaecology and Obstetrics of Saint Petersburg (Von Ott, 1902). In 1940, TeLinde was recognized as the author of one of the first accounts of rigid culdoscopy in The United States (Frenkel et al., 1952). In 1942, Palmer introduced the rigid transvaginal culdoscopy in a supine position (Brosens et al., 2003). In the same year, Decker (1952) invented what became known as the Decker´s culdoscope, a rigid instrument with a light adjacent to the lens at the distal end. Clyman (1963) used a rigid culdoscope to carry out several procedures, such as lysis of adhesions, biopsies and aspirations of ovarian cysts.

In 1999, Watrelot et al. described the fertiloscopy, a minimally invasive technique for investigation of female infertility. It uses a minimally invasive transvaginal access to the pelvic organs and generally combines the following diagnostic procedures: hydrolaparoscopy (or hydropelviscopy), tubal patency test with methylene blue, salpingoscopy, micro-salpingoscopy and hysteroscopy. The use of videoscopic instruments inserted by transvaginal route to explore the pelvic peritoneal cavity is feasible and the technique has been applied in thousands of patients with complication rates below 1% (Gordts et al., 2008). Nohuz et al. (2006) retrospectively evaluated 229 women with primary or secondary infertility without any condition that would justify a laparoscopy and who could benefit from a fertiloscopy (Figures 3 to 5). Two hundred and three (88.6%) procedures were successfully performed, revealing lesions in 58 cases (28.6%).

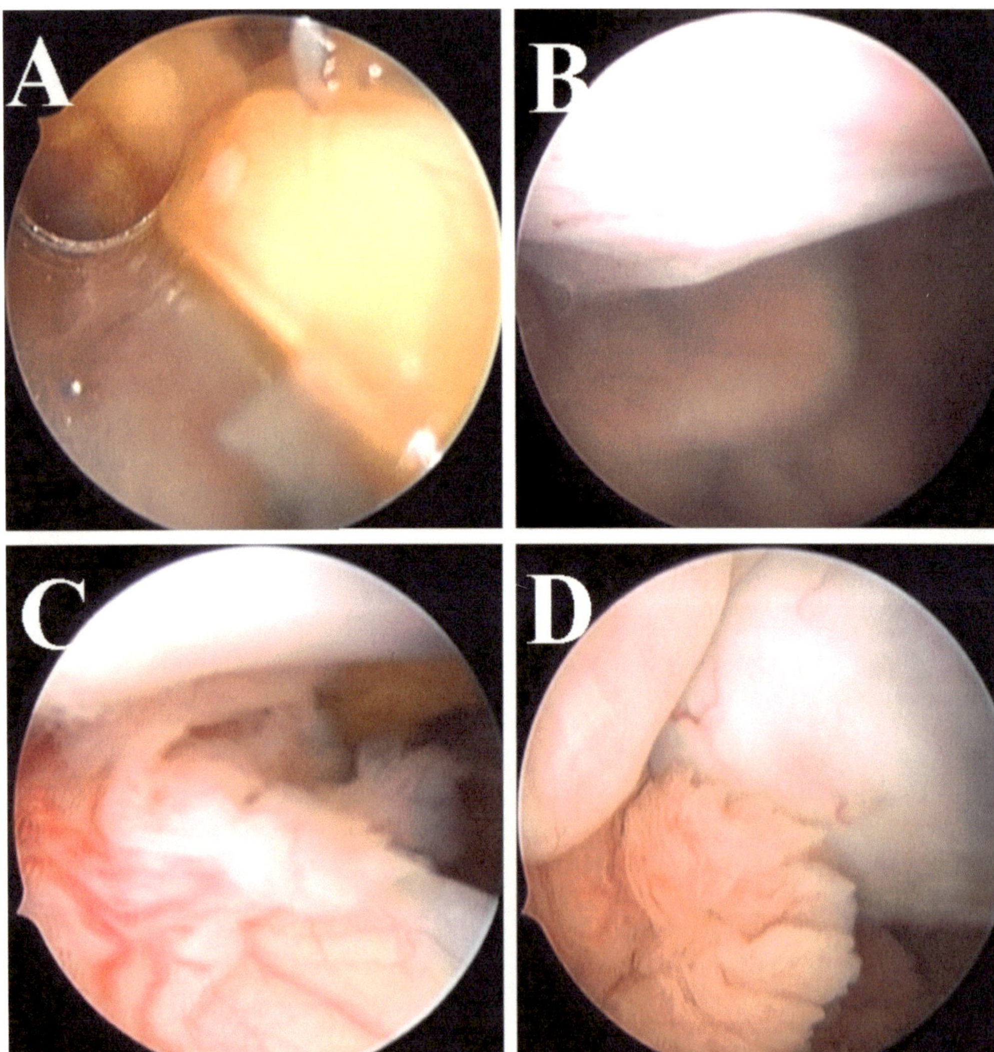

Fig. 3. Fertiloscopy: (A) Transvaginal access. (B) Posterior uterine wall. (C) Left fallopian tube. (D) Right fallopian tube.

Five complications (2.5%) were observed: two involving the rectum, two bleedings and a postoperative salpingitis. The biggest drawback of the rigid endoscope is the inability to explore the entire peritoneal cavity, especially the anterior uterine wall and the peritoneum covering the surface of the bladder and broad ligaments (Hackethal et al., 2011).

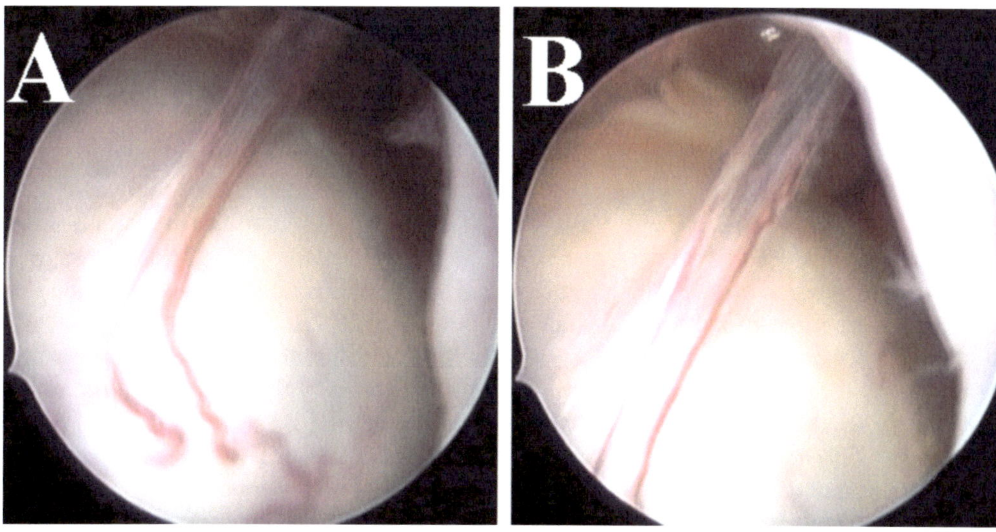

Fig. 4. Identification of adhesion over the left ovary during fertiloscopy.

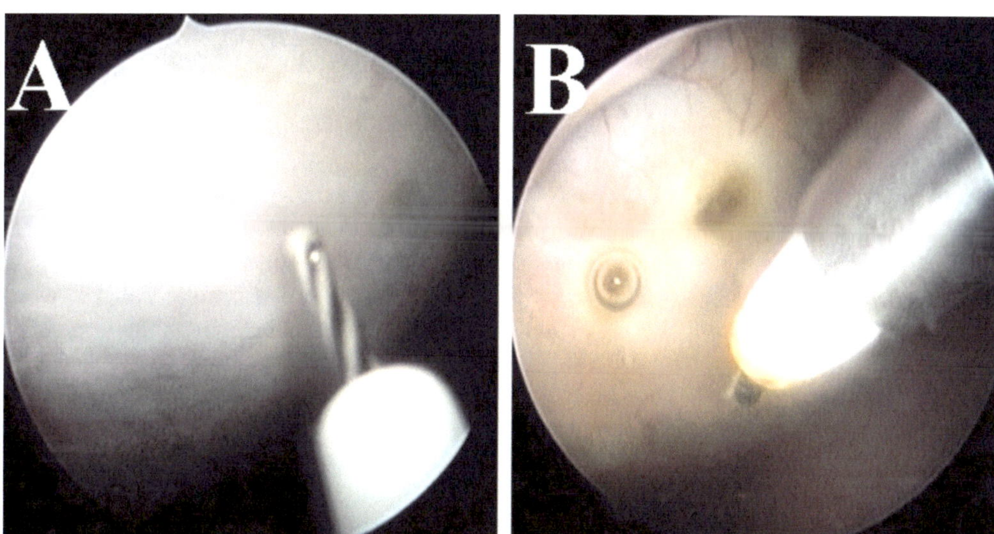

Fig. 5. Ovarian drilling by fertiloscopy.

In 2011, Hackethal et al. tested two new rigid endoscopes that allowed adjustable angles of view for evaluating women via transvaginal surgery: the 10mm rigid endoscope EndoCAMeleon (Karl Storz, Tuttlingen, Germany) that allowed viewing angles ranging from 0 to 120 degrees and the EndoEYE LTF-VH (Olympus, Hamburg, Germany) with a flexible tip that reaches an angle of 100 degrees. It was believed that the use of these new endoscopes could facilitate the surgical access and the visualization of the entire female pelvis. Four patients with infertility (n = 3) and chronic pelvic pain (n = 1) were included in the study. They concluded that these new endoscopes did not allow a good view of the anterior portion of the pelvis to rule out endometriosis or other diseases. For transvaginal surgery with intent to explore the pelvic cavity, non-rigid endoscopes are as easy to manipulate as the rigid endoscopes and provide good visualization of the pelvic anatomy. The obvious disadvantages of rigid endoscopes and its fixed axis of vision have not been overcome by these new endoscopes. The inability of the endoscope be angled back to inspect the pelvic structures undermines the efficiency of the diagnostic evaluation of the patient.

2.3.2 Use of the flexible endoscope

The first description of transvaginal endoscopic surgery was from 2007, when the team of Professor Marescaux in Strasbourg performed a cholecystectomy via hybrid transvaginal access (Marescaux et al., 2007). That same year, several reports of cholecystectomy using this technique were published worldwide (Branco Filho et al., 2007; Dolz et al., 2007; Zorrón et al., 2007). Since then, this access has been used to perform several procedures, including nephrectomy (Branco et al., 2008b; Castillo et al., 2009; Kaouk et al., 2010; Ribal Caparrós et al., 2009), tubal sterilization (Kondo et al., 2009), liver resection (Noguera et al., 2008), sleeve gastrectomy (Fischer et al., 2009; Ramos et al., 2008b), adjustable gastric banding (Michalik et al, 2010), incisional hernia repair (Jacobsen et al., 2010), cancer diagnostic staging (Zorrón et al., 2008), splenectomy (Targarona et al., 2009), retroperitoneoscopy (Zorron et al., 2010a) among others.

More recently, some case series have been published (Alcaraz et al., 2010; Asakuma et al., 2009; Cuadrado-Garcia et al., 2011; Hackethal et al., 2010; Horgan et al., 2009; Lehmann et al., 2010; Niu et al., 2010; Noguera et al., 2009; Noguera et al., 2010; Palanivelu et al., 2008; Pugliese et al., 2010; Ramos et al., 2008a; Sotelo et al., 2010; Zornig et al., 2010a; Zornig et al., 2010b; Zorron et al., 2010b). In China (Niu et al., 2010), cholecystectomies were successfully performed via laparoscopic assisted endoscopic transvaginal surgery. No intra- or postoperative complications were observed. All patients were satisfied with the cosmetic results.

Linke et al. (2010) assessed the feasibility and safety of rigid-hybrid transvaginal NOTES approach in routine practice for symptomatic cholecystolithiasis or acute cholecystitis in a patient population with low selection. One hundred and two consecutive patients were included in the study. Only two patients had conversion to conventional laparoscopic cholecystectomy. There were no intraoperative complications. Two major complications occurred: one stroke and one herniation within the transumbilical access. Minor complications were reported in 13 patients (12.7%) and there were no serious postoperative gynecological findings. At the 6th postoperative week, there were fewer dyspareunia symptoms than preoperatively (p = 0.049). Likewise, Zornig et al. (2010a) reported that by means of rigid laparoscopic instruments, transvaginal cholecystectomy can be routinely performed.

Palanivelu et al. (2008) described the transvaginal approach for endoscopic appendectomy in 6 patients. A totally endoscopic transvaginal appendectomy was successfully performed for one patient. The other five patients were either converted to conventional laparoscopy or aided by a laparoscope. The mean operating time was 103.5 minutes. Hospital stay varied from one to two days. The vaginal wound was examined by the gynecologist and was found to be completely healed within the first (7 days) and second (30 days) follow-up.

Noguera et al. (2010) described 10 women with intra-abdominal infections treated successfully with using hybrid NOTES by transvaginal access. The procedure was performed on an emergency basis by the surgical team on call. The indications for surgery were 6 cases of acute cholecystitis, 2 cases of acute appendicitis, and 2 cases of pelvic peritonitis.

Buesing et al. (2010) performed 14 cases of transvaginal assisted sleeve gastrectomies. Using the transvaginal technique the number of trocars could be reduced by 1-2 and in all cases the resected stomach was retrieved transvaginally. No complications occurred due to the vaginal access.

Alcaraz et al. (2010) evaluated the feasibility of transvaginal NOTES-assisted laparoscopic nephrectomy in female patients with and without renal cancer. Fourteen patients were submitted to the procedure for T1-T3a N0 M0 renal cancer (n=10), lithiasis (n=2), or renal atrophy (n=2). The procedure was completed in all patients. The mean operative time was 132.9 minutes and the mean estimated blood loss was 111.2ml. None of the patients required a blood transfusion and the use of analgesics was low. The mean hospital stay was 4 days. In one case, a major complication (a colon injury) occurred. The patient underwent surgery and a temporary colostomy was performed.

A German NOTES register (Lehmann et al., 2010) included 551 patients on whom surgery was performed in a 14-month period. Cholecystectomy accounted for 85.3% of all procedures. All procedures were performed on women using the hybrid transvaginal technique. Complications occurred in 3.1% of patients and conversion to laparoscopy or open surgery in 4.9%.

Zorron et al. (2010b) reported a multicenter study of 16 centers in 9 countries which included 362 patients who underwent transgastric and transvaginal NOTES. The most common procedures were transvaginal cholecystectomy (66.3%), transvaginal appendectomy (10.2%), transgastric cholecystectomy (8.01%) and transgastric appendectomy (3.87%), accounting for 88.38% of total procedures. The overall rate of complications was 8.84%, including 5.8% of grades I and II complications and 3.04% of grades III and IV complications.

Zornig et al. (2010b) analyzed 108 women who underwent hybrid transvaginal NOTES cholecystectomy with 192 women undergoing laparoscopic cholecystectomy and selected 100 patients in each group for comparison. The duration of the hybrid transvaginal procedure was longer than the conventional laparoscopic cholecystectomy (52 vs. 35 minutes; $p<0.001$). There were no intraoperative complications. There was no statistically significant difference regarding the need for reoperation, wound infections, consumption of analgesics and length of hospital stay. Seventy-five women who underwent hybrid transvaginal surgery and 73 undergoing laparoscopic cholecystectomy had intercourse after surgery with no complaints.

Hensel et al. (2010) performed a retrospective case-controlled study comparing 47 women undergoing transvaginal cholecystectomy with 46 women undergoing conventional laparoscopic cholecystectomy. Women of the former group reported less postoperative pain ($p<0.001$), less nausea or vomiting ($p<0.001$) and a lower analgesic consumption in both opiates ($p<0.001$) and non-opiates ($p<0.001$). Furthermore, the duration of stay in recovery room was shorter in the former group (40 minutes vs. 60 minutes, $p<0.001$). The rate of general and surgical complications was lower in the transvaginal group (1/47) compared to the laparoscopic group (4/46). In 9 women undergoing transvaginal cholecystectomy negligible vaginal bleeding was seen which stopped spontaneously in each case.

3. Preoperative preparation

The transvaginal access requires no special prior preparation. The only important step is the gynecological evaluation preoperatively to rule vulvovaginitis. In the presence of vaginal infections, we recommend antibiotic treatment at least one week before surgery in order to avoid pelvic infectious and its associated complications which result from the introduction of microorganisms into the peritoneal cavity during the development of the transvaginal access.

It is important to obtain the informed consent from the patient, especially in the young and nulliparous women. Although not frequent, the transvaginal access can lead to colpotomy-related dyspareunia postoperatively and only a few studies[66, 83] have evaluated this potential complication with favorable results. In addition, the scar on the posterior vaginal fornix and the posterior cul-de-sac, can lead to the development of which can complicate a future pregnancy in nulliparous women.

The most important point of evaluation and preoperative preparation is the careful selection of patients for transvaginal endoscopic surgery. Although the surgical indications are the same, regardless of the approach being used, some relative and absolute contra-indications must be respected when this new access route is used.

3.1 Contra-indications

The transvaginal endoscopic access cannot be applied to all patients. There is no work showing what would constitute relative and absolute contraindications to the procedure, but based on our experience, we cite the following situations as potential contraindications:

- Deep endometriosis: the patients with severe endometriosis often have their lesions located posterior to the uterus, either in utero-sacral ligaments, in the retrocervical region or in the rectovaginal septum. This prevents access to the pelvic cavity through the posterior fornix of the vagina due to the high risk of iatrogenic injuries of adjacent organs during the creation of the access to the pelvic cavity. Also, the presence of resulting intense inflammatory/fibrotic disease hinders access to the cavity.
- Suspected adnexal lesions: all suspicious adnexal lesions are to be addressed with surgical oncologic principles. The precariousness of endoscopic instruments still makes meticulous surgical gestures difficult using this access. We cannot expose patients to the risk of a possible rupture of a malignant adnexal lesion and consequent contamination of the pelvic cavity with tumor cells.
- Previous pelvic surgery and history of pelvic inflammatory disease: surgical procedures in the pelvic region and previous episodes of pelvic inflammatory disease may lead to the formation of dense adhesions in this region and the instruments currently available for the performance of transvaginal endoscopy does not facilitate the perfect exposure and careful dissection which is required to access areas of the pelvis with large amount of adhesions.
- Complex surgical procedures: the lack of triangulation of the instruments and the endoscope image obtained through the retroflected view (upside down and mirror) do not allow complex surgical gestures can be accomplished.

4. Decision-making, anatomy, and key steps in the operations

Briefly, the important criteria for selecting patients for endoscopic surgery by transvaginal access include:

- Surgical indication for the proposed procedure (independent of the surgical route to be used).
- Female patient.
- Experience of the surgical team with advanced laparoscopic surgery, transvaginal access, and rigid and flexible endoscopic equipment.
- Absence of contraindications to the access.

4.1 Surgical technique

The patient is positioned in the dorsal lithotomy position with the legs in stirrups and the arms tucked at her sides. An orogastric tube and a Foley's catheter are placed. A prophylactic antibiotic (1g of cefazolin) is administered after induction of anesthesia. The surgical field (vaginal cavity) is prepared with povidone iodine or chlorhexidine solution.

The transvaginal access can be performed under direct vision (posterior colpotomy) or guided by laparoscopy.

4.1.1 Transvaginal access by direct visualization (Branco et al., 2008a; Kondo et al., 2009)

A Sims speculum is inserted in the vagina, and the posterior lip of the cervix is grasped by a Pozzi clamp. The vaginal walls are retracted by 2 lateral retractors, and anterior traction is given to the cervix to stretch the posterior fornix. The vaginal mucosa in the posterior cul-de-sac is opened at the cervico-vaginal junction by a semilunar 2.5-cm incision. The posterior margin is grasped by 1 Allis forceps, and sharp dissection is performed with the index finger. The posterior cul-de-sac peritoneum is identified and opened (Figure 6).

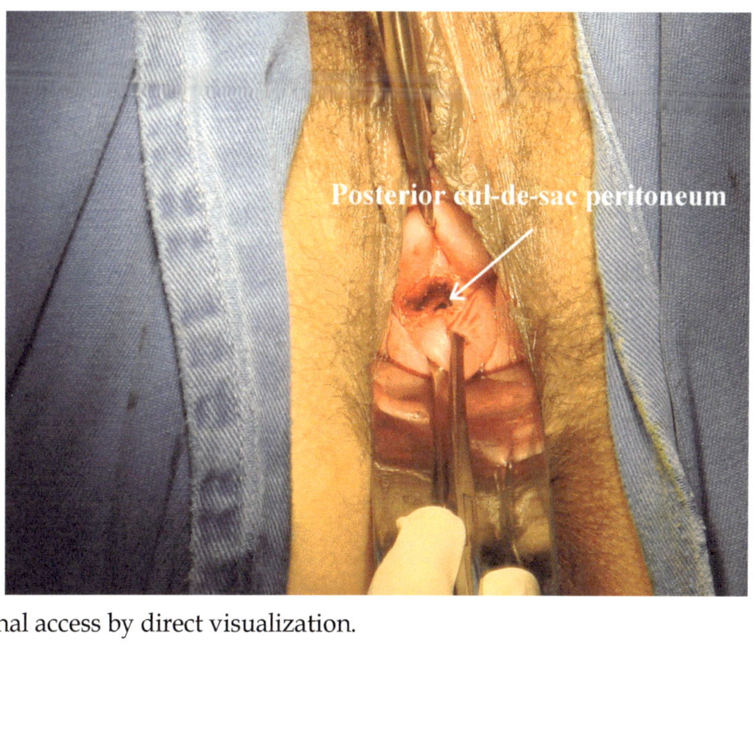

Fig. 6. Vaginal access by direct visualization.

The endoscope is inserted into the pelvic cavity (Figure 7), carbon dioxide insufflation can be achieved via a working channel of the endoscope or through a nasogastric tube connected externally to the endoscope, allowing for the introduction of forceps in each working channel (Figure 8).

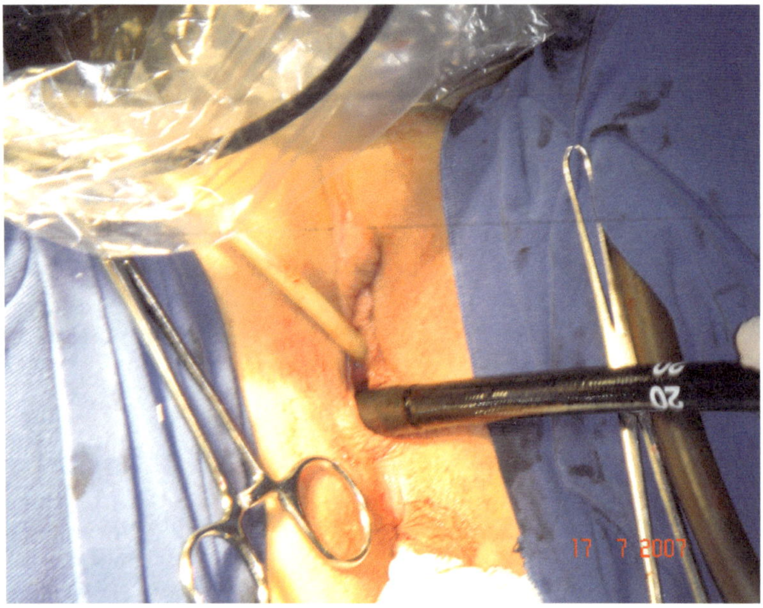

Fig. 7. Introduction of the endoscope through the vaginal cavity.

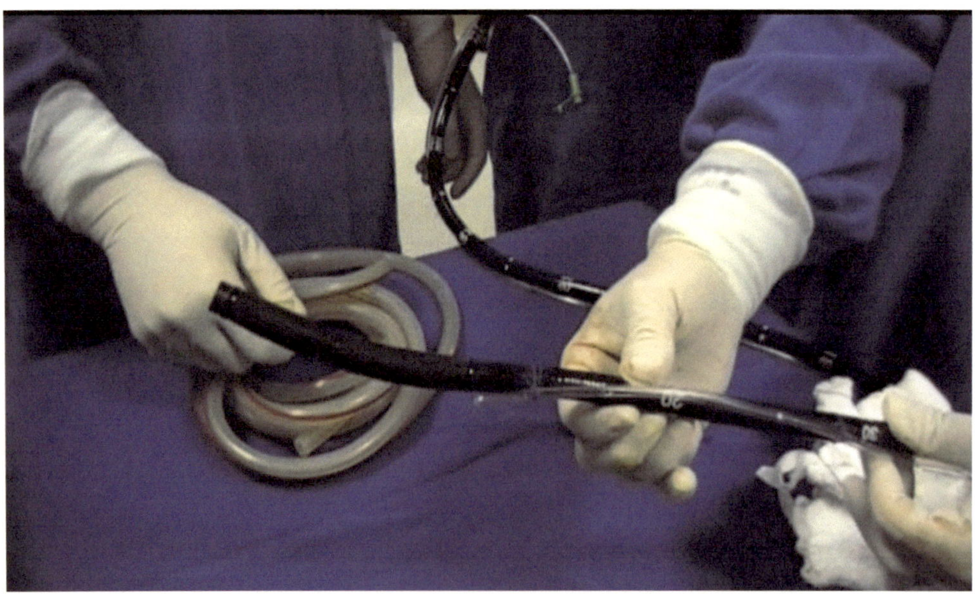

Fig. 8. Preparation of endoscope securing a nasogastric tube to the dual-channel endoscope, through which carbon dioxide was inflated to obtain the pneumoperitoneum.

4.1.2 Transvaginal access via laparoscopic guidance (Zorron et al., 2010b)

The surgeon is placed standing between the patient's legs; the first and second assistants stand on the left and right sides of the patient, respectively. In this setting, 2 visualization systems, one for the abdominal laparoscopic camera and the other for the TV flexible endoscope, are used. The procedure starts with a Veress puncture through an incision in the umbilicus to avoid a visible scar. Pneumoperitoneum is then insufflated through the Veress needle.

A 5-mm trocar is inserted, and a 5-mm laparoscopic optic used to inspect the abdominal cavity. To avoid the risk of injuring pelvic organs, some surgeons perform a thorough examination of the pelvis, looking for adhesions that might prohibit the TV cul-de-sac puncture. In patients who had had a previous hysterectomy, or unknown endometriosis, adhesions obliterating the pouch of Douglas contraindicate the further vaginal insertion of the trocar and conversion to formal laparoscopy is usually indicated. After inventory, a longer 10- to 12-mm laparoscopic trocar is inserted in the vaginal posterior cul-de-sac under laparoscopic guidance (Figure 9). The endoscope is progressed after extraction of the laparoscopic trocar.

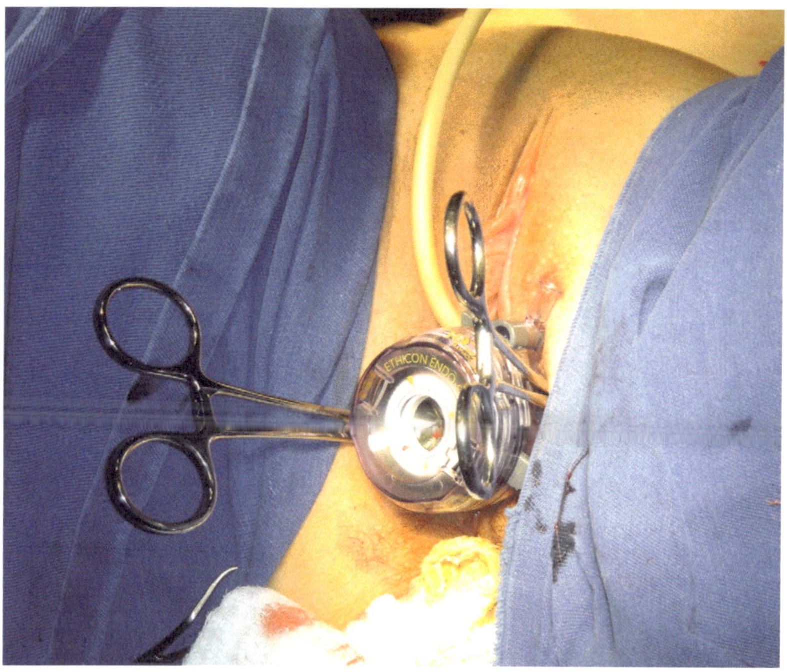

Fig. 9. Placement of transvaginal trocar guided by laparoscopy.

4.1.3 Technical details of the procedure

Technical details of the entire procedure vary according to the surgery to be performed. Here we focused on technical variations that exist specifically for transvaginal NOTES access, regardless of the structure to be operated on.

Four distinct techniques for transvaginal NOTES cholecystectomy have been described by different centers, regarding pure natural orifice surgery or combined hybrid techniques to facilitate efficiency and safety for the procedures (Zorron et al., 2010b):

- Totally NOTES dual scope method (de Sousa et al., 2009): utilizes two endoscopes inserted via the vaginal route (one single-channel gastroscope with the insufflation tube attached and one double-channel colonoscope). The former was used to retract the gallbladder and the latter to perform the cholecystectomy, thus avoiding the necessity of using transabdominal puncture for the introduction of laparoscopic forceps to expose the gallbladder (Figure 10).

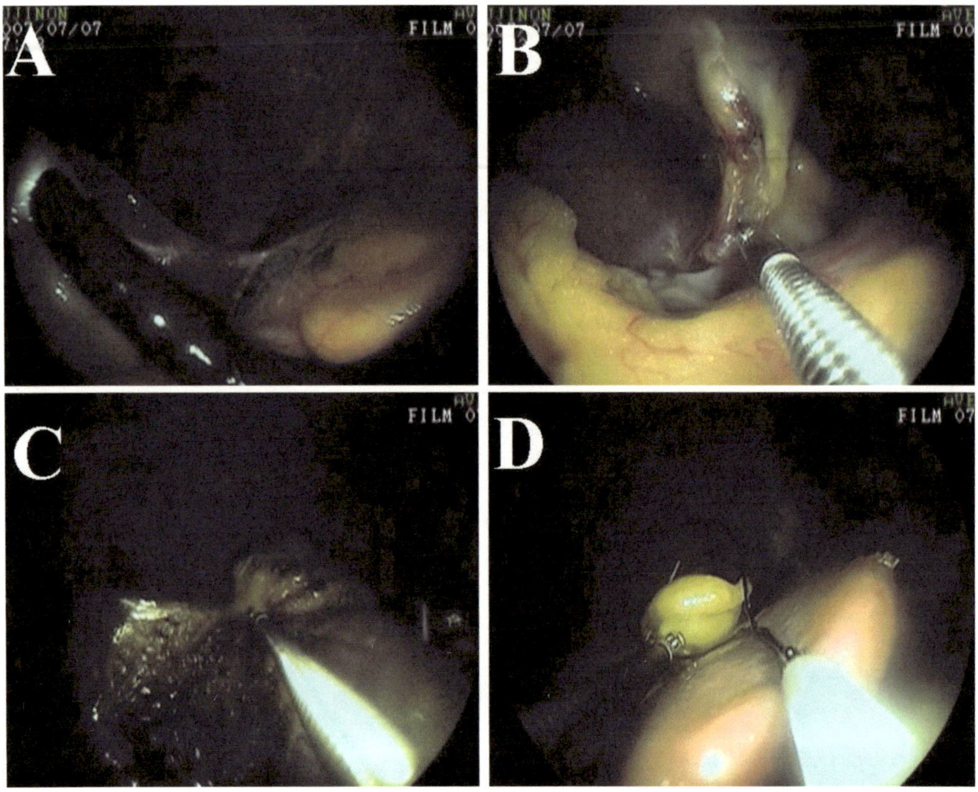

Fig. 10. Totally NOTES cholecystectomy (de Sousa et al., 2009) using two endoscopes. (A) One endoscope is used to retract the gallbladder. (B and C) The second endoscope is used to perform the procedure. (D) The gallbladder is retrieved from the abdominal cavity using an endoscopic polypectomy snare.

- Hybrid NOTES with transvaginal access and abdominal laparoscopy: laparoscopy was used in this technique for purposes such as safe access, visualization, and dissection, usually accomplished by endoscopic instruments or laparoscopy. Avoiding maximally the difficult endoscopic dissection and instrumentation, this method allowed for faster operations in a similar critical laparoscopic view (Figure 11 and 12).
- Transvaginal multipurpose port with flexible surgery: vaginal access and dissection were obtained by a transvaginal port (local adapted trocar) that permitted independent entry of the flexible endoscope (double-channel colonoscope), insufflation channel from a laparoflator, and semiflexible instruments used for retraction, cutting, and clipping using transvaginal laparoscopic titanium clips. Dissection was accomplished by available flexible endoscopic instruments, such as as polipectomy snares and hot-biopsy forceps.

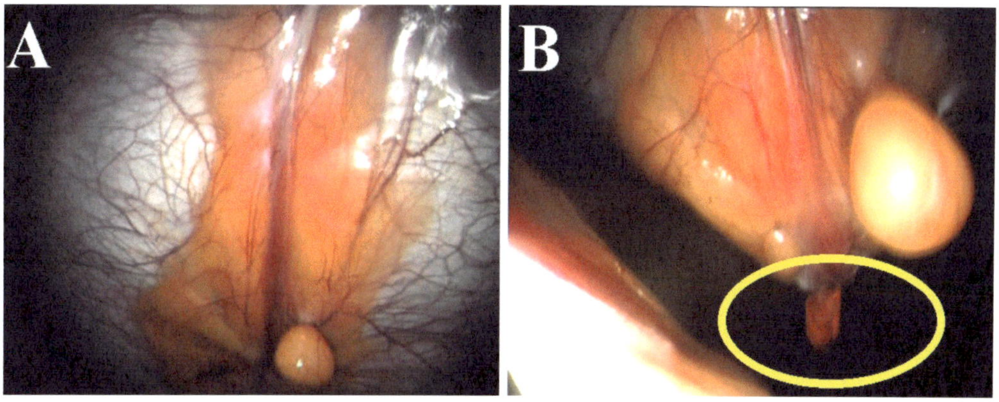

Fig. 11. Placement of a transumbilical trocar (yellow circle) guided by transvaginal endoscopic vision.

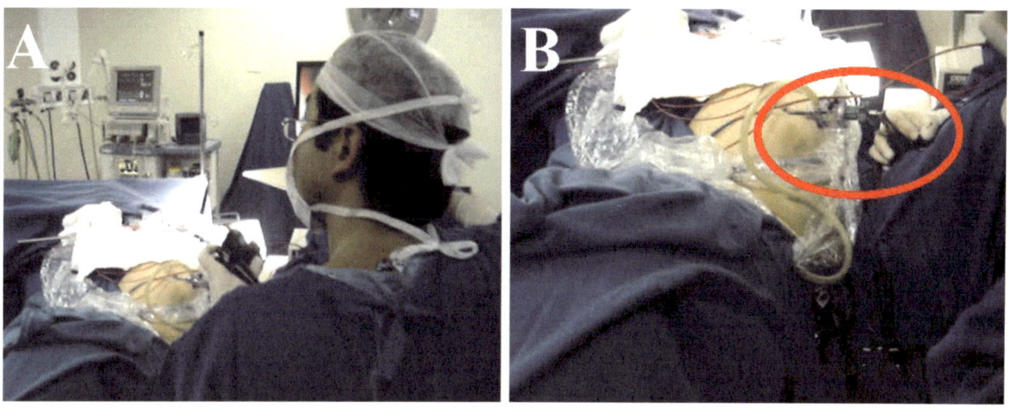

Fig. 12. (A) The surgeon is placed standing between the patient's legs. (B) One conventional laparoscopic instrument (red circle) placed transumbilically (hybrid NOTES).

- Transvaginal trocars (flexible or rigid optic) combined with umbilical minilaparoscopy: pneumoperitoneum was achieved by umbilical Veress needle puncture. After insufflation, opening of the posterior vaginal fornix was performed by direct vision to allow the introduction of a 1- or 2-channel gastroscope in the abdominal cavity. By retroflected view, a specially designed long 10-mm trocar was placed in the vagina, parallel to the endoscope. Two 3-mm trocars were placed transumbilically under direct endoscopic vision. Dissection of Calot's Triangle was performed using endoscopic instruments such as hot-biopsy forceps, polipectomy snares, endoscopic hook, and the umbilical 3-mm instruments. Cystic duct and artery were dissected and clipped using long laparoscopic clipator through the vaginal trocar.

NOTES appendectomies through vaginal access have been performed using direct access to the cavity with or without umbilical laparoscopic assistance. Usually the appendix could be managed without endoscopic retroflection, or using vaginal rigid camera. Although a simple solution would be to perform the dissection through umbilical trocar, most teams used endoscopic dissection with hot-biopsy forceps and polypectomy snare. In case of need for peritoneal lavage due to pus, transvaginal endoscopic aspiration was performed or a laparoscopic irrigator aspirator was used (Zorron et al., 2010b).

For the endoscopic tubal sterilization (Kondo et al., 2009), a uterine manipulator was positioned to facilitate exposure of the tubes for the procedure (Figure 13). The tubes were coagulated and transected using endoscopic instruments inserted through the flexible endoscope with dual working channel (Figure 14).

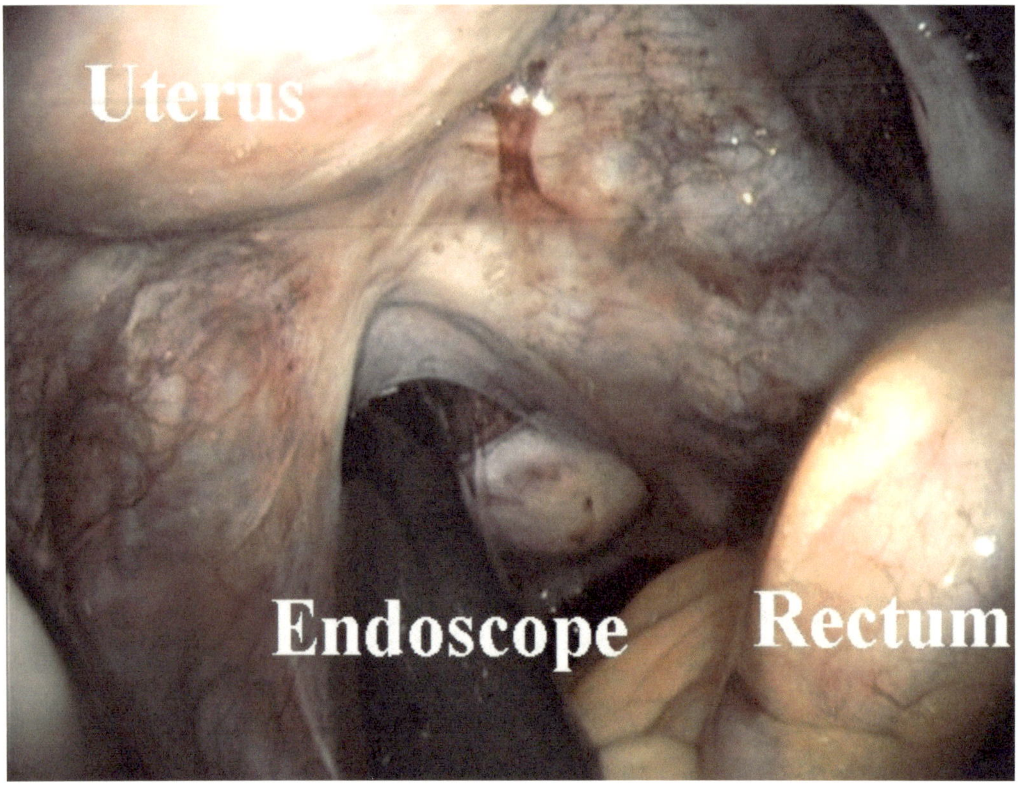

Fig. 13. The manipulation of the uterus using a uterine manipulator allows excellent exposure of the posterior cul-de-sac.

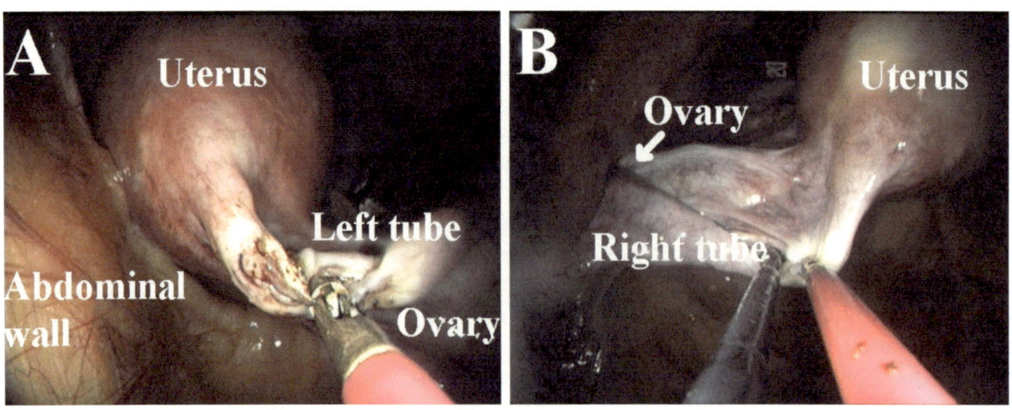

Fig. 14. Transvaginal endoscopic tubal sterilization.

4.1.4 Closure of the vagina

After the procedure, the posterior cul-de-sac and the posterior vaginal fornix are closed with a running 2-0 vicryl suture.

5. Surgical tricks

The presence of an endoscopist in the operating room is of paramount importance in the early learning curve, since he is more familiar with the performance of the maneuvers using the flexible endoscopic equipment.

The use of hybrid technique (endoscopic transvaginal access associated with transabdominal punctures) seems to be a natural transition from the traditional laparoscopic approach to surgery by natural orifices. Some details, which were previously discussed, highlight the measures, which serve to increase the safety of this method and reduce risks to patient:

- Execution of laparoscopic-guided vaginal access: access to the abdominal cavity through the vagina was known long ago by gynecologists (Box et al., 2009), but general surgeons are not familiar with this surgical approach. In this case, we recommend the creation of the pneumoperitoneum through the umbilicus, followed by placement of trocar. With the use of a 5-mm laparoscope and the placement of the patient in maximum Trendelenburg position, the posterior cul-de-sac is exposed. At this surgical step, the placement of a curette through the cervix assists with uterine manipulation (uterine anteversion), allowing to the correct exposure of the posterior cul-de-sac. Thus, one can introduce a trocar through the posterior vaginal fornix under direct vision.
- Hybrid NOTES: hybrid techniques have been used in most case series published to date. The endoscope with two working channels is introduced by vaginal route for the flexible endoscopy forceps and the surgeon uses one or more additional conventional laparoscopy instruments positioned by the transabdominal route for easy handling and checking of structures to achieve triangulation for more complex procedures.
- The use of long rigid endoscope by transvaginal route is also an option for surgery of upper abdomen. In the case of pelvic surgery, requiring a retroflected view, this modification method is not applicable.

6. Postoperative care

The patient is given a clear liquid diet 6 hours after the procedure and a regular diet the following morning. Intravenous dypirone (1 g per 6 hours) is administered for pain relief and usually no supplemental analgesia is necessary.

If the postoperative course is uneventful, patients can be discharged on the first postoperative day. They must be advised to avoid vaginal intercourse for 40 days.

The other postoperative recommendations are inherent to the surgical procedure, varying according to the type of surgery for which the patient was referred.

7. Impact of the technique on modern practice

The use of less aggressive surgical techniques for patients is the goal of modern surgery. The surgical approaches by natural orifices have arisen for this purpose and their role in clinical practice should be established in the future. So far, only a few centers have performed this type of surgery, with promising results.

The transvaginal endoscopic approach has several potential advantages (Dubcenco et al., 2009; Tonouchi et al., 2004):

- Good acceptance by patients, since it leaves no scars on the abdomen.
- Mirrors laparoscopic surgery
- Associated with minimal morbidity.
- Allows viewing of all the pelvic anatomy.
- Minimal postoperative pain.
- Limited postoperative recovery time.
- Prevents hernias in trocar ports and can decrease the formation of intra-abdominal adhesions.

The disadvantages of this method include:

- Inability to use in all patients (see contraindications) and in men.
- Need for a long learning curve.
- Need for prolonged periods of sexual abstinence after the procedure to complete vaginal healing.

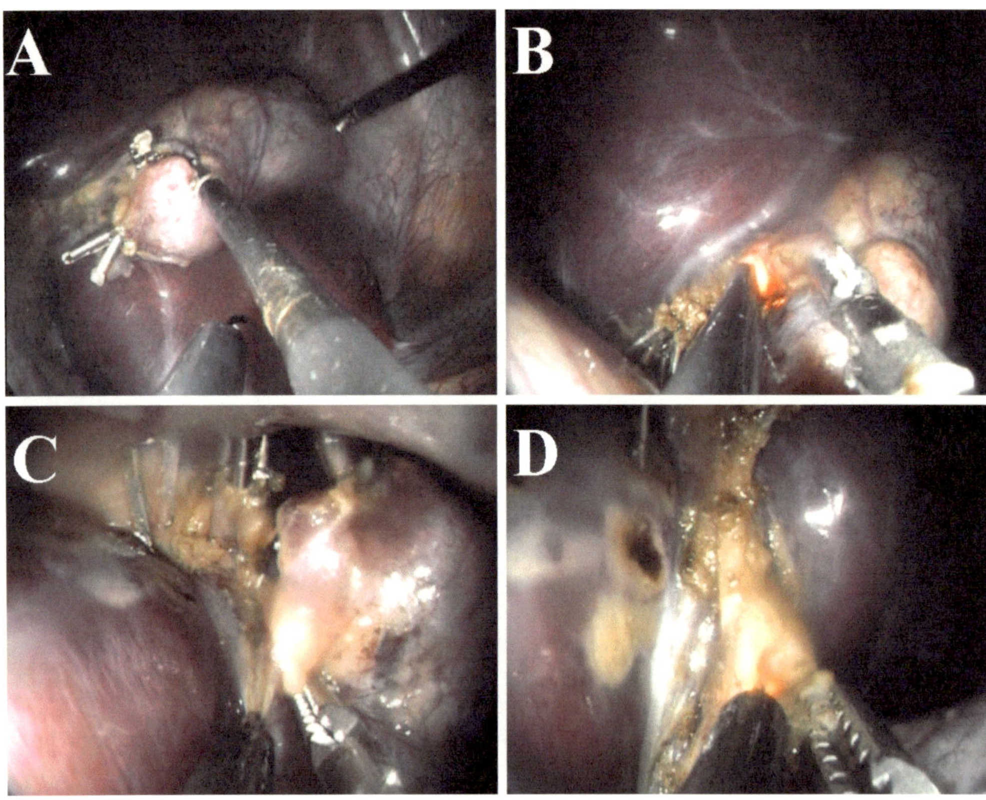

Fig. 15. Hybrid NOTES cholecystectomy. Both endoscopic instruments work in parallel, without triangulation.

7.1 Difficulties

As NOTES involves the use of a flexible scope in a large abdominal cavity, with operating instruments in line with the light source, difficulties associated with poor visibility, maintenance of spatial orientation, maneuverability and grasping are evident. These technical difficulties are well demonstrated in the literature for the transvaginal NOTES (Branco et al., 2008b; Branco Filho et al., 2007; Kondo et al., 2009):

- Flexibility of conventional endoscopes: allows limited control of instruments during surgery.
- Lack of triangulation: the instruments are inserted through the two working channels of the flexible endoscopes, arriving in parallel into the peritoneal cavity, which restricts the movements of the surgeon (Figure 15).
- Lack of stability of the endoscope: the endoscope does not remain stationary within the peritoneal cavity during surgery; thus optimal surgical exposure is constantly lost. Moreover, the commensurate movement of the instruments and the endoscope results in loss of the surgical field of view.
- Retroflected view (U-turn): pelvic surgery is performed with retroflected view, which implies an image upside down and reversed, making difficult the notion of movement of the instruments and the endoscope. It is not always possible to obtain a front view with U-turn, and often a lateral view is obtained, which makes the procedure more laborious (Figure 16). This is not a problem for surgeries of upper abdomen.

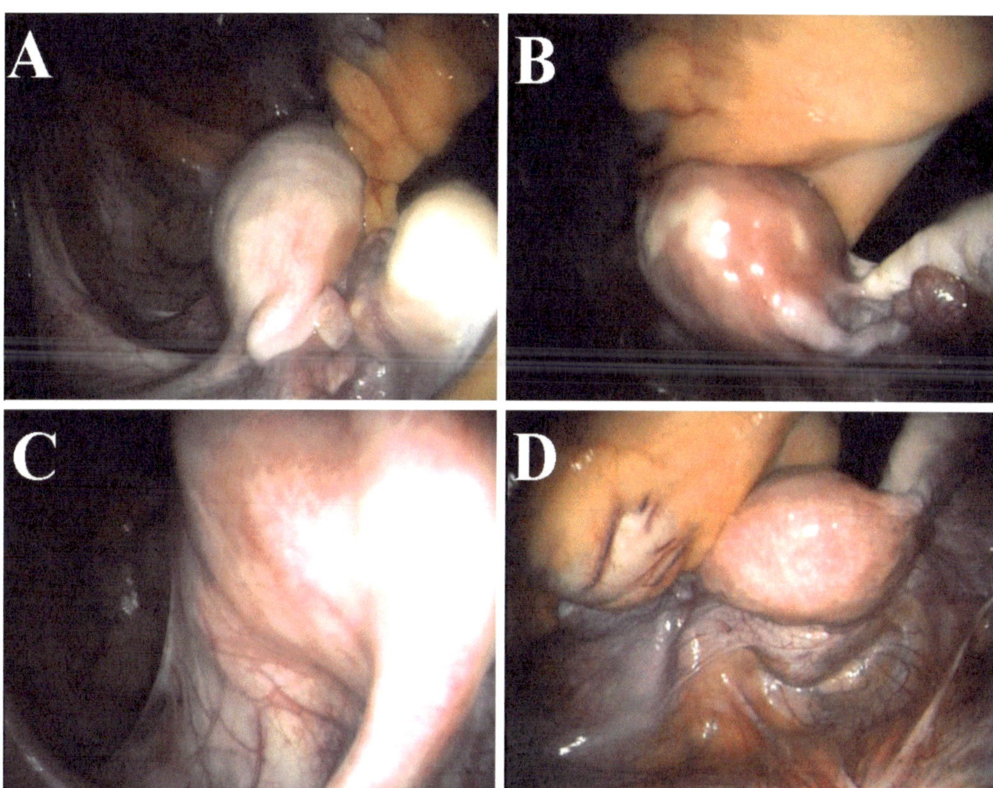

Fig. 16. U-turn to visualize the pelvis. (A to C) The endoscope is turned to inspect the pelvis and the image obtained is lateral. (D) The image is upside down and reversed when the entire pelvis is visualized.

8. Recommendations and conclusions

NOTES using the vagina as an entry point to the peritoneal cavity is very promising and several surgical procedures have been performed using this route. With the development of new instruments and platforms that facilitate handling and stabilization of flexible endoscopes, the surgical approach has the potential to have broad clinical applications in the future.

9. References

Alcaraz, A., Peri, L., Molina, A., Goicoechea, I., García, E., Izquierdo, L. & Ribal, MJ. (2010). Feasibility of transvaginal NOTES-assisted laparoscopic nephrectomy. *Eur Urol*, 57, 2, (Feb 2010), pp. (233-237), ISSN 0302-2838.

Allemann, P., Perretta, S., Asakuma, M., Dallemagne, B., Mutter, D. & Marescaux, J. (2009). NOTES retroperitoneal transvaginal distal pancreatectomy. *Surg Endosc*, 23, 4, (Apr 2009), pp. (882-883), ISSN 1432-2218.

Allemann, P., Perretta, S., Asakuma, M., Dallemagne, B. & Marescaux, J. (2010). NOTES new frontier: Natural orifice approach to retroperitoneal disease. *World J Gastrointest Surg*, 2, 5, (May 2010), pp. (157-164), ISSN 1948-9366.

Aminsharifi, A., Taddayun, A., Shakeri, S., Hashemi, M. & Abdi, M. (2009). Hybrid natural orifice transluminal endoscopic surgery for nephrectomy with standard laparoscopic instruments: experience in a canine model. *J Endourol*, 23, 12, (Dec 2009), pp. (1985-1989), ISSN 0892-7790.

Aron, M., Berger, AK., Stein, RJ., Kamoi, K., Brandina, R., Canes, D., Sotelo, R., Desai, MM. & Gill, IS. (2009). Transvaginal nephrectomy with a multichannel laparoscopic port: a cadaver study. *BJU Int*, 103, 11, (Jun 2009), pp. (1537-1541), ISSN 1464-410X.

Asakuma, M., Perretta, S., Allemann, P., Cahill, R., Con, SA., Solano, C., Pasupathy, S., Mutter, D., Dallemagne, B. & Marescaux, J. (2009). Challenges and lessons learned from NOTES cholecystectomy initial experience: a stepwise approach from the laboratory to clinical application. *J Hepatobiliary Pancreat Surg*, 16, 3, (2009), pp. (249-254), ISSN 1868-6982.

Bessler, M., Stevens, PD., Milone, L., Hogle, NJ., Durak, E. & Fowler, D. (2008). Transvaginal laparoscopic cholecystectomy: laparoscopically assisted. *Surg Endosc*, 22, 7, (Jul 2008), pp. (1715-1716), ISSN 1432-2218.

Bourdel, N., Kondo, W., Botchorishvili, R., Poincloux, L., Niro, J., Rabischong, B., Jardon, K., Pouly, JL., Mage, G. & Canis, M. (2009). Assessment of sentinel nodes for gynecologic malignancies by natural orifices transluminal endoscopic surgery (NOTES): preliminary report. *Gynecol Oncol*, 115, 3, (Dec 2009), pp. (367-370), ISSN 0090-8258.

Box, GN., Bessler, M. & Clayman, RV. (2009). Transvaginal access: current experience and potential implications for urologic applications. *J Endourol*, 23, 5, (May 2009), pp. (753-757), ISSN 0892-7790.

Branco, AW., Branco Filho, AJ., Noda, RW., George, MA., Camargo ,AHLA. & Kondo, W. (2008a). New minimally invasive surgical approaches: transvaginal and transumbilical. *Braz J Video-Sur*, 1, 1, (Jan-Mar 2008), pp. (29-36), ISSN 1983-9901.

Branco, AW., Branco Filho, AJ., Kondo, W., Noda, RW., Kawahara, N., Camargo, AA., Stunitz, LC., Valente, J. & Rangel, M. (2008b). Hybrid transvaginal nephrectomy. *Eur Urol*, 53, 6, (Jun 2008), pp. (1290-1294), ISSN 0302-2838.

Branco Filho, AJ., Noda, RW., Kondo, W., Kawahara, N., Rangel, M. & Branco, AW. (2007). Initial experience with hybrid transvaginal cholecystectomy. *Gastrointest Endosc*, 66, 6, (Dec 2007), pp. (1245-1248), ISSN 0016-5107.

Brosens, I., Campo, R., Puttemans, P. & Gordts, S. (2003). Transvaginal laparoscopy. *Clin Obstet Gynecol*, 46, 1, (Mar 2003), pp. (117-122), ISSN 1532-5520.

Buesing, M., Utech, M., Halter, J., Riege, R., Saada, G. & Knapp, A. (2010). Sleeve gastrectomy in the treatment of morbid obesity : Study results and first experiences with the transvaginal hybrid NOTES technique. *Chirurg*, in press (2010), ISSN 1433-0385.

Castillo, OA., Vidal-Mora, I., Campos, R., Fonerón, A., Feria-Flores, M., Gómez, R. & Sepúlveda, F. (2009). Laparoscopic simple nephrectomy with transvaginal notes assistance and the use of standard laparoscopic instruments. *Actas Urol Esp*, 33, 7, (Jul-Aug 2009), pp. (767-770), ISSN 0210-4806.

Clayman, RV., Box, GN., Abraham, JB., Lee, HJ., Deane, LA., Sargent, ER., Nguyen, NT., Chang, K., Tan, AK., Ponsky, LE. & McDougall, EM. (2007). Rapid communication: transvaginal single-port NOTES nephrectomy: initial laboratory experience. *J Endourol*, 21, 6, (Jun 2007), pp. (640-644), ISSN 0892-7790.

Clyman, MJ. (1963). A new panculdoscope - diagnostic, photographic, and operative aspects. *Obstet Gynecol*, 21, (1963), pp. (343-348), ISSN 0029-7844.

Cuadrado-Garcia, A., Noguera, JF., Olea-Martinez, JM., Morales, R., Dolz, C., Lozano, L., Vicens, JC. & Pujol, JJ. (2011). Hybrid natural orifice transluminal endoscopic cholecystectomy: prospective human series. *Surg Endosc*, 25, 1, (Jan 2011), pp. (19-22), ISSN 1432-2218.

de la Fuente, SG., Demaria, EJ., Reynolds, JD., Portenier, DD. & Pryor, AD. (2007). New developments in surgery: Natural Orifice Transluminal Endoscopic Surgery (NOTES). *Arch Surg*, 142, 3, (Mar 2007), pp. (295-297), ISSN 0004-0010.

de Sousa, LH., de Sousa, JÁ., de Sousa Filho, LH., de Sousa, MM., de Sousa, VM., de Sousa, AP. & Zorron, R. (2009). Totally NOTES (T-NOTES) transvaginal cholecystectomy using two endoscopes: preliminary report. *Surg Endosc*, 23, 11, (Nov 2009), pp. (2550-2555), ISSN 1432-2218.

Decker, A. (1952). Culdoscopy. *Am J Obstet Gynecol*, 63, (1952), pp. (854-859), ISSN 0002-9378.

Dolz, C., Noguera, JF., Martín, A., Vilella, A. & Cuadrado, A. (2007). Transvaginal cholecystectomy (NOTES) combined with minilaparoscopy. *Rev Esp Enferm Dig*. 2007 Dec;99(12):698-702, ISSN 1130-0108.

Dubcenco, E., Assumpcao, L., Dray, X., Gabrielson, KL., Ruben, DS., Pipitone, LJ., Donatelli, G., Krishnamurty, DM., Baker, JP., Marohn, MR. & Kalloo, AN. (2009). Adhesion formation after peritoneoscopy with liver biopsy in a survival porcine model: comparison of laparotomy, laparoscopy, and transgastric natural orifice transluminal endoscopic surgery (NOTES). *Endoscopy*, 41, 11, (Nov 2009), pp. (971-978), ISSN 0013-726X.

Fischer, LJ., Jacobsen, G., Wong, B., Thompson, K., Bosia, J., Talamini, M. & Horgan, S. (2009). NOTES laparoscopic-assisted transvaginal sleeve gastrectomy in humans - description of preliminary experience in the United States. *Surg Obes Relat Dis*, 5, 5, (Sep-Oct 2009), pp. (633-636), ISSN 1550-7289.

Frenkel, DA., Greenem BA. & Siegler, SL. (1952). Technical improvements in culdoscopic examination. *Am J Obstet Gynecol*, 64, (1952), pp. (1303-1309), ISSN 0002-9378.

Gettman, MT., Lotan, Y., Napper, CA. & Cadeddu, JA. (2002). Transvaginal laparoscopic nephrectomy: development and feasibility in the porcine model. *Urology*, 59, 3, (Mar 2002), pp. (446-450), ISSN 0090-4295.

Gordts, S., Campo, R., Puttemans, P., Gordts, SY. & Brosens, I. (2008). Transvaginal access: a safe technique for tubo-ovarian exploration in infertility? Review of the literature. *Gynecol Surg*, 5, 3, (2008), pp. (187-191), ISSN 1613-2076.

Haber, GP., Brethauer, S., Crouzet, S., Berger, A., Gatmaitan, P., Kamoi, K. & Gill, I. (2009). Pure natural orifice transluminal endoscopic surgery for transvaginal nephrectomy in the porcine model. *BJU Int*, 104, 9, (Nov 2009), pp. (1260-1264), ISSN 1464-410X.

Hackethal, A., Sucke, J., Oehmke, F., Münstedt, K., Padberg, W. & Tinneberg, HR. (2010). Establishing transvaginal NOTES for gynecological and surgical indications: benefits, limits, and patient experience. *Endoscopy*, 42, 10, (Oct 2010), pp. (875-878), ISSN 0013-726X.

Hackethal, A., Ionesi-Pasacica, J., Eskef, K., Oehmke, F., Münstedt, K. & Tinneberg, HR. (2011). Transvaginal NOTES with semi-rigid and rigid endoscopes that allow adjustable viewing angles. *Arch Gynecol Obstet*, 283, 1, (Jan 2011), pp. (131-132), ISSN 1432-0711.

Hagen, ME., Wagner, OJ., Swain, P., Pugin, F., Buchs, N., Caddedu, M., Jamidar, P., Fasel, J. & Morel, P. (2008). Hybrid natural orifice transluminal endoscopic surgery (NOTES) for Roux-en-Y gastric bypass: an experimental surgical study in human cadavers. *Endoscopy*, 40, 11, (Nov 2008), pp. (918-924). ISSN 0013-726X.

Hensel, M., Schernikau, U., Schmidt, A. & Arlt, G. (2010). Comparison between Transvaginal and Laparoscopic Cholecystectomy - A Retrospective Case-Control Study. *Zentralbl Chir*, in press, (2010), ISSN 0044- 409X.

Horgan, S., Cullen, JP., Talamini, MA., Mintz, Y., Ferreres, A., Jacobsen, GR., Sandler, B., Bosia, J., Savides, T., Easter, DW., Savu, MK., Ramamoorthy, SL., Whitcomb, E., Agarwal, S., Lukacz, E., Dominguez, G. & Ferraina, P. (2009). Natural orifice surgery: initial clinical experience. *Surg Endosc*, 23, 7, (Jul 2009), pp. (1512-1518), ISSN 1432-2218.

Horváth, S., Gál, I., Rákóczi, I., Jávor, S., Balatonyi, B., Takács, I., Ferencz, A., Ferencz, S. & Wéber, G. (2009). Transvaginal cholecystectomy in animal model: first series in Hungary. *Magy Seb*, 62, 3, (Jun 2009), pp. (120-124), ISSN 0025-0295.

Isariyawongse, JP., McGee, MF., Rosen, MJ., Cherullo, EE. & Ponsky, LE. (2008). Pure natural orifice transluminal endoscopic surgery (NOTES) nephrectomy using standard laparoscopic instruments in the porcine model. *J Endourol*, 22, 5, (May 2008), pp. (1087-1091), ISSN 0892-7790.

Jacobsen, GR., Thompson, K., Spivack, A., Fischer, L., Wong, B., Cullen, J., Bosia, J., Whitcomb, E., Lucas, E., Talamini, M. & Horgan, S. (2010). Initial experience with transvaginal incisional hernia repair. *Hernia*, 14, 1, (Feb 2010), pp. (89-91), ISSN 1265-4906.

Jagannath, SB., Kantsevoy, SV., Vaughn, CA., Chung, SS., Cotton, PB., Gostout, CJ., Hawes, RH., Pasricha, PJ., Scorpio, DG., Magee, CA., Pipitone, LJ. & Kalloo, AN. (2005). Peroral transgastric endoscopic ligation of fallopian tubes with long-term survival in a porcine model. *Gastrointest Endosc*, 61, 3, (Mar 2005), pp. (449-453), ISSN 0016-5107.

Jin, C., Hu, Y., Chen, XC., Zheng, FY., Lin, F., Zhou, K., Chen, FD. & Gu, HZ. (2009). Laparoscopic versus open myomectomy--a meta-analysis of randomized controlled trials. *Eur J Obstet Gynecol Reprod Biol*, 145, 1, (Jul 2009), pp. (14-21), ISSN 0028-2243.

Kalloo, AN., Singh, VK., Jagannath, SB., Niiyama, H., Hill, SL., Vaughn, CA., Magee, CA. & Kantsevoy, SV. (2004). Flexible transgastric peritoneoscopy: a novel approach to diagnostic and therapeutic interventions in the peritoneal cavity. *Gastrointest Endosc*, 60, 1, (Jul 2004), pp. (114-7), ISSN 0016-5107.

Kantsevoy, SV., Jagannath, SB., Niiyama, H., Chung, SS., Cotton, PB., Gostout, CJ., Hawes, RH., Pasricha, PJ., Magee, CA., Vaughn, CA., Barlow, D., Shimonaka, H. & Kalloo, AN. (2005). Endoscopic gastrojejunostomy with survival in a porcine model. *Gastrointest Endosc*, 62, 2, (Aug 2005), pp. (287-292), ISSN 0016-5107.

Kantsevoy, SV., Hu, B., Jagannath, SB., Vaughn, CA., Beitler, DM., Chung, SS., Cotton, PB., Gostout, CJ., Hawes, RH., Pasricha, PJ., Magee, CA., Pipitone, LJ., Talamini, MA. & Kalloo, AN. (2006). Transgastric endoscopic splenectomy: is it possible? *Surg Endosc*, 20, 3, (Mar 2006), pp. (522-525), ISSN 1432-2218.

Kantsevoy, SV., Hu, B., Jagannath, SB., Isakovich, NV., Chung, SS., Cotton, PB., Gostout, CJ., Hawes, RH., Pasricha, PJ., Nakajima, Y., Kawashima, K. & Kalloo, AN. (2007). Technical feasibility of endoscopic gastric reduction: a pilot study in a porcine model. *Gastrointest Endosc*, 65, 3, (Mar 2007), pp. (510-513), ISSN 0016-5107.

Kaouk, JH., Haber, GP., Goel, RK., Crouzet, S., Brethauer, S., Firoozi, F., Goldman, HB. & White, WM. (2010). Pure natural orifice translumenal endoscopic surgery (NOTES) transvaginal nephrectomy. *Eur Urol*, 57, 4, (Apr 2010), pp. (723-726), ISSN 0302-2838.

Keus, F., Gooszen, HG. & van Laarhoven, CJ. (2010). Open, small-incision, or laparoscopic cholecystectomy for patients with symptomatic cholecystolithiasis. An overview of Cochrane Hepato-Biliary Group reviews. *Cochrane Database Syst Rev*, 20, 1, (Jan 2010), p. (CD008318), ISSN 1469-493X.

Kondo, W., Rangel, M., Tirapelle, RA., Garcia, MA., Bahten, LCV., Laux, GL. & Smaniotto, B. (2006). Emprego da laparoscopia em mulheres com dor abdominal aguda. *Rev Bras Videocir*, 4, 1, (2006), pp. (3-8), ISSN 1983-9901.

Kondo, W., Noda, RW., Branco, AW., Rangel, M. & Branco Filho, AJ. (2009). Transvaginal endoscopic tubal sterilization. *J Laparoendosc Adv Surg Tech A*, 19, 1, (Feb 2009), pp. (59-61), ISSN 1092-6429.

Lehmann, KS., Ritz, JP., Wibmer, A., Gellert, K., Zornig, C., Burghardt, J., Büsing, M., Runkel, N., Kohlhaw, K., Albrecht, R., Kirchner, TG., Arlt, G., Mall, JW., Butters, M., Bulian, DR., Bretschneider, J., Holmer, C. & Buhr, HJ. (2010). The German registry for natural orifice translumenal endoscopic surgery: report of the first 551 patients. *Ann Surg*, 252, 2, (Aug 2010), pp. (263-270), ISSN 0003-4932.

Lima, E., Rolanda, C., Pêgo, JM., Henriques-Coelho, T., Silva, D., Osório, L., Moreira, I., Carvalho, JL. & Correia-Pinto, J. (2007). Third-generation nephrectomy by natural orifice transluminal endoscopic surgery. *J Urol*, 178, 6, (Dec 2007), pp. (2648-2654), ISSN 0022-5347.

Linke, GR., Tarantino, I., Hoetzel, R., Warschkow, R., Lange, J., Lachat, R. & Zerz, A. (2010). Transvaginal rigid-hybrid NOTES cholecystectomy: evaluation in routine clinical practice. *Endoscopy*, 42, 7, (Jul 2010), pp. (571-575), ISSN 0013-726X.

Lomanto, D., Chua, HC., Myat, MM., So, J., Shabbir, A. & Ho, L. (2009a). Microbiological contamination during transgastric and transvaginal endoscopic techniques. *J Laparoendosc Adv Surg Tech A*, 19, 4, (Aug 2009), pp. (465-469), ISSN 1092-6429.

Lomanto, D., Dhir, U., So, JB., Cheah, WK., Moe, MA. & Ho, KY. (2009b). Total transvaginal endoscopic abdominal wall hernia repair: a NOTES survival study. *Hernia*, 13, 4, (Aug 2009), pp. (415-419), ISSN 1265-4906.

Madan, AK., Tichansky, DS. & Khan, KA. (2008). Natural orifice transluminal endoscopic gastric bypass performed in a cadaver. *Obes Surg*, 18, 9, (Sep 2008), pp. (1192-1199), ISSN 1708-0428.

Marescaux, J., Dallemagne, B., Perretta, S., Wattiez, A., Mutter, D. & Coumaros, D. (2007). Surgery without scars: report of transluminal cholecystectomy in a human being. *Arch Surg*, 142, 9, (sep 2007), pp. (823-827), ISSN 0004-0010.

Matthes, K., Yusuf, TE., Willingham, FF., Mino-Kenudson, M., Rattner, DW. & Brugge, WR. (2007). Feasibility of endoscopic transgastric distal pancreatectomy in a porcine animal model. *Gastrointest Endosc*, 66, 4, (Oct 2007), pp. (762-766), ISSN 0016-5107.

Michalik, M., Orlowski, M., Bobowicz, M., Frask, A. & Trybull, A. (2010). The First Report on Hybrid NOTES Adjustable Gastric Banding in Human. *Obes Surg*, in press, (2010), ISSN 1708-0428.

Nakajima, K., Takahashi, T., Souma, Y., Shinzaki, S., Yamada, T., Yoshio, T. & Nishida, T. (2008). Transvaginal endoscopic partial gastrectomy in porcine models: the role of an extra endoscope for gastric control. *Surg Endosc*, 22, 12, (Dec 2008), pp. (2733-2736), ISSN 1432-2218.

Nassif, J., Zacharopoulou, C., Marescaux, J. & Wattiez, A. (2009). Transvaginal extraperitoneal lymphadenectomy by Natural Orifices Transluminal Endoscopic Surgery (NOTES) technique in porcine model: feasibility and survival study. *Gynecol Oncol*, 112, 2, (Feb 2009), pp. (405-408), ISSN 0090-8258.

Niu, J., Song, W., Yan, M., Fan, W., Niu, W., Liu, E., Peng, C., Lin, P., Li, P. & Khan, AQ. (2010). Transvaginal laparoscopically assisted endoscopic cholecystectomy: preliminary clinical results for a series of 43 cases in China. *Surg Endosc*, in press, (2010), ISSN 1432-2218.

Noguera, JF., Dolz, C., Cuadrado, A., Olea, JM. & Vilella, A. (2008). Transvaginal liver resection (NOTES) combined with minilaparoscopy. *Rev Esp Enferm Dig*, 100, 7, (Jul 2008), pp. (411-415), ISSN 1130-0108.

Noguera, J., Dolz, C., Cuadrado, A., Olea, J., Vilella, A. & Morales, R. (2009). Hybrid transvaginal cholecystectomy, NOTES, and minilaparoscopy: analysis of a prospective clinical series. *Surg Endosc*, 23, 4, (Apr 2009), pp. (876-881), ISSN 1432-2218.

Noguera, JF., Cuadrado, A., Sánchez-Margallo, FM., Dolz, C., Asencio, JM., Olea, JM., Morales, R., Lozano, L. & Vicens, JC. (2010). Emergency transvaginal hybrid natural orifice transluminal endoscopic surgery. *Endoscopy*, in press, (2010), ISSN 0013-726X.

Nohuz, E., Pouly, JL., Bolandard, F., Rabischong, B., Jardon, K., Cotte, B., Rivoire, C. & Mage, G. (2006). Fertiloscopy: Clermont-Ferrand's experiment. *Gynecol Obstet Fertil*, 34, 10, (Oct 2006), pp. (894-899), ISSN 1297-9589.

Palanivelu, C., Rajan, PS., Rangarajan, M., Parthasarathi, R., Senthilnathan, P. & Prasad, M. (2008). Transvaginal endoscopic appendectomy in humans: a unique approach to NOTES - world's first report. *Surg Endosc*, 22, 5, (May 2008), pp. (1343-1347), ISSN 1432-2218.

Park, PO., Bergström, M., Ikeda, K., Fritscher-Ravens, A. & Swain, P. (2005). Experimental studies of transgastric gallbladder surgery: cholecystectomy and cholecystogastric anastomosis (videos). *Gastrointest Endosc*, 61, 4, (Apr 2005), pp. (601-606), ISSN 0016-5107.

Perretta, S., Allemann, P., Asakuma, M., Dallemagne, B. & Marescaux, J. (2009a). Adrenalectomy using natural orifice translumenal endoscopic surgery (NOTES): a transvaginal retroperitoneal approach. *Surg Endosc*, 23, 6, (Jun 2009), p. (1390), ISSN 1432-2218.

Perretta, S., Allemann, P., Asakuma, M., Cahill, R., Dallemagne, B. & Marescaux, J. (2009b). Feasibility of right and left transvaginal retroperitoneal nephrectomy: from the porcine to the cadaver model. *J Endourol*, 23, 11, (Nov 2009), pp. (1887-1892), ISSN 0892-7790.

Powell, B., Whang, SH., Bachman, SL., Astudillo, JA., Sporn, E., Miedema, BW. & Thaler, K. (2010). Transvaginal repair of a large chronic porcine ventral hernia with synthetic mesh using NOTES. *JSLS*, 14, 2, (Apr-Jun 2010), pp. (234-239), ISSN 1086-8089.

Pugliese, R., Forgione, A., Sansonna, F., Ferrari, GC., Di Lernia, S. & Magistro, C. (2010). Hybrid NOTES transvaginal cholecystectomy: operative and long-term results after 18 cases. *Langenbecks Arch Surg*, 395, 3, (Mar 2010), pp. (241-245), ISSN 1435-2443.

Raman, JD., Bergs, RA., Fernandez, R., Bagrodia, A., Scott, DJ., Tang, SJ., Pearle, MS. & Cadeddu, JA. (2009). Complete transvaginal NOTES nephrectomy using magnetically anchored instrumentation. *J Endourol*, 23, 3, (Mar 2009), pp. (367-371), ISSN 0892-7790.

Ramos, AC., Murakami, A., Galvão Neto, M., Galvão, MS., Silva, AC., Canseco, EG. & Moyses, Y. (2008a). NOTES transvaginal video-assisted cholecystectomy: first series. *Endoscopy*, 40, 7, (Jul 2008), pp. (572-575), ISSN 0013-726X.

Ramos, AC., Zundel, N., Neto, MG. & Maalouf, M. (2008b). Human hybrid NOTES transvaginal sleeve gastrectomy: initial experience. *Surg Obes Relat Dis*, 4, 5, (Sep-Oct 2008), pp. (660-663), ISSN 1550-7289.

Ribal Caparrós, MJ., Peri Cusí, L., Molina Cabeza, A., García Larrosa, A., Carmona, F. & Alcaraz Asensio, A. (2009). First report on hybrid transvaginal nephrectomy for renal cancer. *Actas Urol Esp*, 33, 3, (Mar 2009), pp. (280-283), ISSN 0210-4806.

Sánchez-Margallo, FM., Asencio Pascual, JM., Del Carmen Tejonero Alvarez, M., Sánchez Hurtado, MA., Pérez Duarte, FJ., Usón Gargallo, J. & Sánchez-Gijón, SP. (2009). Training design and improvement of technical skills in the transvaginal cholecystectomy (NOTES). *Cir Esp*, 85, 5, (May 2009), pp. (307-313), ISSN 0009-739X.

Sotelo, R., de Andrade, R., Fernández, G., Ramirez, D., Di Grazia, E., Carmona, O., Moreira, O., Berger, A., Aron, M., Desai, MM. & Gill, IS. (2010). NOTES hybrid transvaginal radical nephrectomy for tumor: stepwise progression toward a first successful clinical case. *Eur Urol*, 57, 1, (Jan 2010), pp. (138-144), ISSN 0302-2838.

Targarona, EM., Gomez, C., Rovira, R., Pernas, JC., Balague, C., Guarner-Argente, C., Sainz, S. & Trias, M. (2009). NOTES-assisted transvaginal splenectomy: the next step in the minimally invasive approach to the spleen. *Surg Innov*, 16, 3, (Sep 2009), pp. (218-222), ISSN 1553-3506.

Tonouchi, H., Ohmori, Y., Kobayashi, M., Kusunoki, M. (2004). Trocar site hernia. *Arch Surg*, 139, 11, (Nov 2004), pp. (1248-1256), ISSN 0004-0010.

Sugimoto, M., Yasuda, H., Koda, K., Suzuki, M., Yamazaki, M., Tezuka, T., Kosugi, C., Higuchi, R., Watayo, Y., Yagawa, Y., Uemura, S., Tsuchiya, H., Hirano, A. & Ro, S. (2009). Evaluation for transvaginal and transgastric NOTES cholecystectomy in human and animal natural orifice translumenal endoscopic surgery. *J Hepatobiliary Pancreat Surg*, 16, 3, (2009), pp. (255-260), ISSN 1868-6982.

Von Ott, D. (1902). Die Beleuchtung der Bauchhohle (Ventroskopie) als Methode bei Vaginaler Coeliotomie. *Abl Gynakol*, 231, (1902), pp. (817-823).

Wagh, MS., Merrifield, BF. & Thompson, CC. (2005). Endoscopic transgastric abdominal exploration and organ resection: initial experience in a porcine model. *Clin Gastroenterol Hepatol*, 3, 9, (Sep 2005), pp. (892-896), ISSN 1542-3565.

Wagh, MS., Merrifield, BF. & Thompson, CC. (2006). Survival studies after endoscopic transgastric oophorectomy and tubectomy in a porcine model. *Gastrointest Endosc*, 63, 3, (Mar 2006), pp. (473-478), ISSN 0016-5107.

Watrelot, A., Dreyfus, JM. & Andine, JP. (1999). Evaluation of the performance of fertiloscopy in 160 consecutive infertile patients with no obvious pathology. *Hum Reprod*, 14, 3, (Mar 1999), pp. (707-711), ISSN 1460-2350.

Zacharopoulou, C., Nassif, J., Allemann, P., Dallemagne, B., Perretta, S., Marescaux, J. & Wattiez, A. (2009). Exploration of the retroperitoneum using the transvaginal natural orifice transluminal endoscopic surgery technique. *J Minim Invasive Gynecol*, 16, 2, (Mar-Apr 2009), pp. (198-203), ISSN 1553-4650.

Zornig, C., Mofid, H., Siemssen, L. & Wenck, CH. (2010a). Transvaginal access for NOTES. *Chirurg;* 81, 5, (May 2010), pp. (426-430), ISSN 1433-0385.

Zornig, C., Siemssen, L., Emmermann, A., Alm, M., von Waldenfels, HA., Felixmüller, C. & Mofid, H. (2010b). NOTES cholecystectomy: matched-pair analysis comparing the transvaginal hybrid and conventional laparoscopic techniques in a series of 216 patients. *Surg Endosc*, in press, (2010), ISSN 1432-2218.

Zorrón, R., Filgueiras, M., Maggioni, LC., Pombo, L., Lopes Carvalho, G. & Lacerda Oliveira, A. (2007). NOTES. Transvaginal cholecystectomy: report of the first case. *Surg Innov*, 14, 4, (Dec 2007), pp. (279-283), ISSN 1553-3506.

Zorrón, R., Soldan, M., Filgueiras, M., Maggioni, LC., Pombo, L. & Oliveira, AL. (2008). NOTES: transvaginal for cancer diagnostic staging: preliminary clinical application. *Surg Innov*, 15, 3, (Sep 2008), pp. (161-165), ISSN 1553-3506.

Zorron, R., Goncalves, L., Leal, D., Kanaan, E., Cabral, I. & Saraiva, P. (2010a). Transvaginal hybrid natural orifice transluminal endoscopic surgery retroperitoneoscopy--the first human case report. *J Endourol*, 24, 2, (Feb 2010), pp. (233-237), ISSN 0892-7790.

Zorron, R., Palanivelu, C., Galvão Neto, MP., Ramos, A., Salinas, G., Burghardt, J., DeCarli, L., Henrique Sousa, L., Forgione, A., Pugliese, R., Branco, AJ., Balashanmugan, TS., Boza, C., Corcione, F., D'Avila Avila, F., Arturo Gómez, N., Galvão Ribeiro, PA., Martins, S., Filgueiras, M., Gellert, K., Wood Branco, A., Kondo, W., Inacio Sanseverino, J., de Sousa, JA., Saavedra, L., Ramírez, E., Campos, J., Sivakumar, K., Rajan, PS., Jategaonkar, PA., Ranagrajan, M., Parthasarathi, R., Senthilnathan, P., Prasad, M., Cuccurullo, D. & Müller, V. (2010b) International multicenter trial on clinical natural orifice surgery - NOTES IMTN study: preliminary results of 362 patients. *Surg Innov*, 17, 2, (Jun 2010), pp. (142-158), ISSN 1553-3506.

9

Diagnostic and Therapeutic Transvaginal Hydrolaparoscopy

Hiroaki Shibahara, Tatsuya Suzuki and Mitsuaki Suzuki
Department of Obstetrics and Gynecology, School of Medicine Jichi Medical University, Tochigi, Japan

1. Introduction

Laparoscopy is the gold-standard procedure for the diagnosis of tubo-peritoneal infertility. However, transabdominal access in laparoscopy is not without major risks, including gastrointestinal injuries [1] and major vascular injuries. [2] In 1998, to minimize the invasiveness of laparoscopy for diagnostic purposes, transvaginal hydrolaparoscopy (THL) was introduced as the first line procedure in the exploration of the adnexal structures in infertile women. [3,4] Demonstration of the advantages of THL, such as the ability to accurately inspect adnexal structures without manipulation, has made it clear that THL is a less traumatic and more suitable outpatient procedure than transabdominal laparoscopy. THL can be performed under local anesthesia of the posterior vaginal fornix. A rigid scope is inserted transavginally through the pouch of Douglas, saline is injected for distension, and a field of vision thereby becomes available. Unlike minimally invasive endoscopic procedures, the natural office surgery is recently called natural office transluminal endoscopic surgery (NOTES). [5]

There are some reports that described the usefulness and prognostic value of diagnostic THL in infertile women. [6-8] Moreover, operative THL such as ovarian drilling for unovulatory women with polycystic ovarian syndrome (PCOS) to induce ovulation has also appeared to be as effective as that by the conventional laparoscopy. [5, 9-13] This procedure is named transvaginal hydrolaparoscopic ovarian drilling (THLOD). THL has also been expected to be useful for adhesiolysis in some limited lesions.

The risk of bowel injury and sepsis by transvaginal access with culdoscopy was higher than that with laparoscopy in old reports. [14] However, the value of direct access to the posterior pelvis at culdoscopy for infertility investigation is well recognized. Although the new technique of THL differs in the use of the dorsal decubitus position for the patient, a small diameter endoscope, and saline solution for peritoneal distension, the principle of THL is similar to that of culdoscopy in that its access is through the posterior fornix.

2. Indication and surgical procedure of THL and THLOD

We have been performing THL for the following five indications: diagnostic THL[7,8] for (i) tubal obstruction and/or peritubal adhesion are suggested by hysterosalpingography (HSG), (ii) serum antibody against *C. trachomatis* is positive, (iii) diagnosis of early-stage endometriosis, (iv) unexplained infertility, and operative THL [10,12-13] for (v) ovarian drilling using Nd:YAG or Holmium laser in infertile women with polycystic ovary syndrome (PCOS).

However, to avoid the major risks of THL, any of the followings are contraindications: i) retroflexed uterus, ii) the past history of pelvic surgery, iii) obstruction of the pouch of Douglas by the rectum or a prolapsed tumor, and iv) acute pelvic inflammatory disease.

THL and THLOD were performed in the lithotomy position as we described previously.[7-8, 10, 12-13, 15-18] Briefly, after premedication, a Hys-cath (Sumitomo Bakelite Co. Ltd., Tokyo, Japan) was inserted into the uterine cavity for use in chromotubation. The uterine cervix was lifted with a tenaculum placed on the posterior lip. Under local anesthesia or general anesthesia, a Veress needle was introduced 1.5 cm below the cervix and inserted into the pelvic cavity (Figure 1a). Approximately 100 ml of normal saline solution is instilled through the cannula in the pouch of Douglas (Figure 1b, 1c). For THL, a 3-mm blunt trocar was inserted by a stab incision in the posterior fornix and a 2.7-mm diameter semirigid endoscope was used at an optical angle of 30° with a flow channel attached to a 3-CCD digital videocamera (Figure 1d). For THLOD, a 5.5-mm blunt trocar is inserted by a stab incision in the posterior fornix. Then a 5.0-mm diameter semirigid endoscope was used with the same technique. The saline irrigation was continued throughout the procedure to keep the bowel and tubo-ovarian structures afloat. The posterior region of the uterus and the bilateral tubo-ovarian structures were carefully observed, and tubal passage was confirmed using indigocarmine. In a few cases, the structure could not be observed due to severe adhesion.[7]

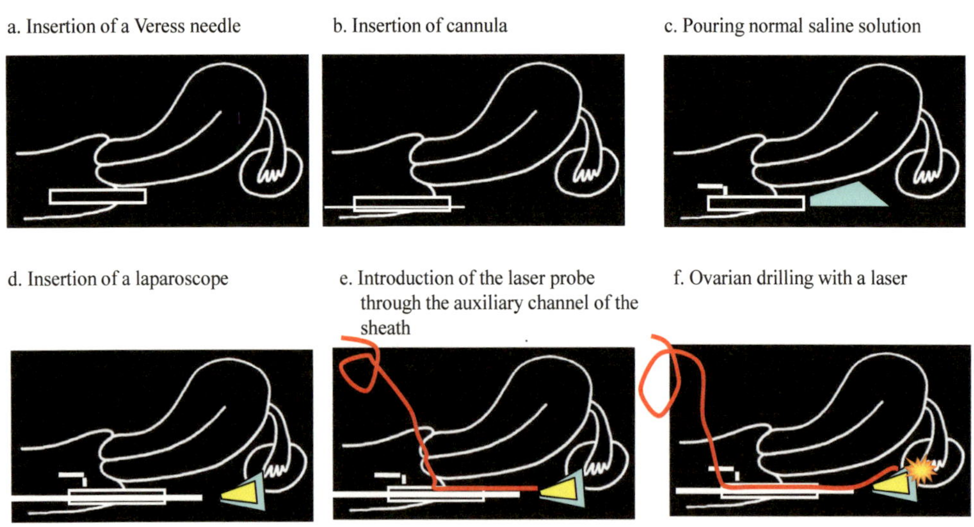

Fig. 1. Procedure for THL and THLOD
The procedure for THL and THLOD are described. a) A Veress needle is inserted into the pelvic cavity. b, c) Normal saline solution is instilled through the cannula in the pouch of Douglas. d) A blunt trocar is inserted by a stab incision in the posterior fornix. Then a semirigid endoscope is used with an optical angle of 30° and a flow channel attached to a 3-CCD digital videocatmera. Tubal passage is confirmed using indigo carmine. e, f) THLOD is performed using a laser to ablate portions of the ovarian cortex.

For THLOD, after careful observation as for diagnostic THL (Figure 2a), ovarian drilling was performed using an Nd:YAG laser (STAGE MY-100, LASER PERIPHERALS LLC, MN, USA) or Holmium laser (VersaPulse, Boston Scientific, MA, USA) to ablate portions of the ovarian cortex (Figure 1e, 1f). A sterile quartz glass fiber measuring 1 mm in core diameter was passed through the operating channel of the laparoscope using a special laser fiber steering device with a deflectable tip (Figure 2b, 2c). The power used ranges up to 10 W. The focused laser beam is used at a distance of 1.5 mm to 3.0 mm to create approximately 40 holes on the surface of each ovary (Figure 2d, 2e, 2f).

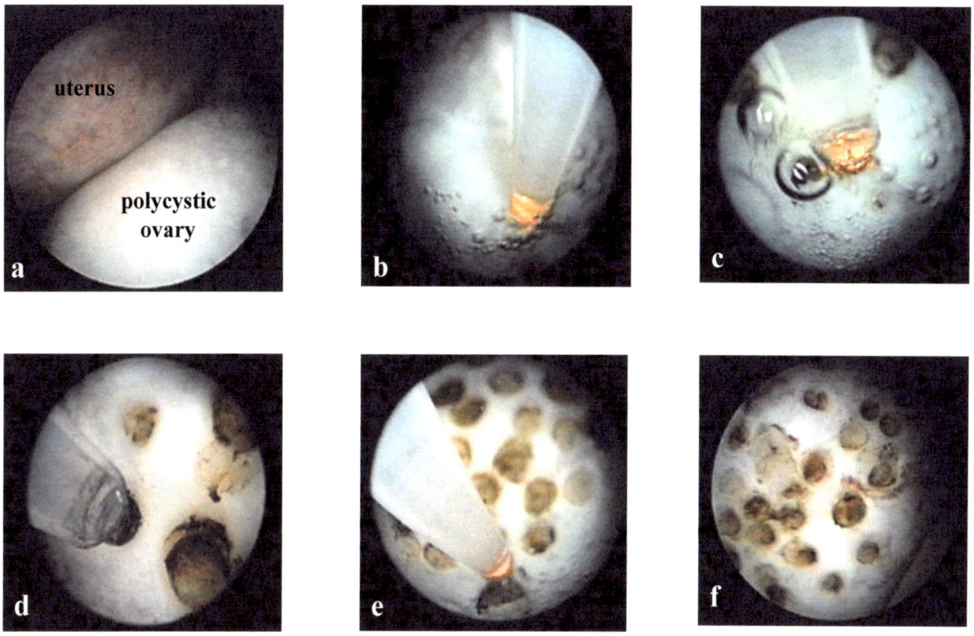

Fig. 2. Performance of THLOD using a laser a)A polycystic ovary behind the uterus is visible through THL. b) Introduction of the laser probe through the auxiliary channel of the sheath. The focused laser beam was used from a distance of 1.5 mm to 3.0 mm. c-e) Approximately 40 holes were made on the ovarian cortex. f) Final phase of ovarian drilling.

3. Visualization of tubo-ovarian structures and salpingoscopy

Assessment of the Fallopian tube represents an integral part for the evaluation of the infertile couple. Because the findings obtained at hysterosalpingography, laparoscopy, or laparotomy are indirect, salpingoscopy has been introduced as an endoscopic examination that can directly evaluate the ampullary tubal mucosa. The standard procedure is transfimbrial salpingoscopy performed at the time of laparoscopy.[19] It is a microendoscopic approach for directly visualizing the tubal mucosa from the ampullary-isthmic junction to the fimbria. Clinical and morphological studies have shown a high correlation between the appearance of the tubal mucosa and the ultimate outcome in terms of pregnancies.[19] Recently, it was suggested that performing salpingoscopy with laparoscopy could significantly increase accuracy in predicting short-term fertility outcome. [20] However, such salpingoscopy under trans-abdominal laparoscopy requires hospitalization and general anesthesia.

In some women, endoluminal examination by salpingoscopy can be simultaneously performed under THL. The transvaginal salpingoscopy under THL is less invasive to infertile women because it does not require hospitalization or general anesthesia. The procedure was first described by Gordts et al.[21] They reported that the fimbriae were visualized in all patients with no obvious pelvic pathology, and cannulation of the distal tubal segment was achieved without manipulation of the tube in 20% before ovulation and 55% in the early luteal phase. Afterward Watrelot et al. [22] reported that salpingoscopies were possible in 19% of women with post-PID lesions without the need to stabilize the tubes. However, salpingoscopies were possible in 41% of those women using a grasp forceps introduced in the operative channel.

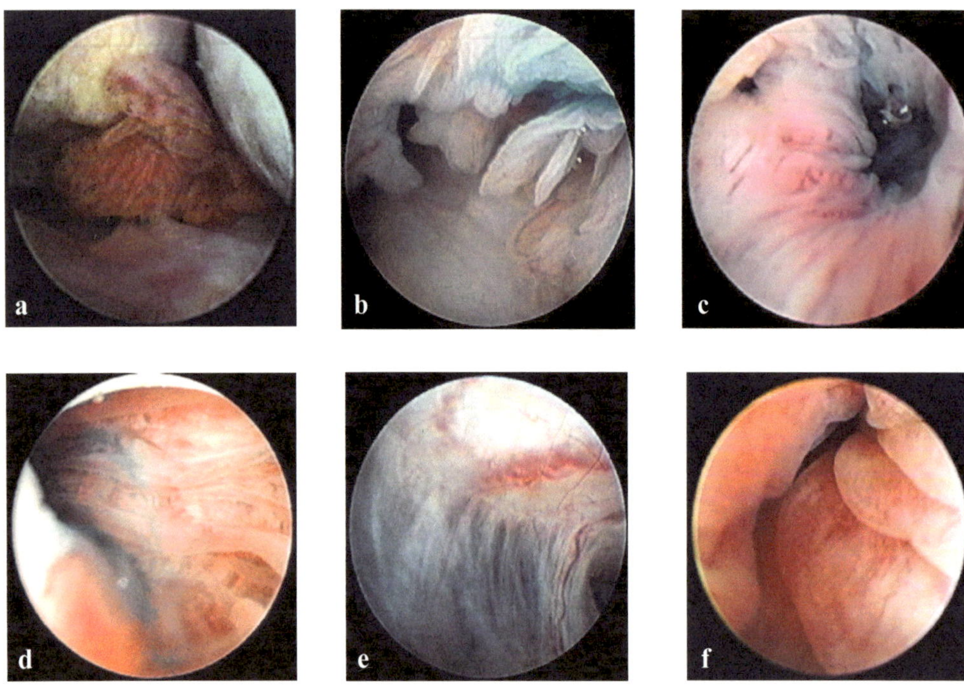

Fig. 3. Visualization of tubo-ovarian structures and salpingoscopy
a)The posterior of the uterus and the bilateral tubo-ovarian structures were carefully observed by THL. The ovary and fimbria are clearly visible. b) Tubal passage was confirmed using indigocarmine. A Hys-cath was inserted into the uterine cavity for the use of chromotubation. c) The endoscope was inserted into the ampulla by the guidance of chromotubation. d) The normal looking tubal mucosa under transvaginal salpingoscopy. e) Unsuccessful salpingoscopy in a case of extensive peritubal adhesion by past *C. trachomatis* infection. f) Endosalpingial edema caused by *C. trachomatis* infection.

We have also been performing salpingoscopy under THL. Consecutive series of 130 infertile women diagnosed tubo-ovarian structures and tubal passage using THL were retrospectively analyzed between May 1999 and November 2003. [17] Access to the pouch of Douglas was achieved in 123 (94.6%) of 130 patients. Twenty-six tubes could not be visualized because of extensive adhesion. Two patients with a history of unilateral salpingectomy and a patient with unicorn uterus were excluded. Therefore, 217 adnexa were clinically evaluated. The posterior of the uterus and the bilateral tubo-ovarian structures were carefully observed (Figure 3a), and tubal passage was confirmed using indigocarmine (Figure 3b).

In 89 (41.0%) of 217 tubes, a salpingoscopy could be performed. The endoscope was inserted from the fimbria by the guidance of chromotubation (Figure 3c) and the distal part of the tubal mucosa could be observed (Figure 3d). To increase the success of salpingoscopy rates, it may be necessary to stabilize the tubes using grasp forceps to introduce an operative channel demonstrated by Watrelot et al.[22]

However, a past history of *C. trachomatis* infection did not seem to influence the success of a salpingoscopy because extensive peritubal adhesion by past *C. trachomatis* infection may disturb visualizing the tubes themselves (Figure 3e). Therefore, we speculate that the successful salpingoscopy rate was similar between women with and without past *C. trachomatis* infection. Typical tubal damages by C. trachomatis infection include verruca and atypical vessel formation, peritubal adhesion, and endosalpingial edema (Figure 3f).

4. Transvaginal Hydrolaparoscopic Ovarian Drilling (THLOD)

Polycystic ovary syndrome (PCOS) is a syndrome of ovarian dysfunction showing cardinal features of hyperandrogenism and polycystic ovarian morphology.[23] It is one of the most common reproductive endocrine disorders in young adult women, showing clinical signs of menstrual disorder, anovulation, hirsutism, acne, and obesity. Frequently, this group of patients present with infertility due to chronic oligoovulation or anovulation. Approximately 15 % of patients with PCOS remain anovulatory despite treatment with clomiphene citrate, and half of patients with PCOS who become ovulatory on this treatment fail to conceive.[24] The alternative of gonadotropin stimulation or surgical treatment is often the next step for the treatment of clomiphene citrate-resistant infertile women with PCOS.

Since Stein and Leventhal reported that all women menstruated regularly post ovarian wedge resection and some of them conceived, [25] ovarian surgery has been used to induce ovulation following unsuccessful medical induction of ovulation. Ovarian surgery has also been indicated in women who hyper-respond to gonadotropin therapy in order to avoid such complications as ovarian hyperstimulation syndrome (OHSS) or multiple gestations.

In recent years, however, because of the rapidly expanding use of techniques involving laparoscopy, surgical treatment has received renewed interest. Laparoscopic ovarian drilling (LOD) by the trans-abdominal approach has been widely used to induce ovulation in women with PCOS after failure of treatment with clomiphene citrate. [26] So far, it has been shown that LOD is effective for inducing ovulation, and the pregnancy rate following LOD seems to be acceptable.

Near the end of the 20th century, THL was developed and it was offered for the operative laparoscopy, especially in women with PCOS for ovarian drilling. This novel technique, THLOD using a laser or bipolar electrosurgery, appears to be an effective minimally invasive procedure to induce ovulation in women with PCOS.[5, 9-13] Fernandez et al.[9,11] have recently reported the feasibility of ovarian drilling by THL for PCOS. They reported the usefulness of THL for the treatment of PCOS by ovarian drilling. They performed ovarian drilling using bipolar electrosurgery by THL in 80 clomiphene citrate-resistant anovulatory women with PCOS. During a mean follow-up of 18.1 months, 73 (91 %) patients recovered regular ovulatory cycles. The cumulative pregnancy rate was 60 % for spontaneous and stimulated cycles, with 40% imputed to drilling alone. [11] It was suggested that THLOD has the same effectiveness as trans-abdominal LOD. It was also reported that there were no complications.

Our group has also been performing THLOD using a laser.[10, 12-13] THLOD has 3 advantages when it was compared with gonadotropin treatments for ovulation induction. Ovulation and pregnancy rates are the same as those for gonadotropin treatments. OHSS and multiple pregnancies are reduced. Furthermore, if ovulation is achieved, the frequency of visiting the outpatient clinic for monitoring the follicular status can be reduced. However, THLOD might have some disadvantages, including the risks of anesthetic and operative complications or possible recurrence of oligoovulatory cycles.

So far, 7 infertile women with PCOS, including 5 women with clomiphene citrate-resistant PCOS and 2 women with the risk of developing OHSS, have undergone THLOD. Except for one patient who dropped out of the study, 6 patients resumed having regular ovulatory cycles without developing OHSS. In 4 (67%) of 6 patients, pregnancies were established; one by timed intercourse during the spontaneous cycle, two by intra-uterine insemination following clomiphene-FSH-HCG treatment, and one by IVF-ET. The pregnancy courses in these patients have been uneventful to this point. There were no intra- or postoperative complications of THLOD.[12]

5. Complications

The risk and outcome of bowel injury during THL were previously reported by Gordts et al.[27] They carried out a multinational retrospective survey based on confidential, self-reported cases from 39 gynecologists in 18 different countries. In their 3667 procedures, a total of 24 bowel injuries were experienced, giving an incidence of 0.65 %.

In our experience, two cases of bowel injury were diagnosed during 168 diagnostic THL procedures. In both cases, the injuries were extraperitoneal and were treated conservatively with antibiotics without major consequences. No complication occurred during THLOD in 9 patients with PCOS. In total, 2 (1.1 %) of 177 cases were diagnosed with bowel injury. [28] In addition to the report by Gordts et al.,[14] we reported our experiences with a review of another series of 549 patients from 9 reported studies published after the year of 2000. [28] Only our study reported bowel injury associated with diagnostic THL. Two (0.35 %) of 565 patients from the 9 studies published after the report of Gordts et al. [27] suffered bowel injury. There is no significant difference of the incidence (0.65 %) of bowel injuries reported by Gordts et al. [27] and that (0.35 %) in the other 9 reports ($P = 0.39$). They also reported that the site of injury involved the extraperitoneal rectum in 21 patients and the rectosigmoid in 3 cases. No leakage of bowel content was reported in their report. Twenty-two (92 %) of the cases were managed expectantly without consequences. These low incidences of major complications should be encouraging for clinicians who have already performed THL as well as those who are now considering introducing THL in their clinics.

As for perforation of the retroflexed uterus, only one case report was obtained.[29] The incidence of perforation of the retroflexed uterus was 0.02 %. In this era of wide use of transvaginal ultrasonography, it is likely that such a complication will seldom occur if clinicians carefully perform transvaginal ultrasonography before judging whether THL is indicated.

To avoid possible bowel injury during THL in patients with appropriate indication and without contraindication, prophylactic use of a laxative and/or enema before the procedure should be considered. Theoretically, it seems that it would be easier to access the pouch of Douglas with less risk if the rectum were not full of stools. Moreover, clinicians should take care when they introduce or re-introduce the Veress needle toward the left pelvic cavity for the anatomical reasons.

6. Conclusion

The usefulness of THL for diagnostic and operative purposes is in no doubt. Moreover, endoluminal assessment by transvaginal salpingoscopy can be simultaneously performed in some infertile women, especially with patent tubes or with regular tubes undergoing THL.
Ovarian surgery for the treatment of PCOS has been shown to be useful in anovulatory infertile women who do not respond to medical induction of ovulation. LOD by the trans-abdominal approach has been used to induce ovulation in women with PCOS after failure of treatment with clomiphene citrate. Following the introduction of THL as the first line procedure for the diagnostic laparoscopy, THLOD was developed as an alternative minimally invasive surgery for PCOS patients.
However, informed consent and careful procedure before and during THL/THLOD should be carried out although they can be done on an outpatient clinic basis.

7. References

[1] Chapron C, Pieere F, Harchaoui Y, et al. Gastrointestinal injuries during gynaecological laparoscopy. Hum Reprod. 1999; 14: 333-337.

[2] Chapron C, Pierre F, Lacroix S, et al. Major vascular injuries during gynecologic laparoscopy. J Am Coll Surg. 1997; 185: 461-465.

[3] Gordts S, Campo R, Rombauts L, et al. Transvaginal hydrolaparoscopy as an outpatient procedure for infertility investigation. Hum Reprod. 1998; 13: 99-103.

[4] Campo R, Gordts S, Rombauts L, et al. Diagnosis accuracy of transvaginal hydrolaparoscopy in infertility. Fertil Steril. 1999; 71: 1157-1160.

[5] Gordts S, Gordts S, Puttemans P, et al. Transvaginal hydrolaparoscopy in the treatment of polycystic ovary syndrome. Fertil Steril 2009; 91: 2520-2526

[6] Darai E, Dessolle L, Lecuru F, et al. Transvaginal hydrolaparoscopy compared with laparoscopy for evaluation of infertile women: a prospective comparative blind study. Hum Reprod. 2000; 15: 2379-2382.

[7] Shibahara H, Fujiwara H, Hirano Y, et al. Usefulness of transvaginal hydrolaparoscopy in investigating infertile women with Chlamydia trachomatis infection. Hum Reprod. 2001; 16: 1690-1693.

[8] Fujiwara H, Shibahara H, Hirano Y, et al. Usefulness and prognostic value of transvaginal hydrolaparoscopy in infertile women. Fertil Steril. 2003; 79: 186-189.

[9] Fernandez H, Alby J-D, Gervaise A, et al. Operative transvaginal hydrolaparoscopy for treatment of polycystic ovary syndrome: a new minimally invasive surgery. Fertil Steril. 2001; 75: 607-611.

[10] Hirano Y, Shibahara H, Takamizawa S, et al. Application of transvaginal hydrolaparoscopy for ovarian drilling using Nd:YAG laser in infertile women with polycystic ovary syndrome. Reprod Med Biol. 2003; 2: 37-40.

[11] Fernandez H, Watrelot A, Alby JD, et al. Fertility after ovarian drilling by transvaginal fertiloscopy for treatment of polycystic ovary syndrome. J Am Assoc Gynecol Laparosc. 2004; 11: 374-378.

[12] Shibahara H, Hirano Y, Kikuchi K, et al. Postoperative endocrine alterations and clinical outcome of infertile women with polycystic ovary syndrome after transvaginal hydrolaparoscopic ovarian drilling. Fertil Steril. 2005; 85: 244-246.
[13] Shibahara H, Hirano Y, Suzuki M. Transvaginal hydrolaparoscopic ovarian drilling for infertile women with polycystic ovary syndrome. Cur Wom Health Rev. 2006; 2: 91-95.
[14] Diamond E. Diagnostic culdoscopy in infertility: a study of 4000 outpatient procedures. J Reprod Med. 1978; 21: 23-28.
[15] Shibahara H, Hirano Y, Ayustawati, et al. Chemokine bioactivity of RANTES is elevated in the sera of infertile women with past Chlamydia trachomatis infection. Am J Reprod Immunol. 2003; 49: 169-173.
[16] Shibahara H, Takamizawa S, Hirano Y, et al. Relationships between Chlamydia trachomatis antibody titers and tubal pathology assessed using transvaginal hydrolaparoscopy in infertile women. Am J Reprod Immunol. 2003; 50: 7-12.
[17] Suzuki T, Shibahara H, Hirano Y, et al. Feasibility and clinical significance of endoluminal assessment by transvaginal hydrolaparoscopy in infertile women. J Minim Invasive Gynecol. 2005; 12: 420-425.
[18] Shibahara H, Suzuki T, Takamizawa S, et al. Role of transvaginal salpingoscopy. (in) Atlas of transvaginal endoscopy. (Ed) Gordts S. Informa Healthcare,. London, UK. 2007, pp 77-84.
[19] Brosens I, Boeckx W, Delattin P, et al. Salpingoscopy: a new pre-operative diagnostic tool in tubal infertility. Br J Obstet Gynaecol 1987; 94: 768-773
[20] Marchino GL, Gigante V, Gennarelli G, et al. Salpingoscopic and laparoscopic investigations in relation to fertility outcome. J Am Assoc Gynecol Laparosc 2001 ; 8; 218-221
[21] Gordts S, Campo R, Rombauts L, Brosens I. Transvaginal salpingoscopy: an office procedure for infertility investigation. Fertil Steril 1998; 70: 523-526
[22] Watrelot A, Dreyfus JM, Andine JP. Evaluation of the performance of fertiloscopy in 160 consecutive infertile patients with no obvious pathology. *Hum Reprod* 1999; 14: 707-711
[23] The Rotterdam ESHRE/ASRM-sponsored PCOS consensus workshop group: Revised 2003 consensus on diagnostic criteria and long-term health risks related to polycystic ovary syndrome (PCOS). Hum Reprod 2004, 19: 41-47.
[24] Nugent D, Vandekerckhove P, Hughes E, Arnot M, Lilford R: Gonadotrophin therapy for ovulation induction in subfertility associated with polycystic ovary syndrome. Cochrane Database Syst Rev 2000; (4): CD000410.
[25] Stein IF, Leventhal ML: Amenorrhea associated with bilateral polycystic ovaries. Am J Obstet Gynecol 1935; 29: 181-191.
[26] Neuwirth RS: A method of bilateral ovarian biopsy at laparoscopy in infertility and chronic anovulation. Fertil Steril 1972; 23: 361-366.
[27] Gordts S, Watrelot A, Campo R, et al. Risk and outcome of bowel injury during transvaginal pelvic endoscopy. Fertil Steril. 2001; 76: 1238-1241.
[28] Shibahara H, Shimada K, Kikuchi K, et al. Major complications and outcome of diagnostic and operative transvaginal hydrolaparoscopy. J Obstet Gynaecol Res 2007; 33: 705-709.
[29] Moore ML, Cohen M, Liu GY. Experience with 109 cases of transvaginal hydrolaparoscopy. J Am Assoc Gynecol Laparosc. 2003; 10: 282-285.

Part 6

Laparoscopic Adnexal Surgery

10

The Role of Laparoscopy and Salpingoscopy in the Assessment of the Fallopian Tube

Koji Nakagawa, Masato Inoue and Rikikazu Sugiyama
Division of Reproductive Medicine, Sugiyama Clinic, Ohara, Setagaya, Tokyo, Japan

1. Introduction

In the field of gynecology, infertility treatment in particular, laparoscopy continues to be the gold standard for the evaluation of mechanical factors affecting the fallopian tubes. However, it cannot be used to directly observe the inner cavity of the fallopian tube. The fallopian tube is more than a passive conduit for gametes and early embryos; it also plays an important role in many reproductive functions such as sperm transport and capacitation, oocyte retrieval and transport, fertilization, and embryo storage. However, there are no reports that relate pregnancy outcomes to conditions inside the fallopian tube. It is, therefore, very important to evaluate the conditions both inside and outside of the fallopian tube.

The fallopian tube is easily damaged by an ascending vaginal infection, or by a uterine infection such as Chlamydia. These types of damage result in impaired fallopian tube function, and subsequently cause mechanical factors that contribute to female subfertility (Mol et al., 1997). Hysterosalpingography (HSG) is the most common test used to evaluate the fallopian tube, due to its safety and low cost. Papaioannou et al. stated that HSG is a reliable test for the diagnosis of proximal and distal obstruction, hydrosalpix and peritubal adhesions (Papaioannou et al., 2007). A recent report indicated that laparoscopy was mandatory after abnormal HSG results in the work-up prior to the start of the infertility treatment (Tanahatoe, 2008), but it cannot be used to directly observe the inner cavity of the fallopian tube.

Salpingoscopy was originally performed during laparotomy for reconstructive tubal surgery to assess the mucosa of the infundibulium and ampulla. A flexible bronchoscope was initially used to improve the images obtained before the introduction of a dedicated, rigid salpingoscope (Papaioannou et al., 2007). Indeed, many clinicians performed salpingoscopy more than a decade ago, and reported abnormal results inside the fallopian tubes (Puttemans et al., 1987; Heylen et al., 1995; Surry & Surry, 1996; Marana et al., 1999; 2003; Marchino et al., 2001). They mainly focused on infertile patients with hydrosalpinges. They performed salpingoscopy during a laparoscopic procedure to repair hydrosalpinges and release patients' tubes from them. One report described normal and abnormal mucosal folds inside fallopian tubes that were damaged by hydrosalpinges (Puttemans et al., 1987). Several reports mentioned results from inside fallopian tubes, but they only described the conditions inside of the fallopian tubes. Salpingoscopy requires special equipment and expertise, making it an expensive proposition. Its risk profile is comparable to laparoscopy, since it is performed simultaneously.

Marhino et al. reported that the prediction of infertility outcomes by laparoscopy could be improved by the concomitant performance of salpingoscopy (Marhino et al., 2001). However, there is no information concerning the accuracy, reliability, prognosis or effectiveness of the procedure. Several studies have reported pregnancy rates after laparoscopy for patients with infertility of unexplained etiology (Cundiff et al. 1995; Nakagawa et al., 2007). However, there are no reports that relate pregnancy outcomes to significant results found inside the fallopian tube. The fertilization between oocyte and sperm is thought to occur at the ampulla of the fallopian tube, and therefore conditions inside of the ampulla are very important. From this point of view, observations from inside the ampulla might be used to predict pregnancy potential.

Assisted reproductive technology (ART) has become a mainstream infertility treatment, but do all patients who received ART treatment need it? It is believed that a significant number of the patients who receive ART treatment have no need for it, but existing infertility screening examination place limitations on the selection of patients who do not need to receive ART treatment, because no examination to evaluate the fallopian tube without HSG is done. Therefore, a new index for evaluation of the fallopian tube is proposed here. In this chapter, the performance of both laparoscopy and salpingoscopy for evaluation of the pelvic cavity and fallopian tube is discussed, with particular attention to the following points: [i] evaluation of the pelvic cavity; [ii] development of a new score for evaluation of the inside of the fallopian tubes (fallopian tube score; F score); and, [iii] the relationship between the F score and pregnancy outcome.

2. Laparoscopy and salpingoscopy

2.1 Procedure for laparoscopy and salpingoscopy

Laparoscopy was performed under general anesthesia. A three-port laparoscopy was used with a 3 mm umbilical port for the scope and two additional 3-mm operating ports. A 3 mm laparoscope was inserted through an umbilical port and connected to a video monitor (Karl-Stortz, Germany). Pneumoperitoneum was established (8-10mmHg). Observation within the pelvic cavity, and complete adhesiolysis and mobilization of the tubes and ovaries was performed if necessary. Tubal patency was checked with indigocarmine. In addition to patency testing, the gross external appearance of the fallopian tube and fimbrial mucosa were assessed with this procedure as well as the presence of peritubal adhesions, pelvic adhesions or lesions of edometriosis, such as bluish spots or red spots. With abnormal results, adhesiolysis, electroablation or resection of endometriotic implants was undertaken to the extent possible. Periadnexal adhesions are one of the main causes of tubal infertility and have a negative impact on the ability to achieve pregnancy. Adhesiolysis and mobilization of the tubes and ovaries, which eliminated effects such as peritubal or salpingo-ovario adhesions, was performed if necessary to evaluate the correlation between salpingoscopic results and their relationship to reproductive outcomes.

After checking the patency of the bilateral tubes, a 2.9 mm salpingoscope (Karl-Stortz, Germany, Fig 1) was inserted through the right port under observational laparoscopy through the umbilical port, and the inner cavity of the fallopian tube was checked. It is particularly worth nothing that two endoscopes were used concurrently for laparoscopy and salpingoscopy, because it is quite difficult to insert a salpingosope into a fallopian tube with no other observation. An atraumatic grasping forceps was applied just behind the fimbriae to hold the tubal wall against the salpingoscope (Fig 2-a), while an infusion of distending saline water was instilled to open up the potential space of the tubal lumen (Nakagawa et al., 2010). A salpingoscope can observe mainly the ampullary portion of the fallopian tube (Fig 2-b).

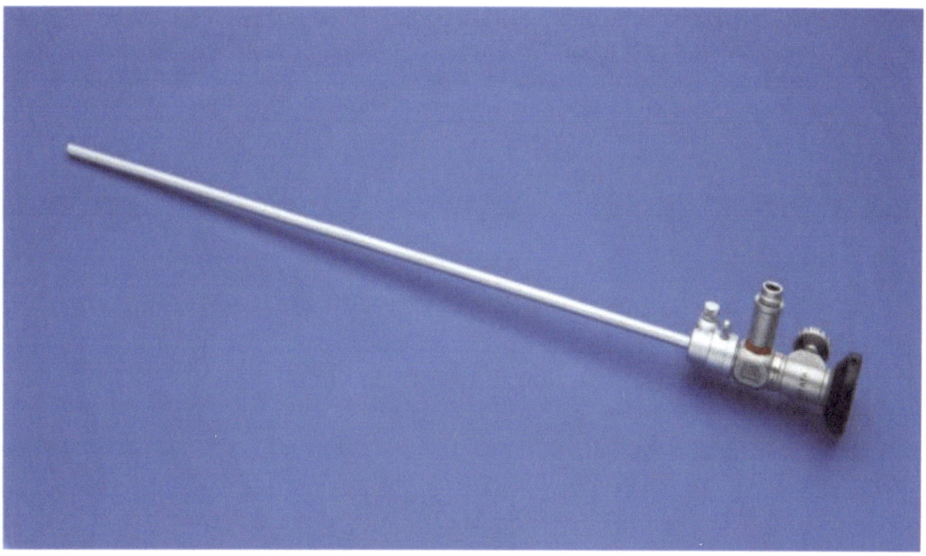

Fig. 1. This rigid scope was used as a salpingoscope (Karl-Stortz, Germany). The diameter was 2.9mm, and maximum magnification was ×60.

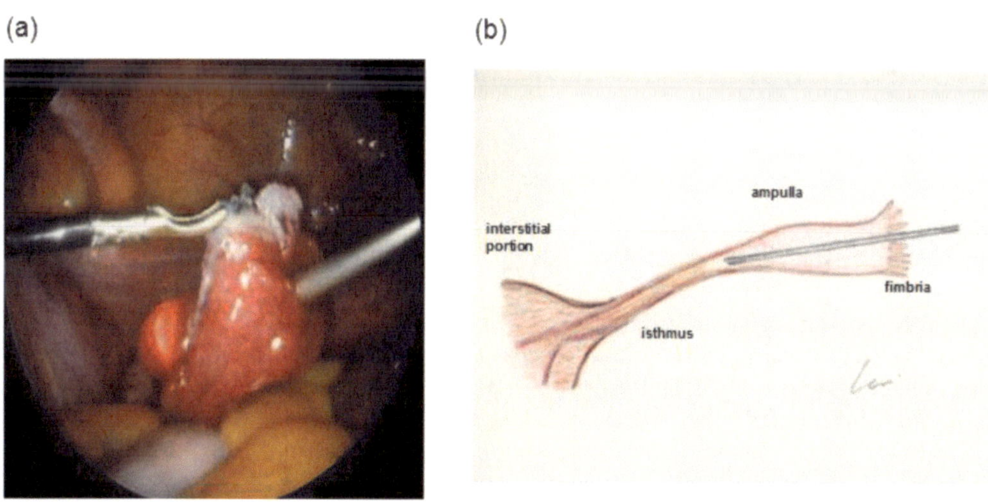

Fig. 2. (a) An atraumatic grasping forceps was applied just behind the fimbriae to hold the tubal wall against the salpingoscope. (b) The salpingoscope can observe mainly the ampullary portion of the fallopian tube.

2.2 Assessment of salpingoscopy

We observed both the right and left tubal lumens with the salpingoscope, paying particular attention to the following six abnormal results: i) adhesions, ii) loss of mucosal folds, iii) rounded edges of mucosal folds, iv) debris, v) foreign bodies, and vi) abnormal vessels.

We used an original classification system for the salpingoscopic results, based on Puttemans' classification (Puttemans et al., 1987). The mucosa of the ampullary segment in normal cases consisted of three to five major folds with secondary folds arising from them, and several minor folds interspaced among them. Examples of normal mucosa are shown in Figure 3-a, and various abnormal results are shown in figure 3-b through 3-g. 'Adhesions' indicated adhesions and/or agglutinations between folds (Fig 3-b). 'Loss of mucosal folds' indicated

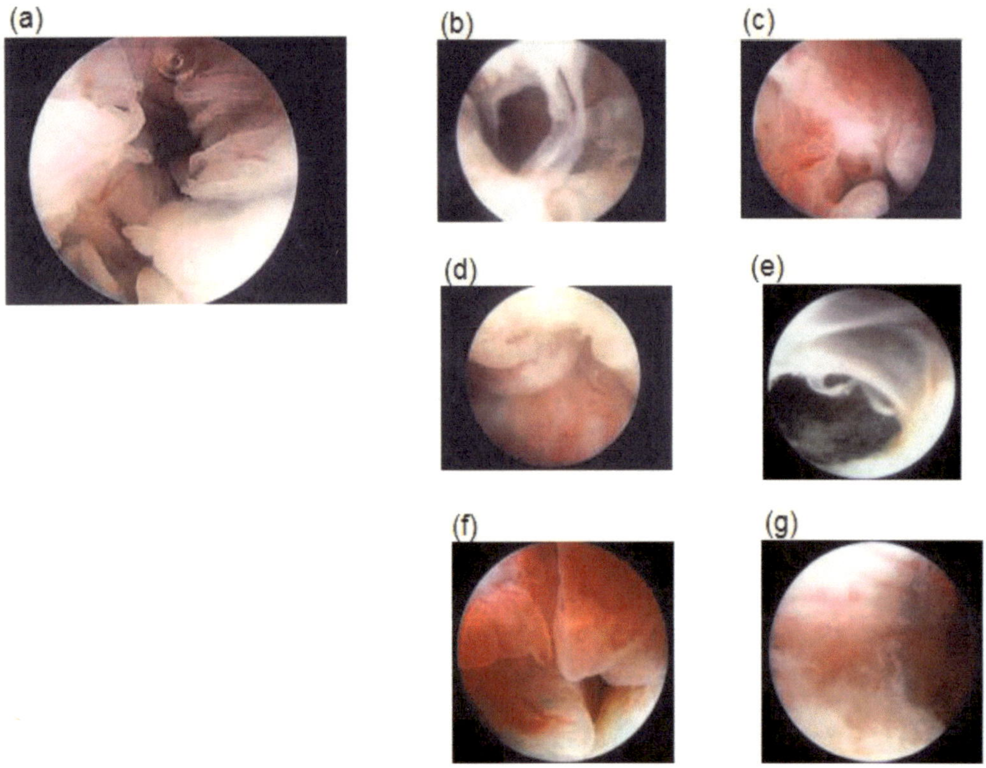

Fig. 3. Normal and abnormal results inside the fallopian tubes detected with the sapingoscope. (a) The mucosa of the ampullary segment in normal cases consisted of 3 to 5 major folds with secondary folds arising from them and several minor folds interspaced among them, and examples of normal mucosa are shown in this figure. (b) 'Adhesions' indicated adhesions and/or agglutinations between folds. (c) 'Loss of mucosal folds' indicated disseminated fold flat areas or a loss of the fold pattern of flattening folds. (d) 'Rounded edges of mucosal folds' indicated the disappearance of the secondary folds. (e) 'Debris' indicated mucus plugs, which were revealed by previous histological examination to consist of a cast of debris containing aggregates of histiocytic-like cells of an endometrial stromal or mesothelial origin. (f) 'Foreign bodies' consisted of oily contrast agents that were used for HSG. (g) 'Abnormal vessels' indicated irregularities of blood vessel diameter.

disseminated fold flat areas or a loss of the fold pattern of flattening folds (Fig 3-c). 'Rounded edges of mucosal folds' indicated the disappearance of the secondary folds (Fig 3-d). 'Debris' indicated mucus plugs, which were revealed by previous histological examination to consist of a cast of debris containing aggregates of histiocytic-like cells of an endometrial stromal or mesothelial origin (Kerin et al., 1991) (Fig 3-e). 'Foreign bodies' consisted of oily contrast agents used for HSG (Fig 3-f). 'Abnormal vessels' indicated irregularities of blood vessel diameters (Fig 3-g).

2.3 F score (fallopian tube score)

After salpingosopy the F score was calculated which was an original score used to evaluate the tubal lumen, expressed as the sum of the abnormal results listed above. Each abnormal result was given one point with a maximum F score of 12 points.

3. Relationship between the F scores and unexplained infertility patients

3.1 Unexplained infertility patients

In the present study unexplained infertility was diagnosed using the following criteria: a) the period of infertility was more than one year; b) the patient's normal menstrual cycle and ovulation was investigated by transvaginal ultrasonography, by estimation of serum progesterone concentrations in the mid-luteal phase; c) the patient showed normal results for genital organs by ultrasonography, and the patency of at least one fallopian tube was confirmed by HSG; d) the patient showed normal values in several hormone analyses (LH, FSH, PRL, E2, P); e) the patient's male partner had normal sperm results (WHO, 1992), and the post-coital test (PCT) was normal; and f) the patient did not achieve pregnancy after more than 6 courses of timed intercourse or intrauterine insemination (IUI). Patients who showed unilateral or bilateral hydrosalpinges or tubal obstruction were excluded, as were patients who had ovarian endometrioma(s) in either ovary. The sera of all patients were checked for anti-chlamydial antibodies before laparoscopy. A total of 227 infertile women who were diagnosed with unexplained infertility and underwent both laparoscopy and salpingoscopy at this clinic were recruited from April 2008 through October 2010 for the present study.

After receiving laparoscopy and salpingoscopy, the patients started infertility treatment as soon as possible, using timed intercourse or intrauterine insemination (IUI). Patients who were in need of ART treatment due to tubal damage were excluded from this evaluation. The patients recruited for the present study were diagnosed with unexplained infertility, and their tubal patency was confirmed by HSG prior to operation. Patients who showed uni- or bilateral hydrosalpinges or tubal obstruction and were in need of ART treatment were excluded from this evaluation, in order to focus on evaluation of the correlation between the salpingoscopic results and the reproductive outcomes. Clinical pregnancy was defined as the development of a gestational sac, as determined by transvaginal ultrasonography after ovulation. The relationship between the F scores and various clinical results and pregnancy rates was analyzed. Data were recorded as the mean ± S.D. or mean ± S.E.M, and were analyzed statistically using the chi- square test. $P < 0.05$ was considered to be statistically significant.

3.2 Patient backgrounds

The backgrounds of the patients who underwent both laparoscopy and salpingostomy due to unexplained infertility are summarized in Table 1. The average age of the patients was

33.8 ± 0.3 years, and the mean duration of infertility was 38.6 ± 0.9 months. The percentage of nullipara was 70.8%, the percentage of patients with positive chlamydial antibodies was 26.4%, and the percentage who showed abnormal HSG results such as peritubal adhesions was 28.9% (table 2 & 3).

3.3 Distribution of F scores

The average F score was 0.9 ± 0.1, and they ranged from 0 to 7. The distribution of the F scores is shown in Figure 4. Slightly more than half (50.7%) of the patients received an F score of 0, and the percentages of patients who received 1, 2, 3 and 4 or more points were 17.2%, 13.2%, 5.3% and 12.8%, respectively.

Number of patients	227
Average age (years)*	33.8 ± 0.2
Duration of infertility (months)*	38.6± 0.9
Percentage of nullipara (%)	70.8
Percentage of patients with positive chlamydial antibodies (%)	26.4
Percentage of patients with abnormal HSG (%)	28.9

*mean±S.E.M

Table 1. Backgrounds of patients who received laparoscopy and salpingoscopy due to unexplained infertility.

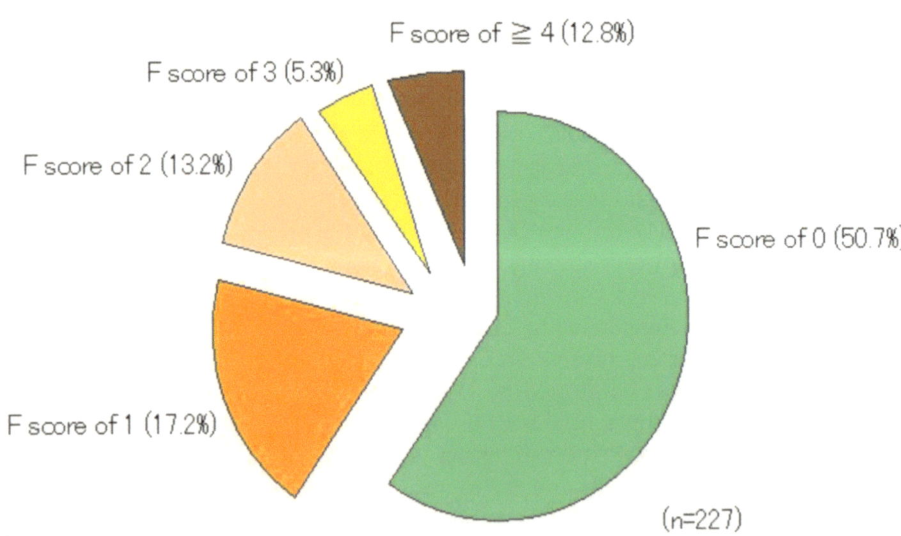

Fig. 4. The distribution of F score is shown in Figure 4. About half (50.7%) of the patients received an F score of 0, and the percentages of patients who received 1, 2, 3 and 4 or more points were 17.2%, 13.2%, 5.3% and 12.8%, respectively.

3.4 Relationship between the F scores and various clinical findings

The average F score of nullipara patients was 1.0 ± 0.2. This was somewhat higher than the scores of patients who had a history of pregnancy (0.5 ± 0.2), but the difference was not statistically significant (Table 2). The average F score of patients with an abnormal HSG was similar to that of patients with normal HSG results (1.2 ± 0.4 and 0.8 ± 0.2, respectively; as shown in table 3). However, the average F score for patients who tested positive for chlamydial antibodies was 1.7 ± 0.4, which was significantly higher than that of patients who tested negative (0.6 ± 0.1, p=0.0003; table 4).

	Pregnancy history		P value
	No gravidity	Pregnant before	
F score	1.0 ± 0.2	0.5 ± 0.2	0.0945

Table 2. The relationship between pregnancy history and F score

	HSG		P value
	normal	abnormal resultss	
F score	0.8 ± 0.2	1.2 ± 0.4	0.3287

HSG: hysterosalpingography

Table 3. The relationship between HSG results and F score

	Chlamydial antibodies		P value
	positive	negative	
F score	1.7 ± 0.4	0.6 ± 0.1	0.0003

Table 4. The relationship between chlamydial antibodies and F score

3.5 Relationship between F scores and pregnancy rates

After evaluation, all patients (n=227) began infertility treatment, and after salpingoscopic evaluation none were in need of ART treatment due to tubal damage. Within a year using either timed intercourse or artificial insemination with the husband's semen, 71 patients achieved pregnancy. The mean duration before achievement of pregnancy after surgery was 111.1 ± 1.2 days. The pregnancy rates of patients with F scores of 0, 1, 2, 3 and 4 or more were 35.9% (42/115), 33.3% (13/39), 33.3% (10/30), 16.7% (2/12), and 13.8% (4/29), respectively. The pregnancy rates for patients with lower F scores (F score ≤2) were significantly higher than the rates for patients with higher F scores (F score ≥3) (table 5, p<0.05).

F score	Number of patients	Number of pregnant patients	Pregnancy rates (%)	
0	115	42	35.9	35.3 [a]
1	39	13	33.3	
2	30	10	33.3	
3	12	2	16.7	14.6
≥4	29	4	13.8	

a: vs the group with F score ≥3

Table 5. The relationship between pregnancy rate and F score.

4. Relationship between F scores and endometriosis-related infertility patients

4.1 Infertility patients with uni- or biilateral endometrioma (s)

From April 2008 through February 2010, there were 94 infertile patients who had unilateral or bilateral endometrioma(s) recruited for the present study. All patients underwent laparoscopic ovarian cystectomy at the clinic. Patients with a history of gynecological operations, other ovarian masses, tubal obstruction or male infertility were excluded from this study. All patients showed regular menstrual cycles, and none of the women received exogenous gonadotropins or clomiphene citrate for ovarian stimulation during the study period. All endometriomas were diagnosed before surgery by magnetic resonance imaging and transvaginal ultrasound. The biaxial diameter of each endometrioma was measured by sonography, and the average was used as the endometrioma size. Informed consent was obtained from all patients and this study was approved by the Institutional Review Board of the Sugiyama Clinic.

An incision was made at the antimesenteric site of the cysts. The cyst was dissected from the ovary by traction and counter traction using a pair of 3 mm atraumatic grasping forceps. Bleeding from the stripped site was stopped by bipolar cauterization of the minimally required area for the shortest possible duration, to avoid thermal damage to the ovarian cortex. None of the operated ovaries were sutured. Tubal patency was checked with indigo carmine. The pelvic cavity was checked for the presence of peritubal and pelvic adhesions and endometriotic lesions, e.g., blue or red spots. Adhesiolysis, electro-ablation, or resection of endometriotic lesions was performed to the extent that these procedures were possible.

After this procedure, salpingoscopic evaluation of the bilateral fallopian tubes was performed as described above. The F scores and several clinical results of these patients (EM group) were compared to those of the unexplained infertility patients who received both laparoscopy and salpingoscopy during the same period (n=133; control group).

4.2 Distribution of F scores among patients with endometrioma(s)

The average F score was 0.3 ± 0.1, with a range of 0 to 4, and was significantly lower than that of the control group (0.8 ± 0.2, $p<0.01$). The distribution of the F scores is shown in Figure 5. About three-fourths (77.6%) of the patients in the EM group received F scores of 0,

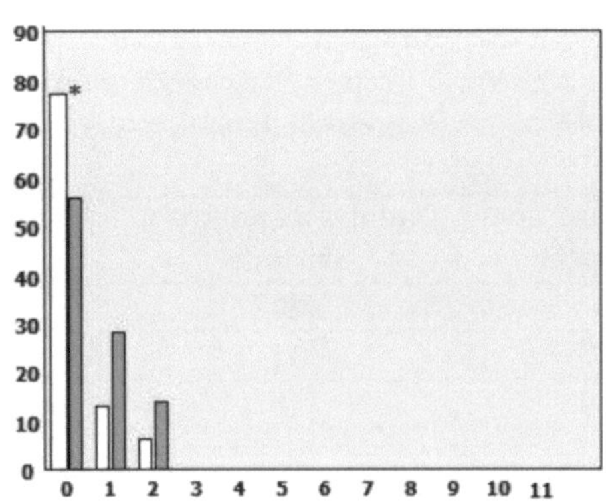

Fig. 5. This figure shows the distribution of F score in the EM group (blank bar) and control groups (dark bar). The percentage of patients with F scores of 0 was significantly lower than in the EM group (77.6%) than in the control group (79/133=59.4%, *$p<0.05$).

and the percentages of patients who received 1, 2, and 3 or more points were 14.9%, 6.4%, and 1.0%, respectively. The percentage of the patients with F scores of 0 in the EM group was significantly lower than that of the patients in the control group (79/133=59.4%, p<0.05).

4.3 Relationship between F scores and pregnancy rates

After laparoscopic cystectomy and salpingoscopy, all patients (n=94) in the EM group began infertility treatment, and 27 patients achieved pregnancy using either timed intercourse or artificial insemination with the husband's semen within 1 year (pregnancy rate= 28.7%). This rate was comparable to that in the control group (46/133=34.6%). In the EM group, the pregnancy rates of patients with F scores of 0, 1, 2 and 3 or more were 21.4% (24/73), 14.9% (3/14), 0% and 0%, respectively. In the control group, the pregnancy rates of patients with F scores of 0, 1, 2 and 3 or more were 36.7% (29/79), 35.7% (10/28), 28.5% (4/14), and 37.5%3 (3/8), respectively (Table 6). The pregnancy rate of patients with F scores of 0 in the EM group was comparable to that in the control group. However, among the patients with F scores of 1, the pregnancy rate in the EM group was significantly lower than that in the control group (p<0.05; Table 6).

F score	EM group	Control	
0	21.4% (24/73)	36.7% (29/79)	n.s.
1	14.9% (3/14)	35.7% (10/28)	P<0.05
2	0	28.5% (4/14)	n.s.
≥3	0	37.5% (3/8)	n.s.

Table 6. The relationship between pregnancy rates and F scores

Based on these results, it is highly possibe that infertility patients with ovarian endometrioma are more likely to have intact fallopian tubes, compared to infertility patients without ovarian endometrioma. Therefore, ovarian endometrioma itself could be one of the main causes of endometriosis-related infertility, and if these patients have abnormal results inside their fallopian tubes, they should receive ART treatment instead of conventional treatment.

5. Relationship between F scores and hydrosalpinges

5.1 Infertility patients with hydrosalpinges and reconstructive surgery

From April 2008 through February 2010, 38 infertile patients with a diagnosis of uni- or bilateral hydrosalpinges were examined by salpingoscopy at the time of resconstructive surgery under laparoscopy. The translaparoscopic salpingoscopy procedure described above was used. Following mobilization of the hydrosalpinx, the tube was opened by a small incision at the site where the scar of the occlusion could be identified. When intact fimbria was confirmed, it was inverted to the outside to prevent it from closing inside, and stitched with thin thread. Bleeding was controlled by endothermic coagulation. A 2.9-mm salpingoscope was used.

After this procedure, salpingoscopic evaluation of the bilateral fallopian tubes was performed as described above. The F scores and several clinical results of these patients (hydro-s group) were compared to those of the patients with unexplained infertility who received both laparoscopy and salpingoscopy during the same period (n=133; control group).

5.2 Distribution of F scores among patients with hydrosalpinges

The average F score was 3.4 ± 0.4, with a range of 0 to 10, and this average was significantly higher than that of the control group (0.8 ± 0.2, $p<0.01$). The distribution of F scores is shown in Figure 6. Only about one- fifth (21.1%) of the patients in the hydro-s group received an F score of 0, and the percentages of patients who showed 1, 2, 3, 4, and 5 or more points were 13.2%, 7.9%, 13.2%, 13.2%, and 31.4%, respectively. The percentage of patients with F scores of 0 was significantly higher in the hydro-s group than in the control group (79/133=59.4%, $p<0.05$). Surprisingly, about one- third of the patients in the hydro-s group received a high F score.

5.3 Relationship between the F scores and pregnancy rates

After laparoscopic reconstructive surgery for hydrosalpinges and salpingoscopy, all patients (n=38) in the hydro-s group began infertility treatment, but only 6 patients achieved pregnancy using either timed intercourse or artificial insemination from the husband's semen within one year (pregnancy rate=15.8%). This rate was significantly lower than that in the control group (46/133=34.6%). The pregnancy rates of patients with F scores of 0, 1, 2, 3, 4, and 5 or more were 12.5% (1/8), 20.0% (1/5), 33.3% (1/3), 20.0% (2/5), 0%, 8.3% (1/12), respectively. In the control group, the rates for patients with F scores of 0, 1, 2, and 3 or more were 36.7% (29/79), 35.7% (10/28), 28.5% (4/14), and 3/8 (37.5%), respectively (Table 7). In the hydro-s group, 4 additional patients achieved pregnancy using ART treatment, and a total of 10 patients achieved pregnancy (pregnancy rate=26.3%). However, in the control group an additional 16 patients achieved pregnancy using ART treatment, and a total of 62 patients achieved pregnancy (pregnancy rate=46.6%).

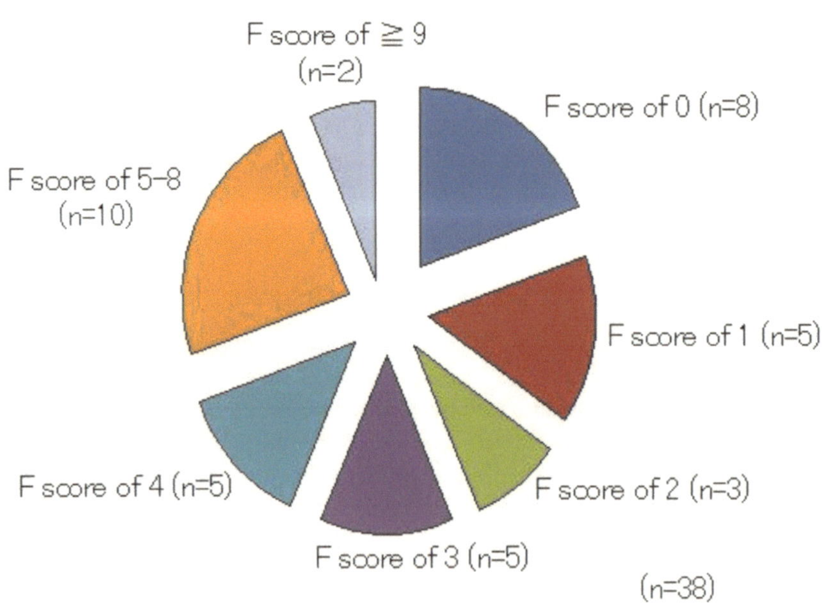

Fig. 6. The distribution of the F scores of patients with hydrosalpinges is shown in Figure 6. About one fifth (21.1%) of the patients received an F score of 0, and the percentages of patients who received 1, 2, 3, 4, and 5 or more points were 13.2%, 7.9%, 13.2%, 13.2% and 31.4%, respectively.

F score	Hydro-s group	Control	
0	12.5% (1/8)	36.7% (29/79)	n.s.
1	20.0% (1/5)	35.7% (10/28)	n.s.
2	33.3% (1/3)	28.5% (4/14)	n.s.
≥3	13.6% (3/22)	37.5% (3/8)	n.s.

Table 7. The relationship between pregnancy rates and F scores

6. Conclusions

Predictions of fertility outcome by laparoscopy can be improved by the concomitant performance of salpingoscopy (Marchino et al., 2001). The two tests probably complement rather than substitute for one another. Salpingoscopy was the first tubal assessment test that to disclose a new world of detailed *in-vivo* images of the actual site of human fertilization. It can clearly demonstrate the presence or absence of anatomical distortions, especially adhesions between, and destruction of, mucosal folds on a micro-endoscopic, i.e. mucosal, level. The proponents of Salpingoscopy argue that it could, and should, direct the infertility investigation and treatment care pathway towards either reconstructive surgery or ART. Lesions of the infundibulum and ampullary segment have been detected in patients with apparently normal tubes upon HSG and laparoscopy (Puttemans et al., 1987).
However, although the presence of ampullary mucosal adhesions has been reported to negatively affect fertility and increase the risk of ectopic pregnancy, mucosal adhesions are not incompatible with normal fertility (Maguiness & Djahanbakhch., 1992) and, unless the damage is severe, there is a poor correlation with histological assessment (Hershlag et al., 1991). Therefore, not enough is known about these lesions, and salpingoscopy remains a research tool.
Essential phenomena of the beginning of life, such as the meeting of between male and female gametes, fertilization, and development, occur inside the fallopian tube. Although in this era ART is the most popular infertility treatment, it is very important and meaningful to focus attention on the results found inside the fallopian tube. According to the data reported here, most of the patients who showed no abnormal results in their pelvic cavity and adnexa could not get pregnant by timed intercourse or IUI when they received high F scores. However, the patients who had no significant results in the fallopian tubes even if significant results were found in the pelvic cavity such as ovarian endometrioma or hydrosalpinges, could expect to achieve pregnancy without using ART treatment. These results indicate that it is very important to focus on conditions inside the fallopian tubes, and the F score might be useful for prediction of the prognosis of infertility treatments andfor treatment selection decisions.

7. References

Cundiff, G.; Carr, BR. & MArshburn, PB. (1995) Infertile couples with a normal hysterosalpingogram. Reproductive outcome and its relationship to clinical and laparoscopic findings. *Journal of Reproductive Medicine*, vol. 40, 19-24.

Hershlag, A.; Seifer, DB.; Carcangiu, ML.; Patton, DL.; Diamond, MP. & DeCherney, AH. (1991) Salpingoscopy: light microscope and electron microscopic correlations. *Obstetrics and Gynecology*, vol. 77, 399-405.

Heylen, SM.; Brosens, IA. & Puttemans, PJ. (1995) Clinical value and cumulative pregnancy rates following rigid salpingoscopy during laparoscopy for infertility. *Human Reproduction*, vol. 10, 2913-2916.

Kerin, JF.; Surry, ES.; William, DB.; Daykhovsky, L. & Grundfest, WS. (1991) Falloscopic observations of endotubal mucus plugs as a cause of reversible obstruction and their histological characterization. *Journal of Laparoendoscopic Surgery*, vol. 1, 103-110.

Maguiness, SD. & Djahanbakhch, O. (1992) Salpingoscopic findings in women undergoing sterilization. *Humun Reproduction*; vol. 7, 269-273.

Marana, R.; Catalano, GF.; Muzii, L. & Mancuso, S. (1999) The prognostic role of salpingoscopy in laparoscopic tubal surgery. *Human Reproduction*, vol. 14, 2991-2995

Marhino, GL.; Gigante, V.; Gennarelli, G.; Mazza, O. & Mencaglia, L. (2001) Salpingoscopie and laparoscopic investigations in relation to fertility outcome. *Journal of the American Association of Gynecological Laparoscopists*, vol.8, 218-221.

Marana, R.; Catalano, GF. & Muzii, L. (2003) Salpingoscopy. *Current Opinion of Obstetrics and Gynecology*, vol. 13, 333-336.

Mol, BW.; Dijkman, B.; Wertheim, P.; Lijmer, J.; van der Veen, F. & Bossuyt, PM. (1997) The accuracy of serum chlamydial antibodies in the diagnosis of tubal pathology: a meta-analysis. *Fertility and Sterility*, vol. 67,1031-1037.

Nakagawa, K.; Ohgi, S.; Horikawa, T.; Kojima, R.; Ito, M. & Saito, H. (2007) Laparoscopy should be strongly considered for examining women with unexplained infertility. *Journal of Obstetrics and Gynecology Research*, vol.33, 665-670.

Nakagawa, K.; Inoue, M.; Nishi, Y.; Sugiyama, R.; Motoyama, K.; Kuribayashi, Y.; Akira, S. & Sugiyama, R. (2010). A new evaluation score that uses salpingoscopy to reflect fallopian tube function in infertile women. *Fertility and Sterility*, vol. 94, 2753-2757.

Puttemans, P.; Brosens, I. & Delattin, P.; Vasquez, G. & Boeckx, W. (1987) Salpingoscopy versus hysperosalpingography in hydrosalpinges. *Humun Reproduction*, vol. 2, 535-540.

Papaioannou, S.; Afnan, M. & Jafettas, J. (2007) Tubal assessment tests: still have not found what we are looking for. *Reproductive BioMedical Online*, vol. 15, 376-382.

Surry, ES. & Surry, MW. (1996) Correlation between salpingoscopic and laparoscopic staging in the assessment if distal fallopian tube. Fertility and Steriliry, vol. 65, 267-271.

Tanahatoe, SJ. (2008) Diagnostin laparoscopy is needed after abnormal hysterosalpingography to prevent over-treatment with IVF. *Reproductive BioMedical Online*, vol.16, 410-415.

WHO. WHO Laboratory Mannual for the Examination of Human Semen and Sperm-Cervical Mucus Interaction. Chembridge University Press. Cambridge, UK. 1992.

Part 7

Laparoscopic Uterine Surgery

11

Reconstructive Endoscopic Myomectomy

Atef M.M. Darwish
Department of Obstetrics and Gynecology,
Woman's Health University Hospital,
Assiut
Egypt

1. Introduction

Myomectomy is an old reconstructive gynecologic operation intended to preserve a functioning uterus suitable for a possible subsequent pregnancy. A lot of the published work on endoscopic myomectomy demonstrates the feasibility of the procedure, highlights the possible advantages, and expresses the skills of the surgeons (1). The question now is not whether the procedure is feasible endoscopically, but whether the endoscopic approach is superior and beneficial to a particular patient as well as cost effective for the community at large (2). Modern practice should be focused on evidence-based medicine (EBM) concept (3).

2. Principles of reconstructive surgery

Reconstructive surgery aims to put genital organs and tissues back together in a way that makes them more functional, and /or with fewer clinical symptoms. It leads to reduce potential problems and side effects from primary surgery and improve patients' quality of life. Early discharge within 24 hours after the procedure with an excellent outcome is a common sequel to reconstructive gynaecologic surgery even if done via laparotomy (2). Nevertheless, reconstructive surgery requires high level of expertise, delicate instruments, fine maneuvers, longer time, and fine energy modalities.

3. Fertility-preserving reconstructive gynecologic surgery

If future fertility is of concern, endoscopic reconstructive gnecologic surgery should follow microsurgical principles (4,5) which include avoidance of serosal insults e.g. tissue trauma, ischemia, hemorrhage, infection, foreign-body reaction, and leaving raw surfaces (6). Other microsurgical principles include minimizing tissue trauma by using atraumatic techniques, meticulous hemostasis, complete excision of abnormal tissues and precise alignment and approximation of tissue planes (7). With this so meticulous reconstruction of the gynecological structures, maximal possibilities of pregnancy without the utilization of other complex procedures of assisted reproduction can be achieved. It has been estimated by some enthusiastic proponents that microsurgery could results in double the pregnancy rate compared conventional macrosurgery (8). However, a recent Cochrane review did not demonstrate any advantage of microsurgery over the conventional approach (6).

Laparoscopic microsurgeons should have enough experience in classical microsurgery as well as highly-developed two-handed laparoscopic skills for intracorporeal knotting (9,10).

4. Reconstructive laparoscopic myomectomy (LM)

The first LM is performed in 1980 when several pedunculated subserous fibroids are removed laparoscopically (11). Since then, several descriptive series (12,13) on LM have been published and these have highlighted several problems associated with the procedure. Long operating times have been reported with some exceeding seven hours (14). This may be related to the need to morcellate the fibroids to facilitate their removal as well as the need for laparoscopic suturing which can be tedious (15). Increased adhesion formation has also been described following this procedure (16). Furthermore, several authors (17-19) have also reported cases of uterine rupture/dehiscence following LM. More attention should be paid to careful uterine repair following this laparoscopic procedure. A large series of pregnancies after LM (20) reported on 100 patients who eventually had deliveries, and recorded only one uterine rupture occurred at the site of the old LM scar (1%; 95% CI, 0.0–5.5%). Although the authors concluded that spontaneous uterine rupture seems to be rare after LM, they caution and re-iterate that particular care must still be given to uterine closure. Data on the risk of recurrence after LM has been published (21) in a series of 622 patients monitored with ultrasonography. They reported a cumulative 10 year recurrence rate of 27%. Although several authors (13,22) have reported pregnancies after LM, there are still no long term data on subsequent fertility following the procedure. Mais et al (23) conducted a prospective RCT comparing early postoperative outcome following LM and laparotomy in 40 patients. They reported less postoperative pain, a shorter hospital stay and a faster rate of recovery after laparoscopy as compared to open surgery. Several authors (11-14,21) have suggested that laparotomy may be preferable to the laparoscopic approach in patients with large multiple myomas, especially in the presence of severe endometriosis. In general, LM is associated with a shorter hospital stay, faster recovery and less blood loss that could be explained in part by the tamponade effect of the pnuemoperitoneum. Patient satisfaction with operative scar after LM is good (24) and as well as fertility satisfaction and reproductive outcome (23).

4.1 Patient selection

Indications include infertility, recent and significant uterine enlargement and symptoms like pelvic pain, pressure, menometrorrhagia and abnormal bleeding (25). Inclusion criteria include age ≤42 years, the presence of at least one symptomatic myoma >3 cm, and a number of myomas equal or less than seven (26). Some authors (27, 28) suggested that no more than three or four myomas with diameters <7–8 cm are to be removed; Nevertheless, the decision should be individualized according to the surgical skills, facilities, age and the pathologic findings (29,30).

4.2 Role of LM in infertility

Whether to perform LM or open microsurgical minilaprotomic myomectomy is a controversial issue. Added to the well documented advantages of laparoscopy, LM is associated with fewer postoperative complications and since no preoperative or intraoperative factors seem to influence the fertility outcome in women with uterine myomas, it is considered as the treatment of choice in infertile patients (31). Those infertile cases with myomata are mostly hyperestrogenic; so laparoscopy will help treat associated lesions particularly endometriosis.

4.3 Preoperative preparation

You should get a consent for either LM or emergency laparotomy whenever required if technical problems or excessive bleeding would be encountered. The size, number, and location of the fibroids as well as the experience of the surgeon all must be factors in the decision to proceed with the laparoscopic approach. Although several suggestions have been made, opinions differ. Whether to use preoperative hormonal preparation or not is still a controversial issue. Some studies reported on significant reduction of the myoma size and introperative blood loss on gonadotrophin-releasing hormone agonist or antagonist. Zullo et al (32) noted that preoperative use of leuprolide acetate decreased estimated blood loss from 172 mL to 132 mL and operating time from 113 minutes to 99 minutes. Felberbaum et al (33) reported on significant preoperative reduction of uterine fibroids in only 16 days by administration of a gonadotrophin-releasing hormone antagonist (Cetrotide). On the other hand, longer operative times, 112 minutes versus 157 minutes, with preoperative GnRH analog use found by Campo and Garcia, are attributed to difficulty in detecting the myoma cleavage plane (34). My practice for a long time is to give patients medorxyprogesterone acetate 15 mg daily for 20 days prior to LM and I notice good surgical field in most of cases.

4.4 Operative technique

LM is usually performed with a standard technique using three suprapubic ports. The uterus is always cannulated to allow the correct exposure of myomas. For pedunculated myomas, the pedicle are secured using a pre-tied or extracorporeally-tied loop and coagulated and transected with bipolar forceps and scissors. For subserous and intramural myomas, serosal incision should be made vertically over the convex surface of the myoma using a monopolar hook, fine needle or one blade of a scissors (Figure 1).

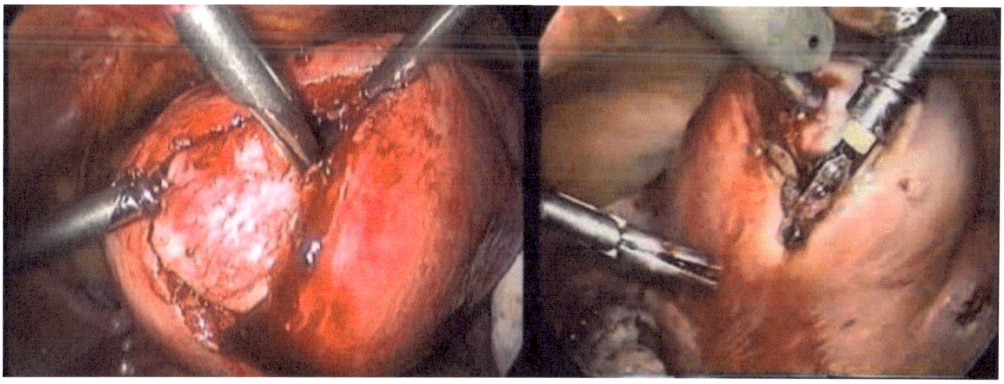

Fig. 1. Uterine incision.

After exposure of the myoma pseudocapsule, grasping forceps is positioned to apply traction to the myoma and expose the cleavage plane (figure 2). An option is to use a 10 mm myoma driller from a midline incision to hold and grasp the myoma firmly against the anterior abdominal wall to facilitate enucleation. Enucleation is carried out by traction on the fibroid and by division with a unipolar hook or needle or mechanical cleavage.

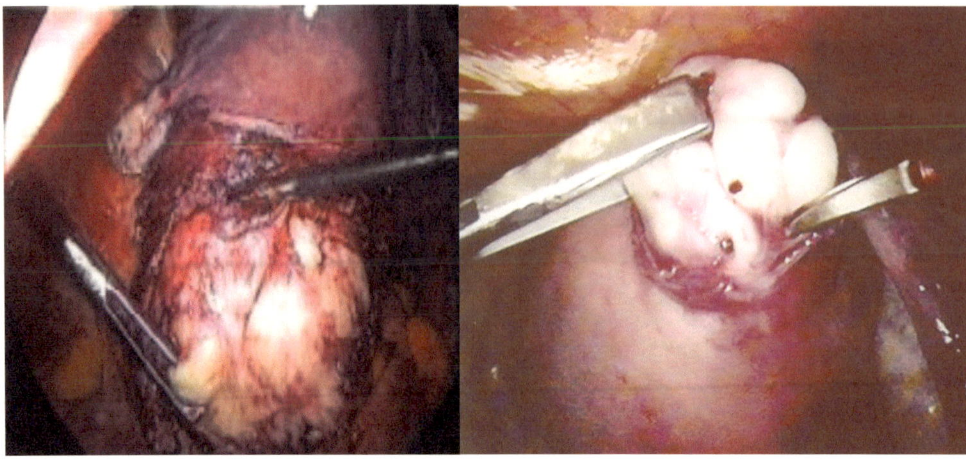

Fig. 2. Myoma enucleation.

Hemostasis during dissection is achieved by bipolar or spray monopolar coagulation. Suturing is usually done along one or two layers including the serosa depending on the depth of incision with interrupted, simple or more frequently cross-stitches tied intracorporeally using 1 or 0 Polyglactin sutures or any delayed absorbable sutures (figure 3).

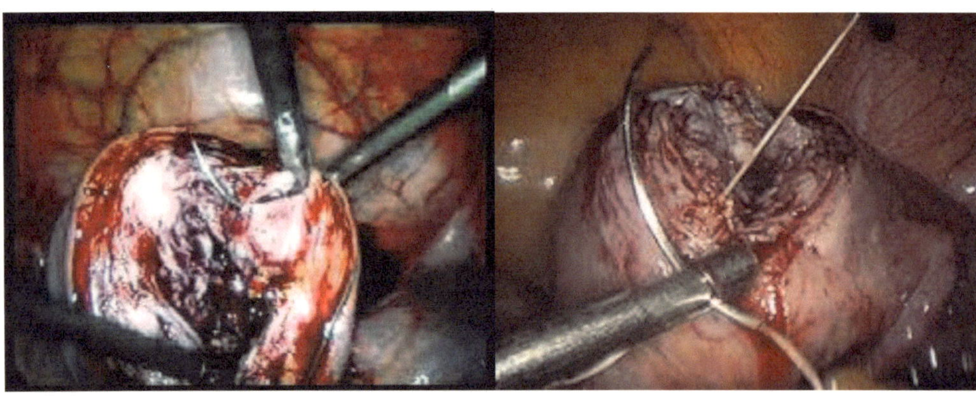

Fig. 3. Closure of the uterine defect with sutures.

A recent study (35) evaluated the use of bidirectional barbed suture and found it significantly shortens the mean duration of surgery.

Morcellation of the myoma is followed by irrigation and placement of adhesion barrier. As a trial to reduce bleeding during LM, Zhao et al (36) tested loop ligation of larger myoma pseudocapsule combined with vasopressin before LM and found it very effective in minimizing bleeding in a randomized controlled trial.

Removal of the fibroids can be performed using morcellation (figure 4), minilaparotomy, or colpotomy Alternatives to these are to destroy the fibroids in place with cryotherapy, bipolar cautery, or laser. No trials have compared these techniques to determine which is the safest or most effective. Chen et al (37) tried simultaneous enucleation and in situ morcellation of myoma and found it convenient. Don't forget to leave an intraperitoneal drain for few hours via an auxillary portal.

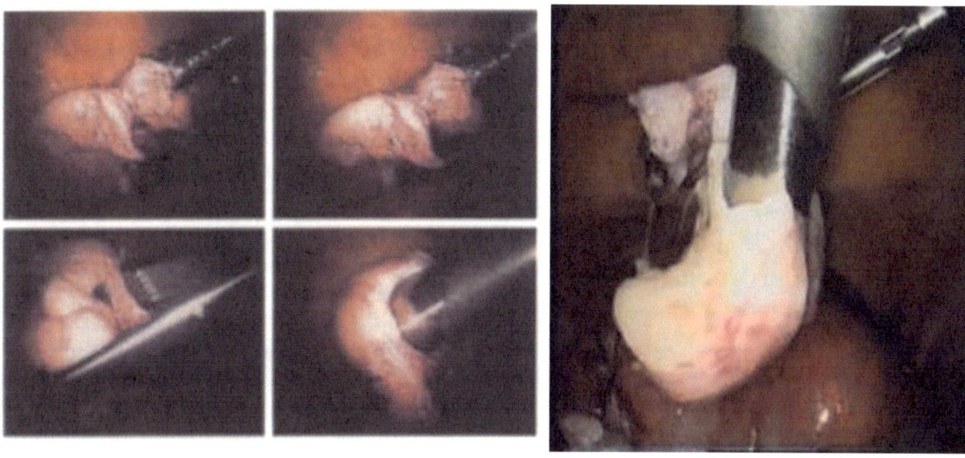

Fig. 4. Morcellation of the myoma.

4.5 Disadvantages of LM

Although LM has been shown to be feasible, the technique is fraught with problems. Furthermore, its place in the treatment of infertile patients still needs to be defined. Laproscopic closure of the uterine incision is performed in a rather simplified manner utilizing just few stitches, unlike conventional open myomectomy. There is a need for meticulously studying the healing pattern of the uterine incision following LM. Integrity of uterine scar is an important consideration for women desiring pregnancy. LM is accused to be a procedure that leaves behind insecure uterine scars as evidenced by reported cases of uterine rupture following LM. Although uterine ruptures during pregnancy have been reported after myomectomies via laparotomy, these are usually sporadic reports (14,15,17, 38-40). Risk factors for uterine rupture after LM may be intramural haematoma formation at the incision site, tissue necrosis because of thermal damage leading to defective scar formation, or incorrect approximation of incision edges leading to healing by secondary intention. Uterine rupture and fistula formation after LM have been reported (14,15,17, 40-42). However, none of these investigators closed the uterine defect in layers. In another series (43), no case of uterine rupture has been reported following pregnancies after LM. The authors have emphasized the importance of avoiding excessive thermal damage and of adequate uterine repair using multiple layer suturing techniques. In cases of deeply embedded myomas, larger than six to seven centimetres in size, LM may be replaced with laparoscopic assisted myomectomy (44). Suturing the myometrium in layers during a LM is also necessary to prevent iatrogenic adenomyosis (45).

4.6 Postoperative care

Like any laparoscopic surgery, LM cases should be monitored. Care of the amount of blood loss in the drainage set. Better to prescribe antibiotics and antipyretics whenever required. Instruct you patient to avoid vagina manipulations or douches if posterior colpotomy is performed. Moreover, she has to avoid sexual intercourse for at least 4 weeks if colostomy is performed. I don't recommend advising pills for contraception as those cases are usually infertile. She has to use a local method for 1-2 months only.

4.7 Follow-up

Our school since 1992 is to follow up cases by both transabdominal and transvaginal ultrasonography to properly evaluate healing of the scar till complete disappearance of the signs of healing.

4.8 Assessment of the integrity of the uterine scar following LM

Various modalities to assess scar healing and strength in the postoperative period have been suggested (46). Ultrasonography is used to detect haematoma formation in the uterine scar. Doppler studies can be used to assess the uterine scar, possibly recognizing the irregularities in the vascular patterns and haematoma formation, which depict poor quality uterine scar. Velocimetric findings at 30th postoperative day may be able to assess the healing process. A high resistance index may suggest abnormal healing and an area of fibrosis (47,48). Hysterosalpingography, despite being non-specific, may be performed to detect the presence of any fistulae (15). Second-look laparoscopy may be carried out between four to eight weeks postoperatively and a methylene blue test is performed to check any uterine fistula. The place of second look laparoscopy has been particularly emphasized in relation to assessment of any postoperative adhesions and its treatment (48,49).

4.9 Impact on reproductive health

Again, those cases are usually hyperestrogenic with evidence of adenomyosis uteri, endometrial htperplasia or endometriosis. So, laparoscopy allows proper assessment of those infertile cases. If an office hysteroscopy is performed prior to LM, this would be considered as one of the keys of success regarding future fertility. Therefore, LM would help solve the infertility problem of those cases. Adding the advantages of laparoscopic surgery with definite lower risk of adhesion formation if compared to laparotomy would favor LM.

4.10 LM versus conventional myomectomy

There is no difference in fertility efficacy outcome if fibroids are removed via laparotomy when compared to laparoscopy (50). Because hematoma formation of measurable size is not normal in wound healing, subsequent uterine rupture may be related to poor wound healing in the presence of hematoma (51). We studied 22 cases that are treated with LM followed by suturing of the incision in two or three layers trying to mimic open myomectomy (52). Moreover, we studied 169 cases treated with conventional open myomectomy with meticulous closure of the incision in multilayers (53). Laparotomy study (53) included many cases with multiple myomata (mean number is 2±0.4) and of varying size (mean size is 216 cm3±61 cm3). Paradoxically, despite having myomata of smaller size with less mean numbers, the laparoscopy study (52) demonstrated higher percentage of hematoma formation in the early postoperative period (74% versus 24% for laparoscopy and laparotomy studies respectively). This highlights the superiority of open microsurgery in terms of meticulous suturing simply because it is technically more feasible than laparoscopic suturing. Continuous training of endoscopists on improving suturing techniques and innovation of easier suturing devices would facilitate thorough laparoscopic multilayer suturing of the myomectomy scar. Nevertheless, the impact of the early postoperative hematoma on wound healing is not clear so far. At 4-6 weeks postoperatively, the incidence of hematoma formation in both studies (52,53) declined markedly (8% at 6 weeks versus 7% at 4 weeks for laparoscopy and laparotomy studies respectively). Thus, the procedure should involve multilayered uterine closure to avoid hematoma formation, weaker scar and subsequent rupture. However, the only way to answer the question as to whether LM can ensure a safe obstetric outcome as open myomectomy, is to perform a large multicenteric comparative trial. LM offers significantly less febrile morbidity, lower transfusion rates, and shorter hospitalization stays if compared to open myomectomy (54). Moreover, it results in shorter operative times and lower postoperative hemoglobin, while hospital stay and pain are less in the laparoscopic group if compared to laparotomic approach (55).

5. Reconstructive hysteroscopic myomectomy (HM)

Submucous myoma may cause abnormal vaginal bleeding, pain, &/or infertility. The incidence of myoma in women with otherwise unexplained infertility is estimated to be 1.0–2.4% (56,57). A systematic review of 11 cohort studies suggests that women with submucous myoma have lower pregnancy rates compared with women with other causes for their infertility (RR 0.30, 95% CI 0.13 to 0.70). HM is not associated with an increase in live birth rate (RR 0.98, 95% CI 0.45 to 2.41) but is associated with a higher pregnancy rate (RR 1.72, 95% CI 1.13 to 2.58) (58). Both HM and polypectomy appeared to enhance fertility compared with infertile women with normal cavities in one study (59). HM currently represents the standard minimally invasive surgical procedure for treating submucous fibroids, with abnormal uterine bleeding and reproductive issues being the most common indications (60,61). Nevertheless, this technique is associated with significant risks of excessive bleeding, prolonged operative time required for cutting the myoma into chips of tissues and extractiing them, risks of fluid overload, and the possibility of incomplete resection and perforation (62). To reduce these risks, more effective patient selection and improved techniques are necessary (63).

5.1 Indications of HM

It is well established and settled that all evidence consider HM as the gold standard and nearly the only line of therapy of submucous myomata of suitable size. The problem is the definition of "suitable size" Most centers consider 2-4 cm as an optimal size. If larger myoma is diagnosed, HM can be tried either on 2 session bases or utilizing our modified technique (see below). An important issue is the association of adenomyosis or intramural myomata. You can excise more than one myoma on the same setting provided the general condition of the patient can tolerate.

5.2 Preoperative preparation of HM

Patient selection is essential to achieve resolution of bleeding symptoms, enhance fertility, and reduce surgical risks. Preoperative imaging with MRI, 3-dimensional ultrasonography or saline-infused sonohysterography (SIS) can provide a map of the uterine myomas and identify the intramural component of the fibroids. The European Society of Hysteroscopy designed a classification system for submucosal fibroids based primarily on this concept (64, figure 5).

- Type 0 fibroids are pedunculated with no intramural component.
- Type I fibroids are sessile submucosal fibroids with less than 50% intramural component.
- Type II fibroids have a greater than 50% myometrial invasion.

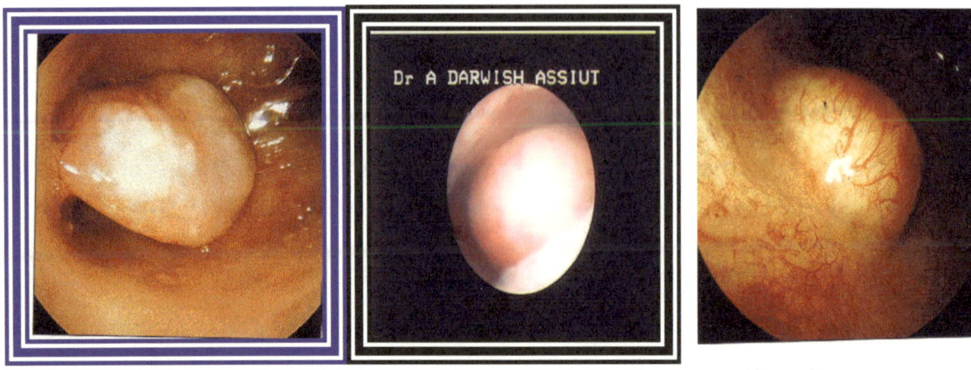

Type 0 Type 1 Type 2

Fig. 5. Classification of submucous myomata.

Incomplete resection of the fibroid is more likely in type II fibroids with more extensive intramural component. Calculated from one study is a 50% chance per procedure of complete resection of type II fibroids, 60% of type I fibroids, and 92% of type 0. After an incomplete resection, the residual intramural component is likely to be expelled into the cavity and a second procedure is often successful. The patient with type II fibroids should be counseled on the risk of failure and the procedure should be performed by experienced hysteroscopic surgeons (65).

Preoperative hormonal preparation of the myoma is a controversial issue. HM should be performed essentially postmenstrual. Preoperative cervical ripening with a prostaglandin analogue has been demonstrated to facilitate cervical dilation. In a controlled randomized study (66), we succeeded to prove that Misoprostol 200 mcg applied vaginally 8-12 hours prior to surgery is well tolerated and can decrease surgical time and reduce the risk of surgical complications.

5.3 Techniques of HM

Myoma resection is usually performed with a loop electrode (figure 6) by shaving the visible portion of the myoma into small pieces. Sometimes, myomas deeply embedded in the myometrium cannot be completely excised. Other techniques for removing the myoma hysteroscopically include using an Nd:YAG laser fiberor electric myoma vaporizer (65).

Various sizes of operating hysteroscopes are now available, but they all include a telescope with a fiberoptic light source and camera. The angle of the telescope is either 0° or an acute angle of 12-30°. The straight visual 0° scope might be helpful with fundal myomas but an angled perspective is more commonly used for fibroid resection. The telescope inserts through an external sheath and internal sheath for continuous outflow and inflow of distension media. The working element of the operating hysteroscope is the resecting loop that is available in many sizes and angles. The electrosurgical energy connected to the loop can be monopolar or bipolar. With the monopolar loops, using nonionic distension media such as glycene 5% or sorbitol 1.5% is necessary. With bipolar loops, both electrodes are within the cavity and normal saline can be used for distending solution. For hysteroscopic myomectomy, various laser types and mechanical loops without electrical energy have also been described (65).

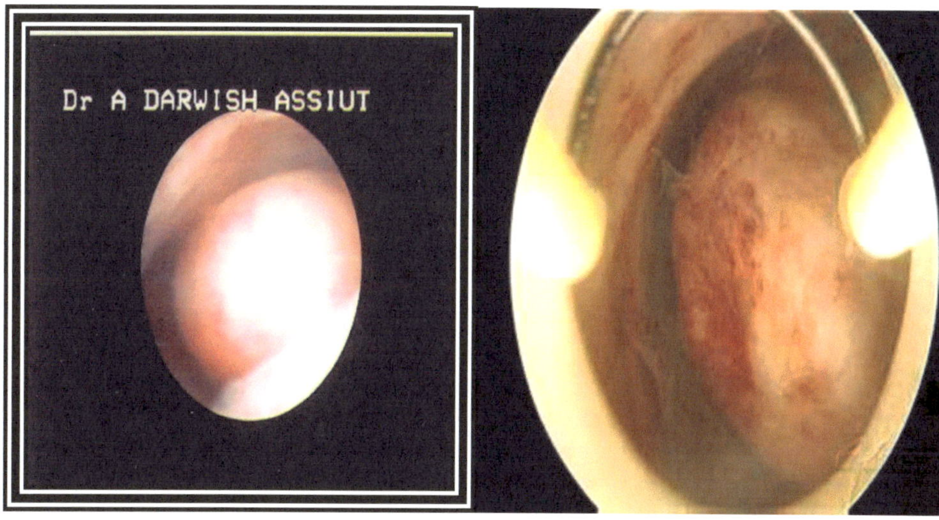

Fig. 6. Myoma cutting with the resectoscope.

There are multiple methods of using the electrosurgical loop to optimize fibroid resection (figure 7). To maintain good visualization, fragments of resected fibroid need to be removed during the procedure. The surgeon may transfer fragments out of the field of resection or retrieve them from the cavity by grasping the tissue with the resecting loop. An intrauterine morcellator has recently been introduced that may improve surgical time by aspirating fibroid fragments through the hysteroscope (65). When applying the monopolar loop, currents as high as 75-150 W are required for smooth tissue cutting. Current should only be applied while the loop is being retracted into the hysteroscope or while the entire resectoscope is being pulled away from the fundus. A combination of the 2 movements is used by the surgeon to safely and effectively slice through the tissue.

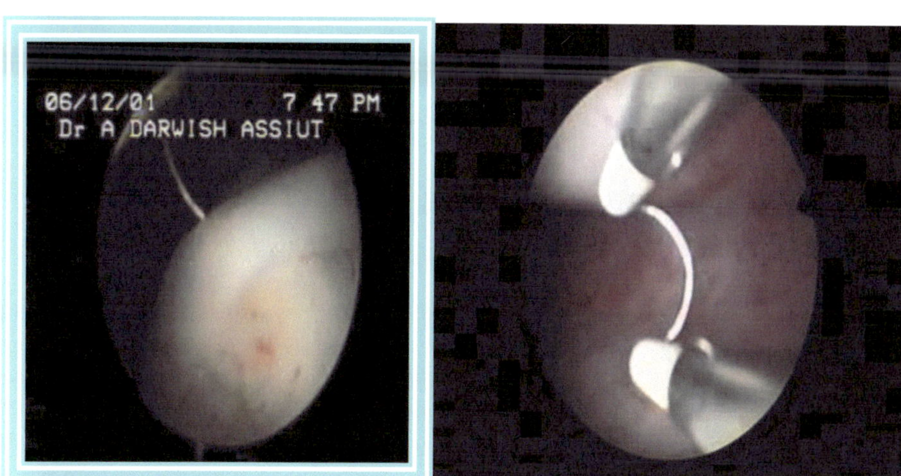

Fig. 6. Resectoscopic myomectomy.

Resection of type 0 fibroids can be accomplished in 1 step by most hysteroscopic surgeons since the border of the fibroid with the endometrium is easily identified (67). Type I and type II fibroids require more surgical expertise as resection of the fibroid extends into the myometrial space. Intraoperative cervical injection of carboprost, a methyl analogue of prostaglandin F2-alpha, has been shown to cause uterine contractions and thereby squeeze the remaining fibroid into the cavity to facilitate a single step. Concomitantly performing laparoscopy with intramuscular injection of prostaglandin F2-alpha is also effective for resection of large fundal fibroids and provides transabdominal visualization (68). In many circumstances, resection of large fibroids with significant intramural component is a 2-step approach since there is often further intracavitary expulsion of the fibroid after the initial surgery. The second procedure can be performed 3-6 weeks later when the residual fibroid has migrated into the submucosal space (69).

5.4 Modified HM for big or intramural myomas: Darwish's technique (70)

All cases should be subjected to office hysteroscopy in the immediate postmenstrual period not preceded by hormonal priming. The objectives are to confirm the sonographic diagnosis of myoma, comment on the number and the size, assess the site of the myoma in relation to the tubal ostia and the uterine walls, detect any pedicle and to estimate the depth of the myoma in relation to the uterine wall. If more than half of the myoma protrudes into the endometrial cavity, the case will be considered a submucous myoma. If the intramural part is more than the intracavitary part, the case will be considered an intramural myoma (type II).

Modified resectoscopic technique starts 8 hours prior to the time of surgery by inserting 200 µg misoprostol intravaginally to allow softening of the cervical canal and the myoma itself. The resectoscope is used to make a deep circumferential incision all around the base of the myoma (figure 7) until complete separation occurs and the myoma became completely free inside the endometrial cavity.

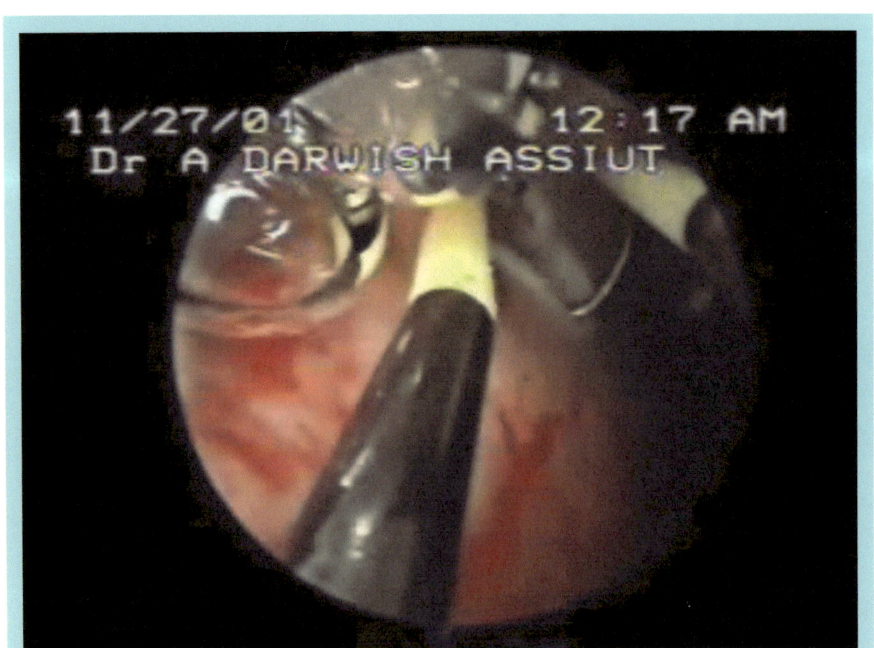

Fig. 7. Circumferential incicion.

This crucial step required changing the angle of the loop electrode into 15 degrees below the horizontal plane to allow easy access to the base. Cutting is made 3-4 mm from the base towards the myoma side to preserve some healthy endometrium for postoperative creeping to cover the row area of the myoma. A specially designed 2 mm myoma driller simulating the laparoscopic myoma driller is introduced alongside the resectoscope under vision. It is a stainless steel wire with a terminal screw. This driller (figure 8) is used to tract the myoma at one side of the endometrial cavity to have an easy access to the base.

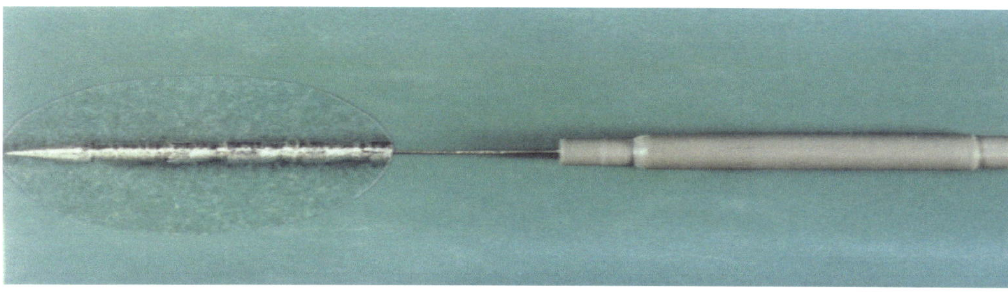

Fig. 8. Hysteroscopic myoma driller

This step is followed by extraction of the whole myoma through the primed cervical canal using a ring forceps. If some difficulty is encountered, the myoma is longitudinally bisected into 2 parts using resectoscopic knife electrode prior to extraction.
If an intramural extension is diagnosed, the following additional steps are done. A vertical linear incision is made over the whole length of the myoma to allow bulging of the myoma into the endometrial cavity i.e. to become a more submucous myoma like opening of the capsule at open myomectomy. IV injection of diluted 0.25 mg ergometrine is given by the anesthiologist to promote uterine contraction in this non-pregnant uterus and to reduce the vascularity. Moreover, minimization of the intrauterine pressure is done to allow most of the myoma to become intracavitary "Myoma shift" as previously described. The base of the myoma is circumfrentially cut with resectoscope using the former mechanical technique.

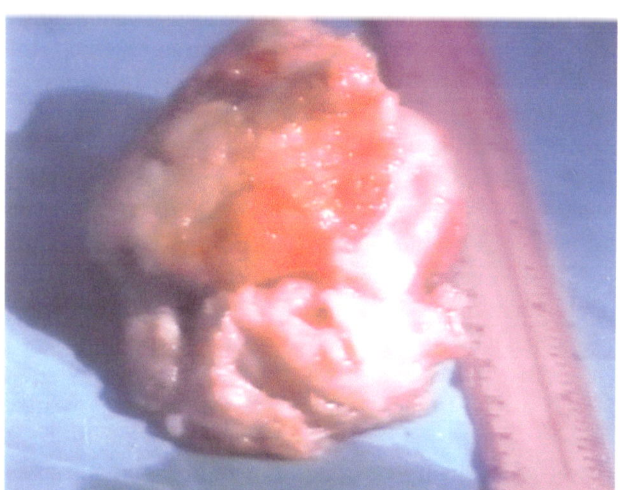

Fig. 9. Postmyomectomy tissue assessment.

The resectoscope is reinserted after extraction of the myoma to ensure complete excision. Operative hysteroscopy is performed using continuous-flow resectoscope after cervical dilatation up to Hegar's 10 utilizing 1.5% glycine as a distending medium. Operative notes should include comment on the feasibility of the operation, operating time calculated from the starting myomectomy until complete extraction of all tissues from the endometrial cavity, amount of fluid used for distending the uterine cavity, possible intraoperative or postoperative complications, and the amount of postoperative blood loss estimated by insertion of an intrauterine balloon at the end of the procedure. All the extracted tissues are evaluated (figure 9). Prophylactic antibiotics are prescribed for all cases.

5.5 Postoperative care

No need for hormonal treatment at all. Sometimes, an intrauterine balloon is left inside the endometrial cavity to control excessive bleeding from the bed of the myoma.

5.6 Limitations of reconstructive HM

It is the most dangerous hysteroscopic procedure due to possible excessive bleeding, prolonged time consumed for cutting the myoma into chips of tissues and their extraction outside the uterine cavity, the risks of fluid overload, possibility of incomplete resection, and liability to perforation. (71). Moreover, there are some studies concerned with the risk of uterine rupture in the subsequent pregnancy (72,73). Most of complications of HM are encountered with large sized myomas, or those with intramural extension (grade 1 or 2 according to the European Society of Hysteroscopy classification). They represent definite nightmare for hysteroscopists even with sufficient experience to the extent that some studies preferred laparoscopic approach in such cases (74). Hysteroscopically, several studies tried to facilitate one-step complete excision. In a case report, succeeful removal of myoma up to 12 cm in one session is reported (75). A modified hysteroscopic approach for big myoma with or without intramural extension has been introduced by our team (70).This technique has been cited and quoted in subsequent publications (76) and comprehensive review articles (77) on this topic. It comprised combined resectoscopic and mechanical approaches to enucleate the myoma in a shorter time with minimal complication rate if compared to the standard morcellation technique. Moreover, it demonstrated some additive perioperative steps that facilitated the procedure like preoperative usage of misoprostol based on a RCT done by our team (66), intraoperative slow IV ergometrine administration, utilization of a novel hysteroscopic myoma driller, and performing a vertical incision on top of deeply impacted intramural myomata. If compared to a study on 44 cases published in the same year (78), the difference would be clear. They performed only circumferential incision at the level of myoma base followed by morcellation technique. They succeeded to perform this procedure in 41 (93. 1%) of 44 women. Of these, 38 (92.6%) had myomas between 2 and 4 cm in diameter and 3 (7.4%) had myomas exceeding 4 cm. Mean operating time is 27 minutes (range 10-45 min). It seems very risky to perform morcellation of a big myoma with high possibility of fluid overload that would obligate the hysteroscopist to stop the procedure based on the recommendation of the anaesthesia team. As a trial to alleviate this risk, one case report is recently published utilizing our previously recommended basal circumferential incision followed by central vaporization, and intraoperative injection of prostaglandin F2alpha (76). Likewise, laser HM guided by laparoscopically assisted intra-abdominal sonohysterography (LHMY-GLAIS) is described in a preliminary study (79).

All these trials would be expected to open the door for more ideas on HM for myomata of considerable size. In this context, innovation of alternative hysteroscopically-guided devices would be promising. Moreover, studies on bipolar resectoscopic myomectomy utilizing saline 0.9% should be encouraged.

5.7 Complications of HM (65)

Complications of hysteroscopic myoma resection include hemorrhage, uterine perforation, damage to the cervix, and excessive absorption of the distention media (usually glycine) into the vascular system, which can cause metabolic disturbances. The most serious potential complication with hysteroscopic myomectomy is excessive absorption of distension media, which can cause pulmonary edema, hyponatremia, cerebral edema, and even death. This is especially true when using nonconducting distension solution with monopolar cautery. A surgeon should also be cautious with saline during resections with bipolar cautery since large volumes of fluid can lead to overload complications. A fluid management system that can accurately calculate the amount of absorbed fluid by measuring the inflow and outflow of distension fluid should be used. Intracervical injection of dilute vasopressin, in addition to reducing the force needed to dilate the cervix, has also been shown to decrease the absorption of distention fluid. In 1991, Corson and Brooks noted 1 case of heavy bleeding that required transfusion and 3 uterine perforations out of 92 patients undergoing hysteroscopic myoma resection. In 1993, Indman noted distension media complications in 2 of 51 women. Intrauterine synechiae can also occur after hysteroscopic myoma resection.

5.8 Impact on the reproductive health

Many studies have assessed fertility rates after hysteroscopic myomectomy and have noted pregnancy rates similar to those after abdominal myomectomy, approximately 60% Again, no studies include expectantly managed control groups (65).

5.9 Poorly evidenced endoscopic myomectomy

Laparoscopically-assisted transvaginal myomectomy has been described for posterior and fundal myomas where a posterior colpotomy is done to allow delivery of myomata and the uterus as well. Uterine reconstruction is then performed by conventional suturing performed transvaginally. The uterus is then replaced into its anatomical position and colpotomy is repaired. A final laparoscopic survey and lavage is performed (80,81). Colposcopic myomectomy is first described by Baggish in 1990s. Thereafter, two case reports with cervical fibroids underwent laser CO_2 excision under colposcopic guidance (82).

5.10 Endoscopic myomectomy prior to IVF/ICSI

The impact of uterine myoma on the outcome of IVF/ICSI is a very controversial topic. Many centers are overdoing myomectomy for nearly all myomata regardless size and site considerations. Contrary, other investigators have shown that fibroids don't exert a deleterious effect. Nevertheless, many studies have provided evidence that uterine myomas have a significant effect on IVF outcomes and there is a large body of evidence that treatment of uterine myomas increases fertility and pregnancy rates, and decreases the rate of pregnancy loss (83). There is no doubt that any cavity-distorting myoma should be removed whether completely submucous or interstitial myoma with submucous encroachment. This highlights the central role of prior hysteroscopy as well as saline infusion solonhysterography (SIS) as previously described (84). Controversy exists for interstitial and subserous myomata. The evidence supports treatment of all very large myomas (>7 cm) (83). Subserosal myomas that are smaller than 7 cm in size and intramural myomas of less than 4–5 cm in diameter appear to have little effect on IVF outcomes. Larger intramural and subserosal myomas present a clinical dilemma and more studies are needed to clarify a definitive plan for management (83). In a prospective controlled study, the distance between the intramural myomas and the endometrial lining did not appear to affect the IVF outcome. An insignificant tendency towards improvement of IVF outcome is found in myomas at more than 5 mm from endometrial lining (85).

6. Keynote points

Uterine myoma may affect fertility according to its size, site and associated pathology. Endoscopic approach has a definite role in its management. HM is the gold standard line of management of submucous myoma of suitable size. LM doesn't seem to be superior to conventional open myomectomy regarding fertility and is characterized by both short and long term drawbacks. Uterine myomata would affect IVF/ICSI outcome whenever disturbing the endometrial cavity or large sized. The impact of other types of myomata on IVF/ICSI deserves further studies.

7. References

[1] Atef M. Darwish. Fertility-enhancing Reconstructive Endoscopic Myomectomy in modern practice. Middle East Fertility Society Journal 2009; Vol. 14, No. 2, 25-29.

[2] Chew S, L C F. An assessment of present day laparoscopic surgery in Gynaecology. Singapore Journal of Obstetrics and Gynaecology 2001;32(1): 1-13.

[3] National Collaborating Centre for Women's and Children's Health. Fertility assessment and treatment for people with fertility problems. RCOG Press. London, 2004, Ch 7,8,9.

[4] Wiedermann R, Hepp H. Selection of patients for IVF therapy or alternative therapy methods. Hum Rep 1989.;4:23-27.

[5] Watson A, Vandekerckhove P, Lilford R. Techiques for pelvic surgery in subfertility. Cochrane Database Syst Rev 2:CD00022, 2000.

[6] Ahmad G, Watson A, Vandekerckhove P, Lilford R. Techniques for pelvic surgery in subfertility.Cochrane Database Syst Rev. 2006 Apr 19;(2):CD000221.

[7] Sauer MV. Tubal infertility. The role of reconstructive surgery. In. Lobo RA, Mishell DR, Paulson RJ, Shoupe D. Infertility, Contraception and Reproductive Endocrinology. Boston, Blackwell Scientific Publications, 4th edition, 1997,Ch 36.

[8] Bateman BG, Nunley JW, Kitchen JD. Surgical management of distal tubal occlusion-are we making progress?. Fertil Steril 1987;48;523.

[9] Gomel V, Taylor PJ (Ed). Fertility-promoting procedures and assisted reproductive technology. In. Diagnostic and Operative Gynaecologic Laparoscopy. St Louis, Mosby-Year Book, Inc., 1995,Ch 15.

[10] Koh CH. Anastomosis of the fallopian tube. In. Tulandi T. Atlas of Laparoscopic and Hysteroscopic Techniques for gynaecologists. 2nd edition, London, W.B. Saunders, 1999. Ch 7.

[11] Semm K, Mettler L. Technical progress in pelvic surgery via laparoscopy Am J Obstet Gynaecol 1980; 138:121-127.

[12] Hasson HM, Rotman C, Rana N, Sistos F, Dmowaki WP. Laparoscopic myomectomy. Obstet Gynaecol 1992; 80:884-888.

[13] Nezhat C, Nezhat F, Silfen SL, Schaffer N, Evans D. Laparoscopic myomectomy. Int J Fertil 1991; 36:275-280.

[14] Harris WJ. Uterine dehiscence following laparoscopic myomectomy. Obstet Gynecol 1992; 80:545-546.

[15] Dubuisson JB, Chavet X, Chapron C, Gregorakis SS, Morice P. Uterine rupture during pregnancy after laparoscopic myomectomy. Hum Reprod 1995; 10:1475-1477.

[16] Friedmann et al. Uterine rupture after laparoscopic Myomectomy. Acta Obstet Gynaecol Scand. 1996; 75: 683-4.

[17] Pelosi M, Pelosi MA. Spontaneous uterine rupture at thirty three weeks subsequent to previous superficial laparoscopic myomectomy. Am. J Obstet. Gynaecol. 1997; 177:1547-49.

[18] Dubuisson JB, Fauconnier A, Deffarges JV, Norgaard C, Kreiker G, Chapron C. Pregnancy outcome and deliveries following laparoscopic Myomectomy. Hum. Repro. 2000; 15: 869-73.

[19] Candiani GB, Fedele L, Parazzini, Villa L. Risks of recurrence after myomectomy. Br. J Obstet Gynaecol 1991; 98:385-389.

[20] Dubuisson JB, Lecuru F, Foulot H. Gonadotrophin-releasing hormone agonist and laparoscopic myomectomy. Clinical Therapeutics 1992; 14:51-55.

[21] Mais V, Ajossa S, Guerriero S, Mascia M, Solla E, Melis GB. Laparoscopic versus abdominal myomectomy: a prospective randomized trial to evaluate benefits in early outcome. Am J Obstet Gynaecol 1996; 174:654-658.

[22] Whittaker MD, Garry R. Patient satisfaction with laparoscopic-assisted removal of large myomas. J Am Assoc Gynaecol Laparosc 1996; 3(4,supplement):S55.

[23] Rossetti A, Sizzi O, Soranna L, Mancuso S, Lanzone A. Fertility outcome: long-term results after laparoscopic myomectomyGynaecol Endocrinol 2001;15(2):129-34.

[24] J Minim Invasive Gynecol. 2011 Jan-Feb;18(1):92-5. Epub 2010 Nov 20. Use of bidirectional barbed suture in laparoscopic myomectomy: evaluation of perioperative outcomes, safety, and efficacy. Einarsson JI, Chavan NR, Suzuki Y, Jonsdottir G, Vellinga TT, Greenberg JA.

[25] Dubuisson, J-B. and Chapron, C. (1996) Uterine fibroids: place and modalities of laparoscopic treatment. *Eur. J. Obstet. Gynecol.*, 65, 91–94.

[26] Donnez, J., Mathieu, P.E., Bassil, S. *et al.* (1996) Laparoscopic myomectomy today. Fibroids: management and treatment: the state of the art. *Hum. Reprod.*, 11, 1837–1840.

[27] Hasson, H.M., Rotman, C., Rana, N. *et al.* (1992) Laparoscopic myomectomy. *Obstet. Gynecol.*, 80, 884–888.

[28] Cittadini, E. (1998) Laparoscopic myomectomy: the Italian experience. *J. Am. Assoc. Gynecol. Laparoscop.*, 5, 7–9.

[29] Palomba S, Zupi E, Falbo, A, et al. A multicenter randomized, controlled study comparing laparoscopic versus minilaparotomic myomectomy: reproductive outcomes. *Fertility and Sterility.* Oct 2007;88:933-941. [Medline].

[30] Di Spiezio Sardo A, Mazzon I, Bramante S, et al. Hysteroscopic myomectomy: a comprehensive review of surgical techniques. *Hum Reprod Update*. Mar-Apr 2008;14:101-19.

[31] Minim Invasive Ther Allied Technol. 2011 Jan 19. Laparoscopic myomectomy in patients with uterine myomas associated with infertility. Hackethal A, Westermann A, Tchartchian G, Oehmke F, Tinneberg HR, Muenstedt K, Bojahr B

[32] Zullo F, Pellicano M, De Stefano R, et al. A prospective randomized study to evaluate leuprolide acetate treatment before laparoscopic myomectomy: efficacy and ultrasonographic predictors. *Am J Obstet Gynecol*. Jan 1998;178(1 Pt 1):108-12.

[33] Felberbaum RE, Küpker W, Krapp M, Gehl B, Ludwig M, Diedrich K.Preoperative reduction of uterine fibroids in only 16 days by administration of a gonadotrophin-releasing hormone antagonist (Cetrotide). Reprod Biomed Online. 2001;3(1):14-18

[34] Campo S, Garcea N. Laparoscopic myomectomy in premenopausal women with and without preoperative treatment using gonadoptropin-releasing hormone analogs. *Human Reproduction*. Jan 1999;14:44-48.

[35] Einarsson JI, Chavan NR, Suzuki Y, Jonsdottir G, Vellinga TT, Greenberg JA. Use of bidirectional barbed suture in laparoscopic myomectomy: evaluation of perioperative outcomes, safety, and efficacy. J Minim Invasive Gynecol. 2011 Jan-Feb;18(1):92-5.

[36] Zhao F, Jiao Y, Guo Z, Hou R, Wang M. Evaluation of loop ligation of larger myoma pseudocapsule combined with vasopressin on laparoscopic myomectomy. Fertil Steril. 2011 Feb;95(2):762-6.

[37] Chen SY, Huang SC, Sheu BC, Chang DY, Chou LY, Hsu WC, Chang WC. Simultaneous enucleation and in situ morcellation of myomas in laparoscopic myomectomy. Taiwan J Obstet Gynecol. 2010 Sep;49(3):279-84.

[38] Golan A, Sandbank O, Rubin A. Rupture of the pregnant uterus. Obstet Gynaecol 1980;56:549-54.

[39] Pelerme GR, Friedman EA. Rupture of the gravid uterus in the third trimester. Am J Obstet Gynaecol 1996;94:571.

[40] Acrangeli S, Pasquarette MM. Gravid uterine rupture after myolysis. Obstet Gynaeco. 1997;89:857

[41] Banas T, Klimek M, Fugiel A, Skotniczny KSpontaneous uterine rupture at 35 weeks' gestation, 3 years after laparoscopic myomectomy, without signs of fetal distress Journal of Obstetrics and Gynaecology Research 2005; 31 (6), 527–530.

[42] Tulandi T, Al-Took S. Endoscopic myomectomy. Laparoscopy and Hysteroscopy. Obstet Gynaecol Clin North Am 1999; 26(1):135-48

[43] Nezhat HC, Nezhat F, Rroemisch M, Seidman DS, Tazuke SI, Nezhat CR Pregnancy following laparoscopic myomectomy: preliminary results. Hum Reprod 1999;14(5):1219-21

[44] Nezhat C, Nezhat F, Bess O, Nezhat CH, Mashiach R. Laparoscopically assisted myomectomy: a report of a new technique in 57 cases. Int J Fertil 1994;39:39-44.

[45] Ostrazenski A: Extensive iatrogenic adenomyosis after laparoscopic myomectomy. Fertil Steril 1998;69(1):143-5.

[46] Garnet J D. Uterine rupture during pregnancy. Obstet Gynaecol 1964; 23:898-902.

[47] Nair S. Contemporary Management of Fibroids. Ann Acad Med Singapore 2003; 32:615-23.

[48] Dubuisson JB, Fauconnier A, Chapron C, Kreiker G,Norgaard C. Second look after laparoscopic myomectomy. Human Reprod 1998;13(8):2102-6.
[49] Bulletti C, Polli V, Glacomucci ,Flamigni C Adhesion formation after laparoscopic myomectomy J Am Gynaecol Laparosc 1996;3(4): 533-6.
[50] Griffiths A, D'Angelo A, Amso N. Surgical treatment of fibroids for subfertility.Cochrane Database Syst Rev. 2006 Jul 19;3:CD003857. Review.
[51] Pun TC, Chau MT, Lam C, Tang G, Leong L. Sonographic evaluation of myomectomy 'scars.' Acta Obstet Gynaecol Scand 1998;77:218.
[52] Keckstein J, Karageorgieva E, Darwish A, Grab D, Paulus W, Tuttlies F. Laparoscopic Myomectomy: Sonographic Follow-Up and Second-Look Laparoscopy for the Evaluation of a New Technique J Am Assoc Gynecol Laparosc. 1994;1(4, Part 2):S16.
[53] Darwish AM, Nasr AM, El-Nashar DA. Evaluation of postmyomectomy uterine scar. J Clin Ultrasound. 2005;26;33(4):181-186.
[54] Seracchioli R, Rossi S, Govoni F, et al. Fertility and obstetric outcome after laparoscopic myomectomy of large myomata: a randomized comparison with abdominal myomectomy. *Hum Reprod.* Dec 2000;15(12):2663-8.
[55] Alessandri F, Lijoi D, Mistrangelo E, et al. Randomized study of laparoscopic versus minilaparotomic myomectomy for uterine myomas. *The Journal of Minimally Invasive Gynecology.* Mar-Apr 2006;13:92-97.
[56] Buttram VC Jr, Reiter RC. Uterine leiomyomata: etiology, symptomatology, and management. Fertil Steril 1981;36:433–45.
[57] Verkauf BS. Myomectomy for fertility enhancement and preservation. Fertil Steril 1992;58:1–15.
[58] Pritts EA. Fibroids and infertility: a systematic review of the evidence. Obstet Gynecol Surv 2001;56:483–91.
[59] Varasteh NN, Neuwirth RS, Brucelevin, Keltz MD. Pregnancy Rates After Hysteroscopic Polypectomy and Myomectomy in Infertile Women. Obstetrics & Gynecology 1999;94:168-171.
[60] McLucas B: Intrauterine applications of the resectoscope. Sur Gynecol Obstet 1991; 172(6):425-430.
[61] Sardo AD, Mazzon I, Bramante S, Bettocchi S, Bifulco G,Guida M, Nappi C HM: a comprehensive review of surgical techniques. Human Reproduction Update 2008; 14(2):101-119.
[62] Pasini A, Belloni C: Intraoperative complications of 697 consecutive operative hysteroscopies. Minerva Ginecol 2001;53(1):13-20.
[63] Hamou J: Electroresection of fibroids. In Endoscopic Surgery for Gynaecologists. Ed by Sutton C and Diamond M. London. Sauhders Co LTD, 1993, Ch41.
[64] Cohen LS, Valle RF. Role of vaginal sonography and hysterosonography in the endoscopic treatment of uterine myomas. *Fertil Steril.* Feb 2000;73:197-204
[65] Marquard KL, Chelmow D. Gynecologic Myomectomy. E Medicine. Aug 6, 2008
[66] Darwish AM, Ahmad AM, Mohammad AM. Cervical priming prior to operative hysteroscopy: a randomized comparison of laminaria versus misoprostol. Hum Reprod 2004; 19(10):2391-2394.
[67] Indman PD. Hysteroscopic treatment of submucous myomas. *Clin Obstet Bynecol.* Dec 2006;49:811-20.

[68] Murakami T, Tachibana M, Hoshiai T, et al. Successful strategy for the hysteroscopic myomectomy of a submucous myoma arising from the uterine fundus. *Fertil Steril.* Nov 2006;86:1513.e19-22. [Medline].

[69] Loffer FD. Removal of large symptomatic intrauterine growths by the hysteroscopic resectoscope. *Obstet Gynecol.* Nov 1990;76:836-40

[70] Darwish A. Modified HM of large submucous fibroids. Gynecol Obstet Invest. 2003;56(4):192-6.

[71] Pasini A, Belloni C: Intraoperative complications of 697 consecutive operative hysteroscopies. Minerva Ginecol 2001;53(1):13-20.

[72] Hamou J: Electroresection of fibroids. In Endoscopic Surgery for Gynaecologists. Ed by Sutton C and Diamond M. London. Sauhders Co LTD, 1993, Ch41.

[73] Stamatellos I, Bontis J. The chance of success decreases whenever an intramural element is present hysteroscopic myomectomy European Clinics in Obstetrics and Gynaecology 2007;1,17-23.

[74] Wang CJ, Soong YK, Lee CL Laparoscopic myomectomy for large intramural and submucous fibroids. Int J Gynaecol Obstet. 2007;97(3):206-7.

[75] Kriplani A, Singh BM, Meena S. One-step hysteroscopic myomectomy: unusual cases and a review of the literature. J Laparoendosc Adv Surg Tech A. 2004;14(6):390-4.

[76] Murakami T, Tachibana M, Hoshiai T, Ozawa Y , Terada Y, Okamura K. Successful strategy for the HM of a submucous myoma arising from the uterine fundus. Fertil Steril. 2006; 86,5,1513.e19-22.

[77] Sardo AD, Mazzon I, Bramante S, Bettocchi S, Bifulco G,Guida M, Nappi C HM: a comprehensive review of surgical techniques. Human Reproduction Update 2008; 14(2):101-119.

[78] Litta P, Vasile C, Merlin F, Pozzan C, Sacco G, Gravila P, Stellia C. A new technique of HM with enucleation in Toto. The Journal of the American Association of Gynecologic Laparoscopists 2003;10,2;263-270.

[79] Kaseki H, Araki T, Valle R. Laser HM guided by laparoscopically assisted intra-abdominal sonohysterography (LHMY-GLAIS): a preliminary report. Journal of Gynecologic Surgery 2001; 17(3): 79-86.

[80] Pelosi MA 3rd, Pelosi MA.Laparoscopic-assisted transvaginal myomectomy. J Am Assoc Gynecol Laparosc. 1997 Feb;4(2):241-6.

[81] Wang CJ, Yen CF, Lee CL, Soong YK. .Laparoscopic-assisted vaginal myomectomy. J Am Assoc Gynecol Laparosc. 2000 Nov;7(4):510-4.

[82] Penna C, Fallani MG, Fambrini M, Galassi D, Basile V, Marchionni M. Cervical myomectomy by laser CO2. Report of two cases. Minerva Ginecol. 2002;54(5):435-8.

[83] Bromer JG, Arici A. Impact of uterine myomas on IVF outcome. Expert Review of Obstetrics & Gynecology 2008;3, 4,515-521.

[84] Darwish AM, Youssef AA. Screening sonohysterography in infertility. Gynecol Obstet Invest. 1999;48(1):43-7.

[85] Aboulghar, M.M., Al-Inany, H.G., Aboulghar, M.A., Serour, G.I., Mansour, R.T. Effect of myomectomy on the outcome of assisted reproductive technologies Middle East Fertility Society Journal 2004; 9 (3), 263-267.

Part 8

Endometriosis

12

Laparoscopy for Diagnosis and Treatment of Endometriosis

Moamar Al-Jefout
Department of Obstetrics & Gynecology, Mutah Medical Faculty, Mutah University, Jordan

1. Introduction

Endometriosis is defined as the presence of endometrial like stroma and glands outside the uterine cavity (Giudice and Kao, 2004). Laparoscopy has been recognized as the gold standard for endometriosis diagnosis and has been used for the surgical treatment of endometriosis. Diagnosis of endometriosis is currently made following laparoscopic inspection of the pelvis, preferably with histological biopsy confirmation (Mettler et al., 2003), although the correlation of biopsy with visual inspection depends on the experience of the endoscopist, inter-observer variability, the technique of excision and the care and experience of the pathologist (Poncelet and Ducarme, 2007). In one recent study, only 67% of lesions identified at laparoscopy as possible endometriosis proved to have the histological features of endometriosis (Stratton et al., 2003). Moreover, visual inspection of the pelvis also has its own limitations, particularly for the diagnosis of atypical and non-peritoneal endometriosis.

Endometriotic lesions can vary in colour, mostly non-black, red, white or like burned powder. In clinical observation the age of a lesion can be estimated from the colour of these lesions. It appears that clear papules are limited to a younger age group (17-31 years), than the red (16-43 years) and black (20-52 years) lesions (Redwine, 1987).

Many studies have clearly shown that there is a substantial delay in endometriosis diagnosis which inevitably has negative effect on quality of life of endometriosis patients (Matsuzaki et al., 2006, Hadfield et al., 1996, Zrubek et al., 1999, Ballard et al., 2006, Stratton, 2006). Ballard et al. demonstrate that the definitive diagnosis of endometriosis is frequently delayed for many years (2006). In a series of patients from southeastern England the mean delay from onset of symptoms to definitive diagnosis was 102 months (9.5 years). Delays usually occurred at every stage in the diagnostic process. An average patient waited for 18 months before been seen by a family doctor. The general practitioner subsequently waited 3 years before referring the patient for a specialized opinion by a gynaecologist, and it takes a further 9 months before the diagnosis is made. This delay is even longer in cases with deep infiltrating endometriosis and advanced endometriosis stage IV (Matsuzaki et al., 2006).

The review by Wykes, C. B showed that there are very few good quality studies in the literature regarding the role of laparoscopy in the diagnosis of endometriosis (Wykes et al., 2004). A negative laparoscopy for endometriosis is helpful and women can be adequately reassured without the need for further testing, while a positive laparoscopy is less informative without histological confirmation. A false positive laparoscopy can hugely affect the woman's quality of life, perception of her own health, fertility and even sexual life.

The aim of surgical management is to remove visible areas of endometriosis and restore anatomy by division of adhesions. Yet, treatment frequently must be individualized. However, distinguishing patients who need no treatment from patients who need intermediate or extensive treatment can be difficult. There are three recognized types of endometriosis: peritoneal endometriosis, ovarian endometriomas and deep adenomyotic nodules of the rectovaginal septum (Nisolle and Donnez, 1997).

Few principles have to be considered regarding the surgical management of endometriosis:

- Severe disease must be treated differently from mild to moderate disease.
- Patients with pain symptoms associated with endometriosis must be approached differently from patients seeking fertility.
- Clinicians and patients should be aware that the expected benefit is depending on operator skills (Vercellini et al., 2009).

Jansen and Russell have shown that peritoneum which looks completely normal does not contain histological features of endometriosis, therefore excision of all abnormally looking peritoneum , deep nodules and ovarian lesions should remove the disease (1986). Yet a downside of this approach is the risk for future adhesion formation.

2. Background

Endometriosis is a common and frequently chronic disease, characterized by the presence of endometrial like-glands and stroma outside the uterine cavity. Endometriosis is still an enigmatic disease as it is still represent itself as a big challenge for patients to coup with the disease and for medical professionals dealing with this category of patients. The challenge is primarily in the diagnostic process of endometriosis as it's clinical features may cross with the clinical features of other conditions such as adenomyosis, interstitial cystitis and irritable bowel syndrome. Another problem with endometriosis diagnosis is the general normalization of pain symptoms by. Moreover, there yet no diagnostic tool with significantly enough specificity and sensitivity for the diagnosis. may be difficult to diagnose, yet may cause considerable distress with pelvic pain and infertility. However, some women will be completely asymptomatic although, having severe stage of the disease incidentally found during laparoscopy for other reasons. Laparoscopy with or without histological confirmation is the gold standard for endometriosis diagnosis. However, there is often a considerable delay in diagnosis of endometriosis, partly because there is no simple tool for effective diagnosis. For many decades, surgical removal of endometriotic lesions was the primary basis for the management of endometriosis and radical removal of ectopic lesions is still the preferred way for most surgeons when dealing with endometriosis (Redwine et al., 2000). However, there is no correlation between findings at laparoscopy and symptoms and prognosis in terms of fertility and recurrence rate (Vercellini et al., 2006). It seems to be that the patient's own preference and plans for her fertility are becoming more important in controlling the management plans (Vercellini et al., 2003).

Medical treatment for endometriosis is mainly for pain symptoms, while medical treatment for infertility purposes has no benefit or may even delay pregnancy, 'more harm than good can be done by drug treatment, because of side effects and the lost opportunity to conceive' (RCOG, 2000). It seems to be that a combined medical and conservative surgical approach is beneficial for most women with endometriosis associated pelvic pain (Davis and McMillan, 2003). Moreover, evidence showed that laparoscopic surgery in terms of excision and or ablation of mild to moderate disease can in fact enhance fertility (Marcoux et al., 1997, Olive and Pritts, 2002). However, an Italian RCT showed that ablation of endometriotic lesions did not markedly improves fertility rates (Parazzini, 1999).

3. Anatomy of the anterior abdominal wall related to laparoscopic surgery for endometriosis

Any surgeon intending to perform laparoscopic surgery for endometriosis must have a complete understanding and a thorough knowledge of the anterior abdominal wall vascular anatomy. This knowledge will reduce vascular complications associated with laparoscopy especially trocar placement. Of particular concern are the superior and inferior epigastric vessels. The superior epigastric artery, one of the terminal branches of the internal thoracic artery, enters the rectus sheath first and then the rectus muscle coursing near its lateral border. This artery and its adjacent vein often can be visualized by transillumination of the abdominal wall with the laparoscope.

Visualization of the ventral abdominal wall laparoscopically will often locate the deep inferior epigastric vessels. The artery, a branch of the external iliac, and its accompanying vein course along the abdominal wall peritoneum just lateral to the rectus muscle until midway between the symphysis pubis and umbilicus, where it blends into the body of the rectus muscle. These vessels may be seen medial to the insertion of the round ligament at the deep inguinal ring. Therefore, placement of the trocar lateral to the deep inguinal ring and lateral border of the rectus muscle will avoid injury to these vessels.

If placement of the trocar is too far laterally, branches of the superficial circumflex iliac vessels may be injured. Again, transillumination of the anterior abdominal wall by using the laparoscope will assist in avoiding these vessels.

As a general guideline, the superficial and inferior epigastric vessels are located approximately 5.5 cm from the midline. The superficial circumflex iliac vessels are approximately 7 cm from the midline. Theoretically, a "safe area" would be 8 cm above the symphysis pubis and 8 cm from the midline. If transillumination is not effective due to a thick abdominal wall, the surgeon may consider insertion of a spinal needle through the abdominal wall at the selected trocar insertion site. If no bleeding is observed after removal of the needle, the location is likely safe for trocar placement.

4. Delay in diagnosis of endometriosis

Many studies have clearly shown that there is a substantial delay in endometriosis diagnosis which inevitably has negative effect on quality of life of endometriosis patients (Matsuzaki et al., 2006, Hadfield et al., 1996, Zrubek et al., 1999, Ballard et al., 2006, Stratton, 2006). Ballard et al. demonstrate that the definitive diagnosis of endometriosis is frequently delayed for many years (2006). In a series of patients from southeastern England the mean delay from onset of symptoms to definitive diagnosis was 102 months (9.5 years). Delays usually occurred at every stage in the diagnostic process. An average patient waited for 18 months before been seen by a family doctor. The general practitioner subsequently waited 3 years before referring the patient for a specialized opinion by a gynaecologist, and it takes a further 9 months before the diagnosis is made. This delay is even longer in cases with deep infiltrating endometriosis and advanced endometriosis stage IV (Matsuzaki et al., 2006).

The fundamental question about such delays is whether they matter. The work of Ballard et al. suggests that they do. The absence of a specific diagnosis left patients fearful of what was wrong with them and unable to communicate about their problems to others, particularly their employers. Learning of the correct diagnosis was associated with positive experiences in terms of reassurance about the absence of more sinister problems and in improving access to social support and accurately tailored treatment.

An open, mutually understanding relationship between doctor and patient is necessary if the diagnosis is to be made without undue delay (Kennedy, 1991) thus improving the chances of getting better results in treatment and compliance.

5. Laparoscopy as the gold standard for the diagnosis of endometriosis

5.1 Laparoscopy as gold standard

Laparoscopy (figure 2) in endometriosis is based on the visualization of superficial implants, endometriomas, adhesion distribution, bowel disease and ureteric disease. In doubtful cases, biopsies showing glands and stroma have been the basis of the diagnosis. Endometriotic lesions can vary in colour, mostly non-black, red, white or like burned powder. In clinical observation the age of a lesion can be estimated from the colour. It appears that clear papules are limited to a younger age group (17-31 years), than the red (16-43 years) and black (20-52 years) lesions (Redwine, 1987).

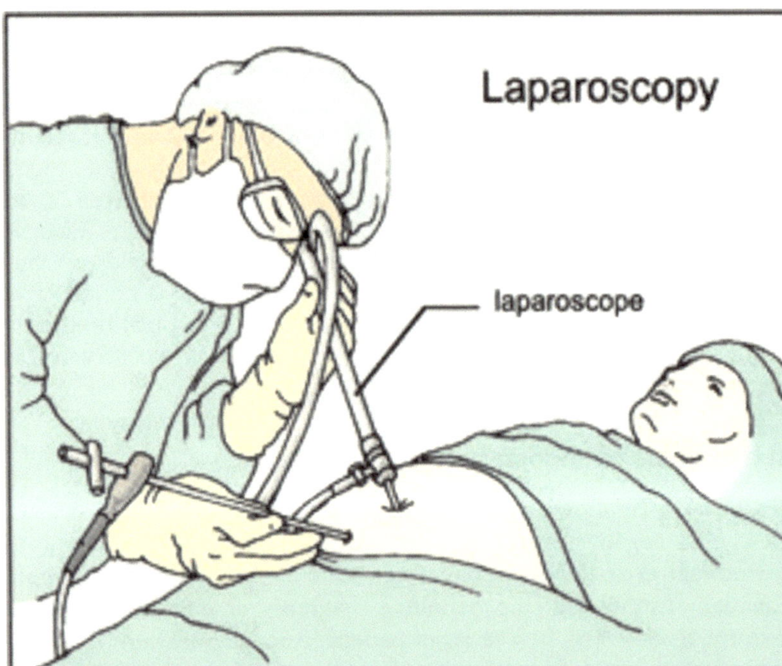

Fig. 1. Laparosocpy

In some cases asymptomatic women endometrial implants have been found in biopsies from normal peritoneum, resulting in the suggestion that mild endometriosis is not a disease and that all women have this mild form of endometriosis (Koninckx, 1994, Evers, 1994).

In the years 1994-1996 378,100 women with pelvic/abdominal pain underwent ambulatory diagnostic laparoscopy for pelvic pain. This figure excluded women undergoing laparoscopy as an in-patient procedure and represents 34% of the 1.1 million diagnostic laparoscopies performed in the U.S. during that period (Natuzzi et al., 1993).

One-third of all diagnostic laparoscopies revealed endometriosis, one-third revealed no visible pathology, and the remaining one-third demonstrated a variety of other gynecologic conditions (Howard, 1993). Thus, two-thirds of all patients who undergo this invasive diagnostic procedure will not have endometriosis. To avoid false negative endometriotic lesion biopsy a multiple biopsy approach was proposed (Kazanegra et al., 2008).

The review by Wykes, C. B showed that there are very few good quality studies in the literature regarding the role of laparoscopy in the diagnosis of endometriosis (Wykes et al., 2004). A negative laparoscopy for endometriosis is helpful and women can be adequately reassured without the need for further testing, while a positive laparoscopy is less informative without histological confirmation (Wykes et al., 2004). A false positive laparoscopy can hugely affect the woman's quality of life, perception of her own health, fertility and even sexual life. Recently other diagnostic tools been proposed for the diagnosis of endometriosis such as blood markers and most recently an endometrial biopsy looking for nerve fibres in the functional layers been proposed (Al-Jefout et al., 2007, Al-Jefout et al., 2009), however, more studies are needed for further confirmation.

5.2 Risks of laparoscopy

As an invasive surgical procedure, laparoscopy still carries occasional risks of injuring vessels, ureter or intestine. An estimated risk of death of 0.1/1000 mainly due to vascular injuries and the risk of injury to bowel, bladder, or blood vessel of 2.4%, of whom two-thirds will require a laparotomy and this concern is still a significant contributor to the delay in diagnosis (Hadfield et al., 1996, Arruda et al., 2003, Brosens et al., 2003, Ballard et al., 2006, Schenken, 2006).

5.3 Laparoscopic conscious pain mapping

Laparoscopic conscious pain mapping was first described when it was used for laparoscopic evaluation of the appendix(Almeida et al., 1998). Pelvic pain mapping during laparoscopy performed under conscious sedation can provide useful information about visceral and somatic sources of chronic pelvic pain (Steege, 1998). Conscious laparoscopic pain mapping has been proposed as a way to improve information derived from laparoscopic evaluations in gynaecology even in an office set up (Howard, 2000, Almeida and Val-Gallas, 1998, Howard, 2003). Conscious pain mapping can be done with reasonable success in women with prior surgical evaluations and treatments for chronic pelvic pain. Chronic visceral pain syndrome, adhesions, and endometriosis were the most common diagnoses (Howard et al., 2000) Although, long term results needs to be verified in larger scale studies(Tytherleigh et al., 2004).

5.4 Transvaginal hydrolaparoscopy (THL)

In order to avoid the risks accompanied with laparoscopy a new diagnostic procedure trans-vaginal hydro-laparoscopy (Figure 2) has been proposed as an office based procedure (Gordts et al., 2000, Campo et al., 1999). Because it is done under local anaesthetic; the risks of general anaesthesia are avoided. The use of saline for visualization gives surgeons more sensitivity for identifying adhesions (Brosens et al., 1999). Use of this technology resulted in a 50% increase in finding peri-ovarian adhesions in comparison with conventional laparoscopy. THL also gives the surgeons and the patients more options in planning future treatment plans.

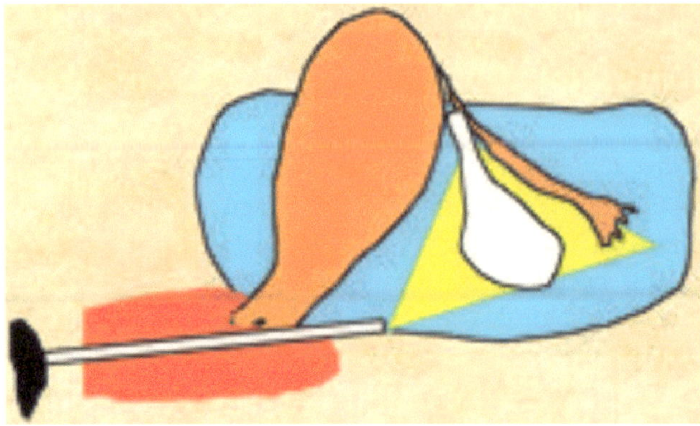

Fig. 2. Hydrolaparosocpy

6. Laparoscopy for the staging of endometriosis

6.1 Historical background of endometriosis classification

Wicks and Larson proposed the first classification of endometriosis (1949) which was based on pathological and histological examination of the endometriotic lesions. The next step was a proposed system based on macroscopic evidence of the disease (Huffman, 1951). However, this staging system did not include adhesions. The next staging system included the adhesions and for the first time guidelines were proposed to determine which patients should be treated medically and which ones surgically (Riva et al., 1962). Beecham suggested a new classification which recorded the medical data of patients(1966). It was not until 1973 that the first acceptable classification appeared and was known as the Acosta classification (Acosta et al., 1973). It was the first classification to take into account the size of the lesions, scarring and fibrosis around the implants, as well as all adhesions. However, this system did not clarifys if the lesions were uni- or bilateral and did not provide any prognosis about recurrence.

6.2 The perfect classification, is there such a thing?

Endometriosis is one of the most studied diseases in gynaecology, yet the mechanisms underlying the development of endometriosis are not understood. Nor is there understanding of the relationship between the clinical picture in terms of infertility and pain symptoms with the extent of the disease. Despite numerous clinical studies and intensive research, there are still no convincing answers to these questions and probably will not be for many years to come. The perfect classification should give clinicians the ability to correctly anticipate the prognosis for conception, relief of pelvic pain and the risk of recurrence. A perfect classification should also use common medical terminology, which clinicians from all over the world can interpret in the same way.

7. The reivised american society of reproductive medicine (rASRM) previously (rAFS)

The American fertility Society proposed a new classification which was at that time simple and the most informative (1979). Now a widely used classification of endometriosis (renamed as the revised American Society for Reproductive Medicine (rASRM) (Figure 1)

includes number, size and location of endometrial implants, endometriomas and if present adhesions. It is based (1) on the appearance, size, and depth of peritoneal and ovarian implants; (2) on the presence, extent and type of lesions: red (red, red-pink, and clear), white (white, yellow-brown, and peritoneal defects) and black (black and blue); (3) on the presence, extent, and type of adnexal adhesions and the degree of cul-de-sac obliteration. This helped to establish the stage of the disease as Stage I(minimal disease), Stage II (Mild disease), Stage III (Moderate disease) and Stage IV (Severe disease.
In a following meeting of the AFS this classification was revised after some comments from many experts and now it is widely for in the diagnosisof endometriosis (1985).

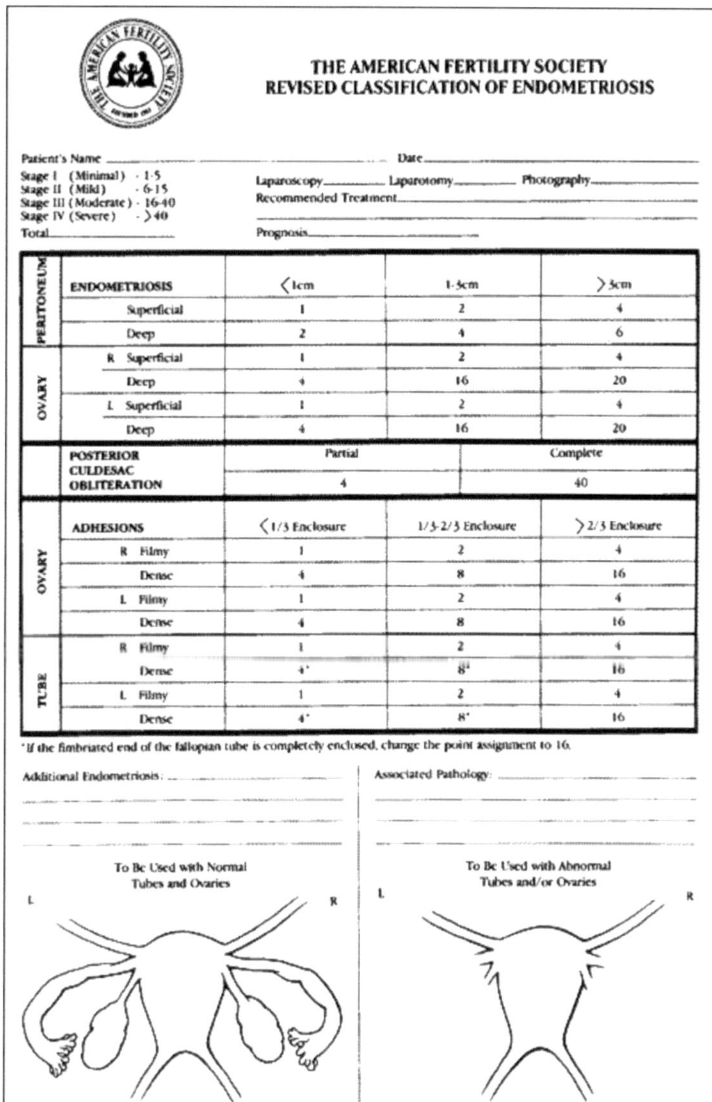

THE AMERICAN FERTILITY SOCIETY
REVISED CLASSIFICATION OF ENDOMETRIOSIS

Patient's Name ________ Date ________

Stage I (Minimal) - 1-5
Stage II (Mild) - 6-15
Stage III (Moderate) - 16-40
Stage IV (Severe) - >40
Total ________

Laparoscopy ________ Laparotomy ________ Photography ________
Recommended Treatment ________
Prognosis ________

PERITONEUM	ENDOMETRIOSIS	<1cm	1-3cm	>3cm
	Superficial	1	2	4
	Deep	2	4	6
OVARY	R Superficial	1	2	4
	Deep	4	16	20
	L Superficial	1	2	4
	Deep	4	16	20
	POSTERIOR CULDESAC OBLITERATION	Partial		Complete
		4		40
OVARY	ADHESIONS	<1/3 Enclosure	1/3-2/3 Enclosure	>2/3 Enclosure
	R Filmy	1	2	4
	Dense	4	8	16
	L Filmy	1	2	4
	Dense	4	8	16
TUBE	R Filmy	1	2	4
	Dense	4*	8*	16
	L Filmy	1	2	4
	Dense	4*	8*	16

*If the fimbriated end of the fallopian tube is completely enclosed, change the point assignment to 16.

Additional Endometriosis: ________ Associated Pathology: ________

Fig. 3. Revised classification of endometriosis according to American Society for Reproductive Medicine.

7.1 Advantages of rASRM

The rASRM requires thorough description of the lesions and their extent, so in order to complete the classification form clinicians need to be thorough in their inspection of the abdominal cavity, thus enabling them to decrease false positive results at laparoscopies. Finally, this system can be used electronically to analyse the data later on

7.2 Disadvantages of rASRM

The American Fertility Society classification does not reflect the intensity of endometriosis-associated symptoms, probably underestimating the most active forms of this disease, and does not facilitate tracking the likely natural progression of the disease (Marana et al., 1991).

7.2.1 The ENZIAN-Score

German Authors tried to substitute the rASRM by the ENZIAN-Score which was proposed as a new system to stage and classify deep infiltrating endometriosis. The endometriotic nodules are assigned to different subgroups depending on their localization and expansion. The authors of this system claimed that the still used r ASRM (rAFS)-score is of no clinical significance especially in patients with severe intestinal endometriosis (Tuttlies et al., 2005).

7.3 Peritoneal endometriosis surgical management

7.3.1 Minimal or mild disease

The severity of pain symptoms in minimal disease are found not to be correlated with findings at laparoscopy (Chene et al., 2008). Surgical approaches like resection of peritoneal endometriosis; or monopolar electrocoagulation/ablation may be used. In the early stages, surgical treatment seems to reduce pain symptoms as effective as by drug therapy (Boing and Kimmig, 2007, Golfier and Sabra, 2007, Frishman and Salak, 2006). In the resection technique the peritoneum is incised near the lesion using a monopolar electrode and is dissected bluntly, separating healthy tissue from endometriotic tissue. Resection seems to be more efficient than diathermy coagulation, yet, it is more difficult, increases the time of the operation, and the cost (Martin and O'Conner, 2003). Monopolar electrocoagulation is done by applying a monopolar electrode to the visible endometriotic lesion. Extra care must be taken when treating the lateral pelvic side wall to avoid thermal damage to the ureter. To minimize this thermal effect, the peritoneum on the pelvic side wall could be opened and dissected to allow visualization of the ureter. Alternatively, 'hydroprotection' can be used. This involves injection of 0.9% saline under the diseased peritoneum, which elevates the peritoneum, allowing safe vaporization or diathermy.

For peritoneal endometriotic implants, a power setting of 40–50 W (laser CO_2) is usually used using a continuous firing mode (Donnez et al., 2004). To date, only one double-blind, RCT has been reported that examined the effect of laparoscopic treatment of endometriosis on pain (Sutton et al., 1994). This study has shown that laser excision of endometriosis significantly improves pain symptoms.However, this study has been criticized because the investigators performed semaltenously laparoscopic uterine nerve ablation and laser excision of the endometriosis and hence we cannot know which treatment has resulted in the pain relief. Sutton et al (1997) in a follow up study reported that 90% of responders had a pain relief for 1 year after laser excision, while 29% of patients had progressive disease and the same percentage (29%) had spontaneous regression. Finally, pain symptoms reported to be improved with the use of Helica TC (thermal coagulator) in women with stages I and II endometriosis. However, this approach requires further evaluation as part of randomized controlled trials (Nardo et al., 2005).

Laparoscopic uterine nerve ablation (LUNA) and presacral neurectomy were also suggested as a treatment of pain symptoms. LUNA was found beneficial for dysmenorrhoea not associated with endometriosis (Johnson et al., 2004), while presacral neurectomy was found to reduce pain symptoms in endometriosis without significant side effects (Garcia Leon et al., 2003, Zullo et al., 2004).

7.3.2 Ovarian endometriomas

Surgical laparoscopic management of ovarian endometriomas can involve stripping of the cyst lining or laser vaporization of the internal wall of the cyst. If laser used, the depth of this vaporization may be superficial and only the glandular epithelium and the adjacent stroma have to be vaporized (Brosens et al., 1996).

Operative laparoscopy should be the first choice for management of ovarian endometrioma whenever possible (Ruhlmann et al., 1996) and seems to be effective in alleviating pain associated with ovarian endometriomas (Yoshida et al., 2002). Medical therapy alone has not generally been effective in reducing endometrioma size and formed adhesions (Donnez and Nisolle, 1991).

7.3.3 Deep infiltrating endometriosis (DIE)

Deep endometriosis has been defined as endometriosis infiltrating deeper than 5 mm under the peritoneum (Koninckx and Martin, 1994). Unfortunately, the current classification of endometriosis is unsuccessful in predicting the major clinical outcomes, including pain symptoms (Vercellini et al., 2006).

In a retrospective study on 225 women with pelvic pain symptoms and DIE the anatomic locations of DIE implants and specific pain symptoms were recorded (including severe dysmenorrhoea, deep dyspareunia, non-cyclical chronic pelvic pain, painful defecation during menstruation, urinary tract symptoms, and gastrointestinal symptoms)(Fauconnier et al., 2002). There was an association between the frequency of severe dysmenorrhoea and DIE in the Douglas pouch adhesions, between the frequency of dyspareunia and DIE of uterosacral ligaments. The frequency of non-cyclical chronic pelvic pain was higher when it involved the bowel. The frequency of painful defecation during menstruation was higher when DIE involved the vagina; lower urinary tract symptoms were more frequent when DIE involved the bladder. The authors concluded that the types of pelvic pain can be broadly related to the anatomic location of DIE. Although, this study was retrospective, yet it gave good evidence of the correlation between locations of DIE and pain symptoms. Deep lesions need to be excised rather than vaporized (Koninckx and Martin, 1994). Coagulation, bipolar electrosurgery, argon laser, Potassium-Titanyl-Phosphate, (KTP) laser are also inadequate for management of lesions larger than 2 mm.

Operative laparoscopy in terms of complete excision of the disease is efficient for the treatment of painful symptoms related to deep endometriosis infiltrating uterosacral ligaments (Chopin et al., 2005). The segments of the rectum involved in the disease must be freed, leaving the deep endometriotic nodule attached to the posterior wall of the vagina. Resection of the whole lesion requires the posterior wall of the vagina to be resected and the vagina is usually opened (Chapron et al., 2001), whereas ureterolysis is often unnecessary.

Because laparoscopic excision of deep bowel lesions has been associated with a residual of pelvic pain, laparotomy may sometimes be needed. Moreover, a new combined vaginal-laparoscopic-abdominal approach was compared with laparoscopy, laparotomy and laparoscopy followed by laparotomy for bowel resection or laparoscopy followed by vaginal bowel resection for rectovaginal endometriosis. The new approach allows intra-operative digital bowel palpation to assess bowel infiltration and reduce unnecessary bowel resections and found to minimize complication rate, re-hospitalization rate, and hospitalization time (Zanetti-Dallenbach et al., 2008).

Surgeons have been treating endometriosis using several approaches; either by laparoscopic excision, ablation or removal of endometriomata and endometriosis associated adhesions.

The laparoscopic approach seems to have more favorable outcome than open approach in terms of quality of surgery and patients acceptance. Laparoscopic surgical management is now recognized as the best approach for endometriosis associated infertility treatment followed by assisted reproductive techniques. However, for endometriosis associated pain symptoms there is no general consensus regarding the best way of dealing with these symptoms. The problems of comorbidity and recurrence is still a problem and under great debate.

7.4 Infertility and endometriosis

Infertility is common in endometriosis sufferers and is generally manifested as a reduced monthly chance of conceiving (reduced fecundability). Nevertheless, even in severe cases of endometriosis spontaneous successful conception and delivery of a healthy baby often occur. Despite enormous studies about the relationship between endometriosis and subfertility, this relationship still controversial issue. The main problems in those studies, that they don't have a defined patient population, clinical features arising from different endometriosis types are not well defined and the fact that scientists investigating endometriosis are lacking enough clinical data about patients they are studying. They just deal with tissues blindly.

However, an association between endometriosis and infertility has repeatedly been reported in the literature, but an absolute cause-and-effect relationship has yet to be confirmed (Mahutte and Arici, 2002). Many mechanisms have been proposed to cause fertility problems in endometriosis. These include altered folliculogenesis (Doody et al., 1988), leading to ovulatory dysfunction and low quality oocytes, as well as luteal phase defects (Grant, 1966), impaired fertilization (Wardle et al., 1985), and abnormal embryogenesis (Garrido et al., 2002), abnormalities in peritoneal fluid (Minici et al., 2008), eutopic endometrium and immunological abnormalities (Akoum et al., 2006).

It seems that not one mechanism is responsible for the reduced fecundability in endometriosis it is rather a complex of several mechanisms rather than one mechanism. The problem of conflicting results in different studies about infertility in endometriosis may be due to the lack of proper characterization of patient population, the defects imbedded in the current classification of endometriosis and the difficulty of elimination of other factors that affect fertility such as sperm quality and different interpretation by different laboratories.

8. References

Acosta, A. A., Buttram, V. C., Jr., Besch, P. K., Malinak, L. R., Franklin, R. R. & Vanderheyden, J. D. (1973) A proposed classification of pelvic endometriosis. *Obstet Gynecol,* 42, 19-25.

Akoum, A., Metz, C. N., Al-Akoum, M. & Kats, R. (2006) Macrophage migration inhibitory factor expression in the intrauterine endometrium of women with endometriosis varies with disease stage, infertility status, and pelvic pain. *Fertil Steril,* 85, 1379-85.

Al-Jefout, M., Andreadis, N., Tokushige, N., Markham, R. & Fraser, I. (2007) A pilot study to evaluate the relative efficacy of endometrial biopsy and full curettage in making a diagnosis of endometriosis by the detection of endometrial nerve fibers. *American Journal of Obstetrics and Gynecology,* 197, 578.e1-578.e4.

Al-Jefout, M., Dezarnaulds, G., Cooper, M., Tokushige, N., Luscombe, G. M., Markham, R. & Fraser, I. S. (2009) Diagnosis of endometriosis by detection of nerve fibres in an endometrial biopsy: A double blind study. *Human Reproduction,* 24, 3019-3024.

Almeida, O. D., Jr. & Val-Gallas, J. M. (1998) Office microlaparoscopy under local anesthesia in the diagnosis and treatment of chronic pelvic pain. *J Am Assoc Gynecol Laparosc,* 5, 407-10.

Almeida, O. D., Jr., Val-Gallas, J. M. & Rizk, B. (1998) Appendectomy under local anaesthesia following conscious pain mapping with microlaparoscopy. *Hum Reprod,* 13, 588-90.

Arruda, M. S., Petta, C. A., Abrao, M. S. & Benetti-Pinto, C. L. (2003) Time elapsed from onset of symptoms to diagnosis of endometriosis in a cohort study of Brazilian women. *Hum Reprod,* 18, 756-9.

Ballard, K., Lowton, K. & Wright, J. (2006a) What's the delay? A qualitative study of women's experiences of reaching a diagnosis of endometriosis. *Fertil Steril,* 86, 1296-301.

Beecham, C. T. (1966) Classification of endometriosis. *Obstet Gynecol,* 28, 437.

Boing, C. & Kimmig, R. (2007) [Surgical management of endometriosis--an overview]. *Gynakol Geburtshilfliche Rundsch,* 47, 124-31.

Brosens, I., Campo, R. & Gordts, S. (1999) Office hydrolaparoscopy for the diagnosis of endometriosis and tubal infertility. *Curr Opin Obstet Gynecol,* 11, 371-7.

Brosens, I. A., Van Ballaer, P., Puttemans, P. & Deprest, J. (1996) Reconstruction of the ovary containing large endometriomas by an extraovarian endosurgical technique. *Fertil Steril,* 66, 517-21.

Brosens, J., Timmerman, D., Starzinski-Powitz, A. & Brosens, I. (2003) Noninvasive diagnosis of endometriosis: the role of imaging and markers. *Obstet Gynecol Clin North Am,* 30, 95-114, viii-ix.

Campo, R., Gordts, S., Rombauts, L. & Brosens, I. (1999) Diagnostic accuracy of transvaginal hydrolaparoscopy in infertility. *Fertil Steril,* 71, 1157-60.

Chapron, C., Jacob, S., Dubuisson, J. B., Vieira, M., Liaras, E. & Fauconnier, A. (2001) Laparoscopically assisted vaginal management of deep endometriosis infiltrating the rectovaginal septum. *Acta Obstet Gynecol Scand,* 80, 349-54.

Chene, G., Jaffeux, P., Lasnier, C., Aublet-Cuvelier, B., Matsuzaki, S., Jardon, K., Mage, G., Pouly, J. L. & Canis, M. (2008) [Are there anatomical and clinical correlations between minimal and deep endometriosis? First results of Auvergne's Registry of Endometriosis]. *Gynecol Obstet Fertil,* 36, 17-22.

Chopin, N., Vieira, M., Borghese, B., Foulot, H., Dousset, B., Coste, J., Mignon, A., Fauconnier, A. & Chapron, C. (2005) Operative management of deeply infiltrating endometriosis: results on pelvic pain symptoms according to a surgical classification. *J Minim Invasive Gynecol,* 12, 106-12.

Davis, C. J. & Mcmillan, L. (2003) Pain in endometriosis: effectiveness of medical and surgical management. *Curr Opin Obstet Gynecol,* 15, 507-12.

Donnez, J. & Nisolle, M. (1991) Laparoscopic management of large ovarian endometrial cyst: use of fibrin sealant. *J Gynecol Surg,* 7, 163-6.

Donnez, J., Pirard, C., Smets, M., Jadoul, P. & Squifflet, J. (2004) Surgical management of endometriosis. *Best Pract Res Clin Obstet Gynaecol,* 18, 329-48.

Doody, M. C., Gibbons, W. E. & Buttram, V. C., Jr. (1988) Linear regression analysis of ultrasound follicular growth series: evidence for an abnormality of follicular growth in endometriosis patients. *Fertil Steril,* 49, 47-51.

Evers, J. L. (1994) Endometriosis does not exist; all women have endometriosis. *Hum Reprod,* 9, 2206-9.

Fauconnier, A., Chapron, C., Dubuisson, J. B., Vieira, M., Dousset, B. & Breart, G. (2002) Relation between pain symptoms and the anatomic location of deep infiltrating endometriosis. *Fertil Steril,* 78, 719-26.

Frishman, G. N. & Salak, J. R. (2006) Conservative surgical management of endometriosis in women with pelvic pain. *J Minim Invasive Gynecol,* 13, 546-58.

Garcia Leon, F., Oviedo Ortega, G., Reyes Cuervo, H., Ibarrola Buenabad, E. & Von Der Meden, W. (2003) [Presacral neurectomy and uterine nerve ablation in chronic pelvic pain. Laparoscopic management. A comparative study.]. *Ginecol Obstet Mex,* 71, 137-42.

Garrido, N., Navarro, J., Garcia-Velasco, J., Remoh, J., Pellice, A. & Simon, C. (2002) The endometrium versus embryonic quality in endometriosis-related infertility. *Hum Reprod Update,* 8, 95-103.

Giudice, L. C. & Kao, L. C. (2004) Endometriosis. *Lancet,* 364, 1789-99.

Golfier, F. & Sabra, M. (2007) [Surgical management of endometriosis]. *J Gynecol Obstet Biol Reprod (Paris),* 36, 162-72.

Gordts, S., Campo, R. & Brosens, I. (2000) Office transvaginal hydrolaparoscopy for early diagnosis of pelvic endometriosis and adhesions. *J Am Assoc Gynecol Laparosc,* 7, 45-9.

Grant, A. (1966) Additional sterility factors in endometriosis. *Fertil Steril,* 17, 514-9.

Hadfield, R., Mardon, H., Barlow, D. & Kennedy, S. (1996a) Delay in the diagnosis of endometriosis: a survey of women from the USA and the UK. *Hum Reprod,* 11, 878-80.

Howard, F. M. (1993) The role of laparoscopy in chronic pelvic pain: promise and pitfalls. *Obstet Gynecol Surv,* 48, 357-87.

Howard, F. M. (2000) The role of laparoscopy as a diagnostic tool in chronic pelvic pain. *Baillieres Best Pract Res Clin Obstet Gynaecol,* 14, 467-94.

Howard, F. M. (2003) Chronic pelvic pain. *Obstet Gynecol,* 101, 594-611.

Howard, F. M., EL-MINAWI, A. M. & SANCHEZ, R. A. (2000) Conscious pain mapping by laparoscopy in women with chronic pelvic pain. *Obstet Gynecol,* 96, 934-9.

Huffman, J. W. (1951) External endometriosis. *Am J Obstet Gynecol,* 62, 1243-52.

Jansen, R. P. & Russell, P. (1986) Nonpigmented endometriosis: clinical, laparoscopic, and pathologic definition. *Am J Obstet Gynecol,* 155, 1154-9.

Johnson, N. P., Farquhar, C. M., Crossley, S., Yu, Y., Van Peperstraten, A. M., Sprecher, M. & Suckling, J. (2004) A double-blind randomised controlled trial of laparoscopic uterine nerve ablation for women with chronic pelvic pain. *BJOG,* 111, 950-9.

Kazanegra, R., Zaritsky, E., Lathi, R. B., Clopton, P. & Nezhat, C. (2008) Diagnosis of stage I endometriosis: comparing visual inspection to histologic biopsy specimen. *J Minim Invasive Gynecol,* 15, 176-80.

Kennedy, S. (1991) What is important to the patient with endometriosis? *Br J Clin Pract Suppl,* 72, 8-10; discussion 11-3.

Koninckx, P. R. (1994) Is mild endometriosis a condition occurring intermittently in all women? *Hum Reprod,* 9, 2202-5.

Koninckx, P. R. & Martin, D. (1994a) Treatment of deeply infiltrating endometriosis. *Curr Opin Obstet Gynecol,* 6, 231-41.

Mahutte, N. G. & Arici, A. (2002) New advances in the understanding of endometriosis related infertility. *J Reprod Immunol,* 55, 73-83.

Marana, R., Muzii, L., Caruana, P., Dell'acqua, S. & Mancuso, S. (1991) Evaluation of the correlation between endometriosis extent, age of the patients and associated symptomatology. *Acta Eur Fertil,* 22, 209-12.

Marcoux, S., Maheux, R. & Berube, S. (1997) Laparoscopic surgery in infertile women with minimal or mild endometriosis. Canadian Collaborative Group on Endometriosis. *N Engl J Med,* 337, 217-22.

Martin, D. C. & O'conner, D. T. (2003) Surgical management of endometriosis-associated pain. *Obstet Gynecol Clin North Am,* 30, 151-62.

Matsuzaki, S., Canis, M., Pouly, J. L., Rabischong, B., Botchorishvili, R. & Mage, G. (2006a) Relationship between delay of surgical diagnosis and severity of disease in patients with symptomatic deep infiltrating endometriosis. *Fertil Steril,* 86, 1314-6; discussion 1317.

Mettler, L., Schollmeyer, T., Lehmann-Willenbrock, E., Schuppler, U., Schmutzler, A., Shukla, D., Zavala, A. & Lewin, A. (2003) Accuracy of laparoscopic diagnosis of endometriosis. *JSLS,* 7, 15-8.

Minici, F., Tiberi, F., Tropea, A., Orlando, M., Gangale, M. F., Romani, F., Campo, S., Bompiani, A., Lanzone, A. & Apa, R. (2008) Endometriosis and human infertility: a new investigation into the role of eutopic endometrium. *Hum Reprod,* 23, 530-7.

Nardo, L. G., Moustafa, M. & Gareth Beynon, D. W. (2005) Laparoscopic treatment of pelvic pain associated with minimal and mild endometriosis with use of the Helica Thermal Coagulator. *Fertil Steril,* 83, 735-8.

Natuzzi, E. S., Ursell, P. C., Harrison, M., Buscher, C. & Riemer, R. K. (1993) Nitric oxide synthase activity in the pregnant uterus decreases at parturition. *Biochem Biophys Res Commun,* 194, 1-8.

Nisolle, M. & Donnez, J. (1997) Peritoneal endometriosis, ovarian endometriosis, and adenomyotic nodules of the rectovaginal septum are three different entities. *Fertil Steril,* 68, 585-96.

Olive, D. L. & Pritts, E. A. (2002) The treatment of endometriosis: a review of the evidence. *Ann N Y Acad Sci,* 955, 360-72; discussion 389-93, 396-406.

Parazzini, F. (1999) Ablation of lesions or no treatment in minimal-mild endometriosis in infertile women: a randomized trial. Gruppo Italiano per lo Studio dell'Endometriosi. *Hum Reprod,* 14, 1332-4.

Poncelet, C. & Ducarme, G. (2007) [Endometriosis: good practice rules for diagnostic laparoscopy]. *J Gynecol Obstet Biol Reprod (Paris),* 36, 135-40.

Rafs (1979) Classification of endometriosis. . *Fertil Steril,* 32, 633-4.

Rcog (2000) The investigation and management of endometrioisis. *Giudelines.* London, RCOG Press

Redwine, D., Mann, C. H. & Wright, J. T. (2000) Evidence on endometriosis. Elitism about randomised controlled trials is inappropriate. *BMJ,* 321, 1077-8.

Redwine, D. B. (1987a) Age-related evolution in color appearance of endometriosis. *Fertil Steril,* 48, 1062-3.

Riva, H. L., Kawasaki, D. M. & Messinger, A. J. (1962) Further experience with norethynodrel in treatment of endometriosis. *Obstet Gynecol,* 19, 111-7.

Ruhlmann, C., Vetrano, R., Bernaldo, D. G., Basso, F., Rolla, E. & Delger, R. (1996) Comparison of Laparoscopic versus Conventional Treatment of Ovarian Endometrioma. *J Am Assoc Gynecol Laparosc,* 3, S44.

Schenken, R. S. (2006) Delayed diagnosis of endometriosis. *Fertil Steril,* 86, 1305-6; discussion 1317.

Society, A. F. (1985) Revised American Fertility Society classification of endometriosis: 1985. *Fertil Steril,* 43, 351-2.

Steege, J. F. (1998) Superior hypogastric block during microlaparoscopic pain mapping. *J Am Assoc Gynecol Laparosc,* 5, 265-7.

Stratton, P. (2006a) The tangled web of reasons for the delay in diagnosis of endometriosis in women with chronic pelvic pain: will the suffering end? *Fertil Steril,* 86, 1302-4; discussion 1317.

Stratton, P., Winkel, C., Premkumar, A., Chow, C., Wilson, J., Hearns-Stokes, R., Heo, S., Merino, M. & Nieman, L. K. (2003) Diagnostic accuracy of laparoscopy, magnetic resonance imaging, and histopathologic examination for the detection of endometriosis. *Fertil Steril,* 79, 1078-85.

Sutton, C. J., Ewen, S. P., Whitelaw, N. & Haines, P. (1994) Prospective, randomized, double-blind, controlled trial of laser laparoscopy in the treatment of pelvic pain associated with minimal, mild, and moderate endometriosis. *Fertil Steril,* 62, 696-700.

Sutton, C. J., Pooley, A. S., Ewen, S. P. & Haines, P. (1997) Follow-up report on a randomized controlled trial of laser laparoscopy in the treatment of pelvic pain associated with minimal to moderate endometriosis. *Fertil Steril,* 68, 1070-4.

Tuttlies, F., Keckstein, J., Ulrich, U., Possover, M., Schweppe, K. W., Wustlich, M., Buchweitz, O., Greb, R., Kandolf, O., Mangold, R., Masetti, W., Neis, K., Rauter, G., Reeka, N., Richter, O., Schindler, A. E., Sillem, M., Terruhn, V. & Tinneberg, H. R. (2005) [ENZIAN-score, a classification of deep infiltrating endometriosis]. *Zentralbl Gynakol,* 127, 275-81.

Tytherleigh, M. G., Fell, R. & Gordon, A. (2004) Diagnostic conscious pain mapping using laparoscopy under local anaesthetic and sedation in general surgical patients. *Surgeon,* 2, 157-60.

Vercellini, P., Crosignani, P. G., Abbiati, A., Somigliana, E., Vigano, P. & Fedele, L. (2009) The effect of surgery for symptomatic endometriosis: the other side of the story. *Hum Reprod Update,* 15, 177-88.

Vercellini, P., Fedele, L., Aimi, G., De Giorgi, O., Consonni, D. & Crosignani, P. G. (2006a) Reproductive performance, pain recurrence and disease relapse after conservative surgical treatment for endometriosis: the predictive value of the current classification system. *Hum Reprod,* 21, 2679-85.

Vercellini, P., Fedele, L., Pietropaolo, G., Frontino, G., Somigliana, E. & Crosignani, P. G. (2003) Progestogens for endometriosis: forward to the past. *Hum Reprod Update,* 9, 387-96.

Wardle, P. G., Mitchell, J. D., Mclaughlin, E. A., Ray, B. D., Mcdermott, A. & Hull, M. G. (1985) Endometriosis and ovulatory disorder: reduced fertilisation in vitro compared with tubal and unexplained infertility. *Lancet,* 2, 236-9.

Wicks, M. J. & Larson, C. P. (1949) Histologic criteria for evaluating endometriosis. *Northwest Med,* 48, 611-3.

Wykes, C. B., Clark, T. J. & Khan, K. S. (2004a) Accuracy of laparoscopy in the diagnosis of endometriosis: a systematic quantitative review. *Bjog,* 111, 1204-12.

Yoshida, S., Harada, T., Iwabe, T. & Terakawa, N. (2002) Laparoscopic surgery for the management of ovarian endometrioma. *Gynecol Obstet Invest,* 54 Suppl 1, 24-7; discussion 27-9.

Zanetti-Dallenbach, R., Bartley, J., Muller, C., Schneider, A. & Kohler, C. (2008) Combined vaginal-laparoscopic-abdominal approach for the surgical treatment of rectovaginal endometriosis with bowel resection: a comparison of this new technique with various established approaches by laparoscopy and laparotomy. *Surg Endosc,* 22, 995-1001.

Zrubek, H., Sikorski, M., Nasser, M., Stachowicz, N. & Chil, A. (1999a) [Endometriosis in adolescents and young women. Can we afford to delay the diagnosis?]. *Ginekol Pol,* 70, 264-9.

Zullo, F., Palomba, S., Zupi, E., Russo, T., Morelli, M., Sena, T., Pellicano, M. & Mastrantonio, P. (2004) Long-term effectiveness of presacral neurectomy for the treatment of severe dysmenorrhea due to endometriosis. *J Am Assoc Gynecol Laparosc*, 11, 23-8.

Part 9

Laparoscopic Management of Gynecologic Malignancies

13

Two-Port Access Staging Laparoscopy for Gynecologic Cancers

Jiheum Paek[1] and Sang Wun Kim[2]
[1]*Department of Obstetrics and Gynecology, Ajou University School of Medicine, Suwon,*
[2]*Division of Gynecologic Oncology, Department of Obstetrics and Gynecology, Yonsei University College of Medicine, Seoul, Korea*

1. Introduction

In gynecologic cancer surgery, objectives of the surgery include optimal debulking, proper surgical staging, direct exploration by operators, and less operative morbidity (1). Comprehensive operation determines surgical stage and is important in guiding adjuvant chemotherapy. Due to these specific characteristics of gynecologic cancer operation, just surgical approaches by laparotomy have been performed for treatment of gynecologic cancers regardless of stage and kind of cancers merely until a few years ago. However, with improvements in surgical expertise with optimal instrumentation, the interests of minimally invasive surgery have increased. As a result, laparoscopic operations have become a commonly utilized approach instead of laparotomy in the gynecologic field. Recently, many surgeons have tried to reduce the number and size of ports in laparoscopic surgery for reducing morbidity and better cosmetic outcome. Compared with conventional laparoscopy, single-port access (SPA) surgery or laparoendoscopic single-site surgery (LESS) is expected to offer reduced postoperative pain (2) and better cosmetic results and, because it involves fewer trocars, may help avoid operative complications related to trocar insertion. Despite these advantages, SPA surgery has systemic limitations, including a crush between instruments or between instruments and endoscope, a limited amount of instruments, and the limited mobility of straight laparoscopic instruments because surgical instruments work through only one port. These technical problems cause lower accuracy of the operation compared to conventional laparoscopy and longer operation time. Consequently, there was few report of minimally invasive approach for a gynecologic cancer. Recently, although minimally invasive surgeries for gynecologic cancers have been attempted, it is still difficult to perform these surgical approaches widely due to the technical difficulties, despite the development of optimal instruments.
Based on these considerations, we tried to perform appropriate staging operation with minimal skin incisions using two-port access (TPA) system. The ultimate goal of the TPA system was to perform a proper cancer operation with less invasive access and to complement the technical limitations of SPA surgery.

2. Surgical techniques

The authors have reported a pilot study of 12 patients underwent TPA staging laparoscopy (1). This system consisted of a single multi-channel port system at the umbilicus and an ancillary 5-mm trocar in the suprapubic area (Fig. 1).

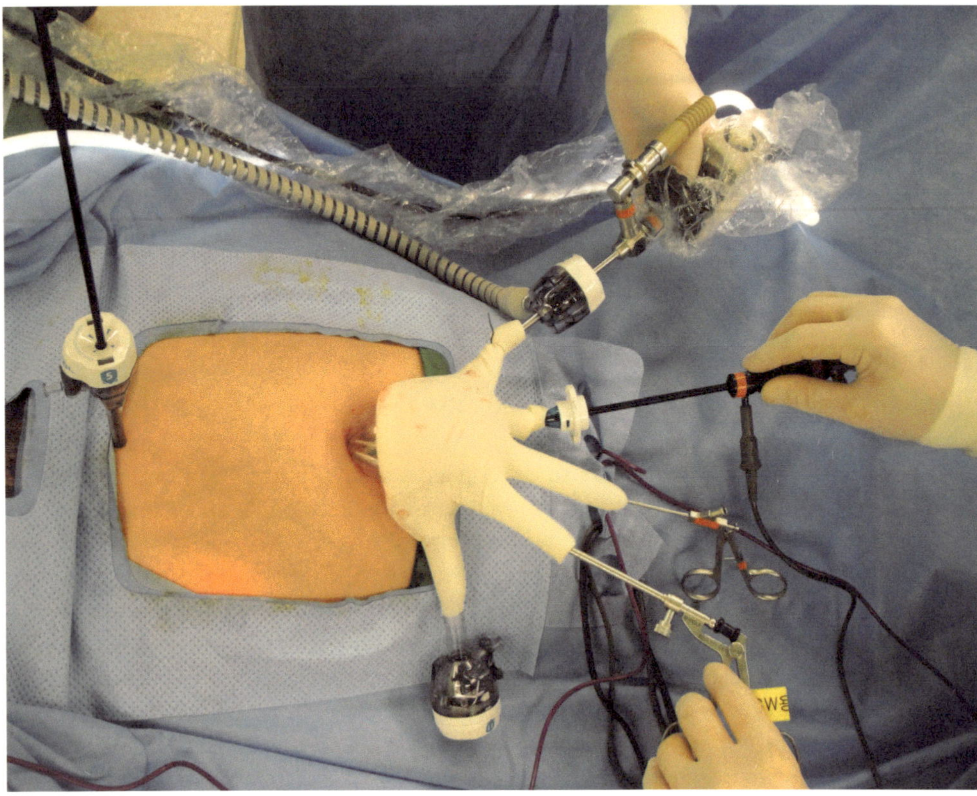

Fig. 1. Two-port system consists of a single multi-channel port system at the umbilicus and an ancillary 5-mm trocar in the suprapubic area.

TPA staging laparoscopy was performed for various gynecologic cancers from May 2009 in our institute. The inclusion criteria were patients who had newly diagnosed untreated gynecologic cancers and needed lymph node dissection for surgical staging and treatment. Procedures included endometrial cancer staging, ovarian cancer staging, and radical hysterectomy. All patients underwent pelvic lymph node dissection (PLD) and paraaortic lymph node dissection (PALD). In most of them, upper PALD extended to the renal vein level was performed. For a single multi-channel port system, after making a 1.5-cm vertical intra-umbilical skin incision, the Alexis® wound retractor (Applied Medical, CA, USA) is inserted into the peritoneal cavity through the umbilicus. A 7½ surgical glove is fixed to the outer ring of the wound retractor. After making small incisions in the finger tip portions of the glove, two 5-mm trocars and one 11-mm trocar are inserted. Another 5-mm trocar in the suprapubic area is used as the assistant port for the procedures and ventilating CO_2 gas. A rigid 30-degree, 5-mm, 45 cm length endoscope is used. Surgical instruments used are bipolar forceps, monopolar scissors, atraumatic forceps, toothed grasper, laparoscopic needle holder, a suction-irrigation system, Harmonic Ace™ (Ethicon Endo-surgery, Ohio, USA) and the LigaSure Atlas™ (Covidien, CO, USA). A RUMI uterine manipulator is placed with a KOH colpotomizer system (Cooper Surgical, CT, USA).

For the pelvic lymph node dissection, the retroperitoneal space is developed by incising peritoneum lateral to the infundibulopelvic ligament from the pelvic brim to the round ligament using a monopolar hook. The paravesical and pararectal spaces are identified. After the pelvic vessels and bilateral ureters are identified, pelvic lymph nodes are isolated and removed by incising tissue that is lateral and parallel to the external iliac artery extending from the bifurcation of the common iliac artery to the point where the deep circumflex iliac vein crossed over the external iliac artery. Then, lymphatic tissues in the obturator fossa and on the internal iliac vessels are dissected (Fig. 2).

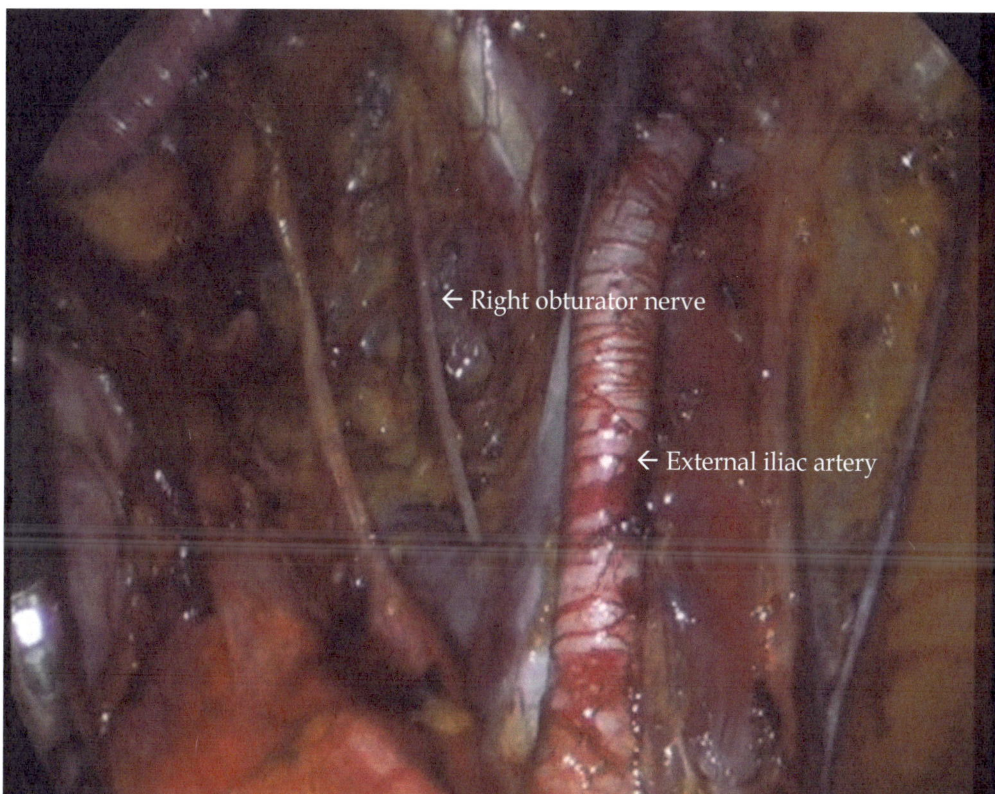

Fig. 2. Two-port laparoscopic staging; intraoperative view of right pelvic lymphadenectomy.

For the radical hysterectomy, the uterine vessels are dissected at their origins from the internal iliac vessels. The vesicocervical space is developed inferiorly and laterally. The medial edge of the divided uterine vessels is then pulled medially, and the ureter is completely freed from the retroperitoneal bed to the entry into the bladder by a complete dissection of the vesicouterine ligament (Fig.3). The cardinal ligament is transected at the medial wall of the internal iliac vessels. The anterior parametrium is transected near the bladder wall and the posterior parametrium including the uterosacral ligament is divided midway from its origin of the uterus to the sacrum until the bulge from the colpotomizer second lower ring in the vagina was reached. After completely detaching the uterus from the vagina, the uterus is extracted through the vagina. Pneumoperitoneum is maintained with a surgical glove filled with normal saline. A 40 mm round-bodied needle is introduced through the 11-mm port and we perform the closure of vaginal cuff intracorporeally with a 1-0 Vicryl continuous running suture.

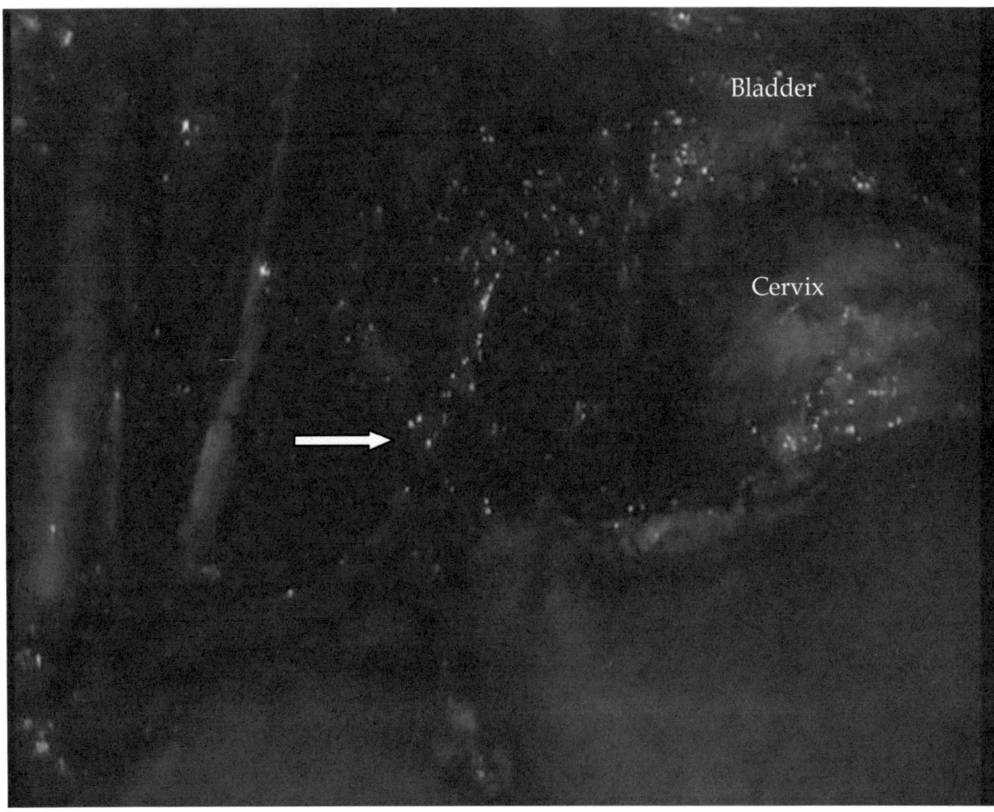

Fig. 3. Two-port laparoscopic radical hysterectomy; the left ureter (arrow) is completely freed from the retroperitoneal bed to the entry into the bladder.

Paraaortic lymph node dissection is performed using a monopolar hook and a Harmonic Ace™. The peritoneal incision extends from the aortic bifurcation up to the transverse duodenum. After the inferior mesenteric artery and bilateral ureters are isolated, lymphatic tissues on the paraaortic, paracaval and presacral space are carefully dissected (Fig. 4, 5). For Infracolic omentectomy in ovarian cancer, the infracolic omentum is divided along its superior border just adjacent to the transverse colon using Harmonic Ace™. The resected omentum is extracted through the vagina with the uterus after the hysterectomy. The drainage bag is connected through the 5-mm port in the suprapubic area. After hemostasis, the single multi-channel port and ancillary port are removed and the umbilical fascia and subcutaneous tissue is approximated with 2-0 Vicryl sutures.

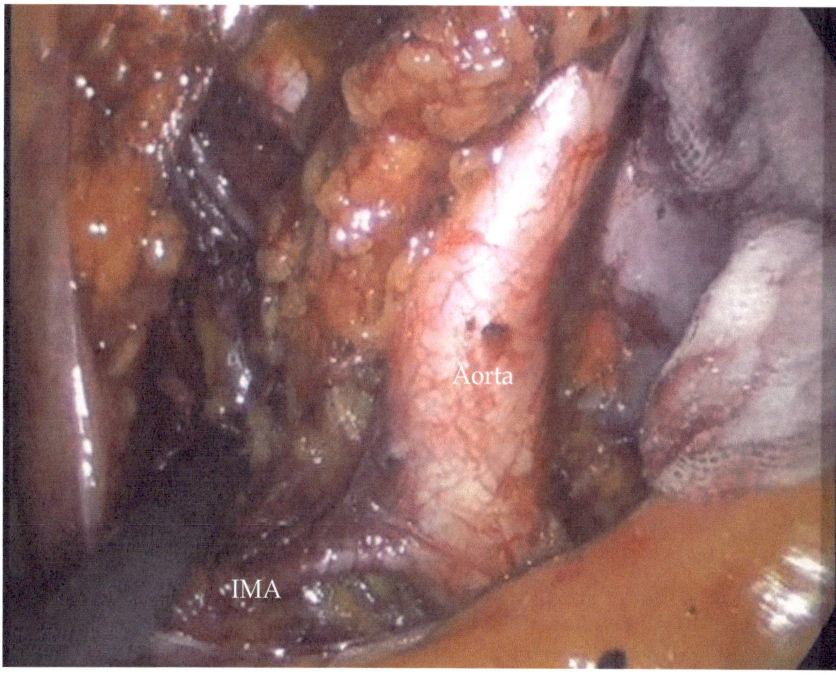

Fig. 4. Two-port laparoscopic staging; intraoperative view of left lower paraaortic lymphadenectomy.

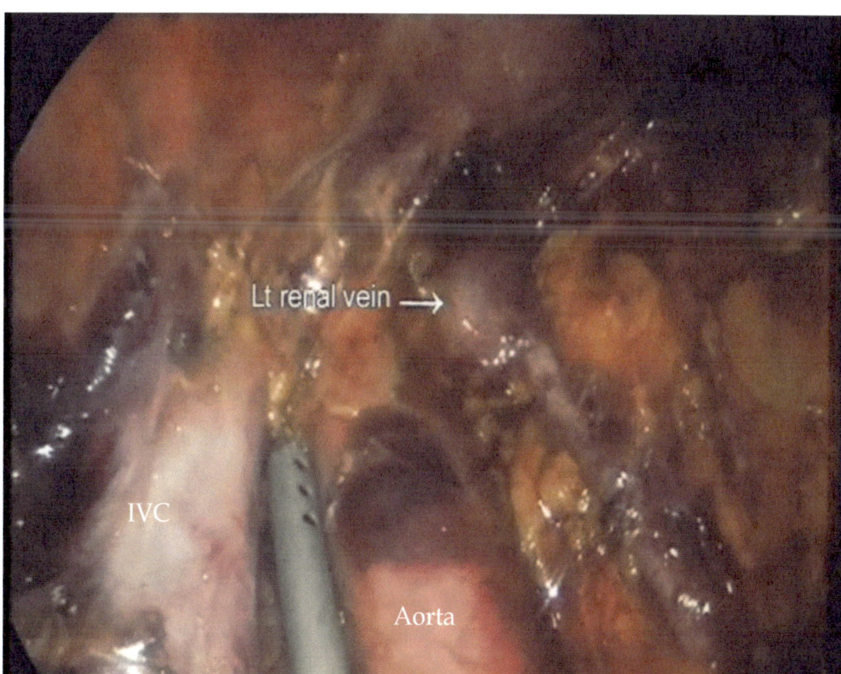

Fig. 5. Two-port laparoscopic staging; intraoperative view of upper paraaortic lymphadenectomy.

3. Surgical outcomes

To date, more than 60 patients underwent TPA staging laparoscopy. Of these, we performed type III radical hysterectomy in 14 patients and type II (modified) radical hysterectomy for 3 patients. All operations were completed laparoscopically with no conversion to laparotomy. The mean patient age and body mass index were 49.3 (standard deviation, 13.0) years and 23.0 (SD, 3.5) kg/m^2, respectively. The mean operating time was 251.8 (SD, 69.1) minutes. The mean estimated blood loss was 144.9 (SD, 13.5) mL. The median number of lymph nodes obtained was 36 (SD, 13.5). The mean postoperative pain scores using a validated visual analogue pain scale after 6, 24, and 48 hours were 3.3, 3.1, and 2.7, respectively. The mean postoperative hospital stay was 6.4 (SD, 2.6) days. There were no intraoperative complications requiring further management.

4. Discussion

For benign gynecologic diseases, minimally invasive surgeries have already been considered as a popular approach, including SPA or LESS. This surgical trend does not occur in surgeries for only benign disease. In 2009, Fader and Escobar presented the first 13 cases of LESS for the treatment of various gynecologic oncology conditions (3). Since then, they showed that single-port risk-reducing salpingo-oophorectomy and staging operations were feasible in patients with cancerous conditions (4, 5). With the development of optimal instrumentation, it seems that efforts to perform minimally invasive surgery for gynecologic cancers will be continued. Although this surgical approach is new and innovative, this still remains incomplete for performance of complete cancer operation. For cancer operations, operators must have surgical skills to perform PLD or PALD. However, to date, the SPA system has limitations for traction of soft tissues, the ureter, and the bowel. This surgical action is essential for lymph node dissection. Therefore, we tried to perform a proper staging laparoscopy using the two-port technique. This system involves less invasive access, enabling operators to minimize the skin incision and the occurrence of complications from port insertion as compared to conventional or multi-port laparoscopy.

In our system, the most important role of the ancillary 5-mm port in the suprapubic area is traction from an assistant (Fig. 1). In order to minimize the scar, a 2 or 3-mm instrument may be used without trocar insertion (6). The operator can grasp tissues or push them aside slightly using these instruments. However, they are so flexible that an assistant cannot perform counter-traction of tissues against the operator. Additionally, it is difficult to maintain traction for a long time and to perform traction of fine tissues. Especially for PALD, we were able to remove lymphatic tissues safely without injury of organs with traction through a 5-mm port. An additional 5-mm port in the suprapubic area is also useful for ventilation of CO_2. For the SPA system, non-ventilated air often obstructs the operator's view, complicating the procedure and leading delays in operating time. Another role of the additional 5-mm port is to perform the main action for the upper PALD. For the upper PALD, the operator exchanges his position from left to right side of patient. The assistant holds the endoscope and instrument for traction through multi-channel port at the umbilicus. At that time, the operator holds a grasper or dissector in his left hand at the umbilicus and the instrument for the main action, such as a Harmonic Ace™ or bipolar forcep, in his right through the 5-mm port in the suprapubic area. The operator's change of position can prevent the mirror effect on his view. Furthermore, a blunt injury by the tip of the instrument can be avoided because the angle between the Harmonic Ace™ and the large vessel is not sharp but parallel through the 5-mm port in the suprapubic area (Fig. 6). Finally, we insert drainage through the ancillary 5-mm port after completion of all procedures.

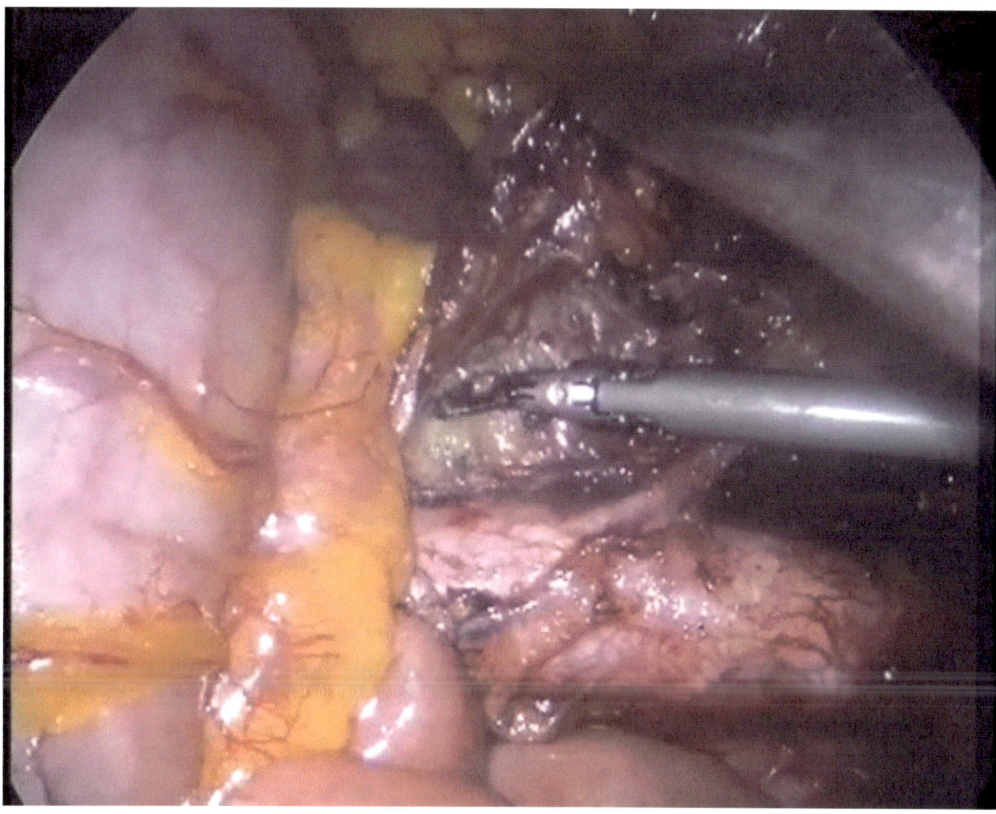

Fig. 6. A blunt injury by the tip of the instrument can be avoided because the angle between the Harmonic Ace™ and the large vessels is parallel.

Compared to commercial umbilical multi-port systems, our homemade system using surgical gloves has several advantages for performing staging operations. First, another 2- or 3-mm instrument can be added for traction. At that time, the total number of used instruments is five, including an endoscope. Also, the surgical gloves are somewhat flexible, so that the surgeon can overcome the limitation of range of motion that occurs in the small umbilical incision. Because we performed PLD and PALD after hysterectomy and closure for the vaginal cuff, the glove port system was useful for removal of lymphatic tissues or the omentum (Fig. 7).

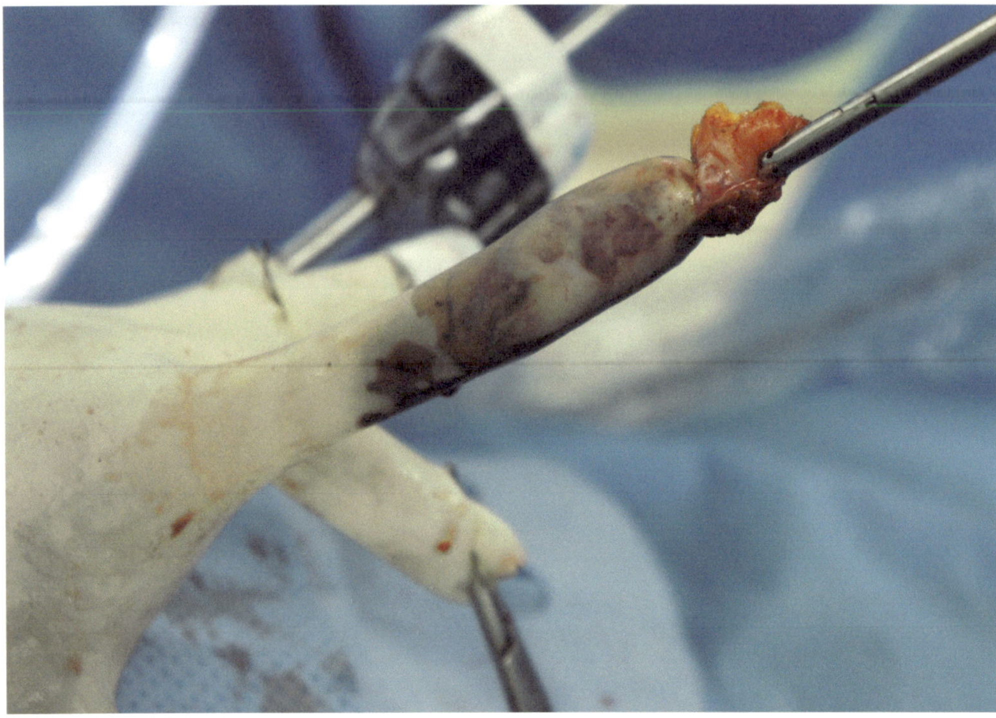

Fig. 7. Removal of lymphatic tissues through the hole of the surgical gloves.

In addition, upper PALD extending to the renal vein level was performed, although we had some troubles due to difficulty in traction of the bowel and limited angle of laparoscopic view. However, we were able to overcome this problem by using a 5-mm sized laparoscopic articulating fan retractor (Tekno Medical, Germany) through the multi-port at the umbilicus (Fig. 8).

Although operating time in TPA surgery was not short, it gradually decreased with the experiences for this surgical approach. The median number of lymph nodes resected in our study was 36, and this number is sufficient compared to the results of other studies with a conventional laparoscopic or robotic approach (7-9). For pain analysis, we showed that TPA staging laparoscopy had tolerable postoperative pain. Pain after laparoscopy is multi-factorial. Mouton et al. recommended the following for reduction of pain after laparoscopy: inject port sites with local anesthesia at the start of the operation; keep intra-abdominal pressure during pneumoperitoneum below 15 mmHg, avoiding pressure peaks and prolonged insufflation; use humidified gas at body temperature if available; use nonsteroidal anti-inflammatory drugs at the time of induction; attempt to evacuate all intraperitoneal gas at the end of the operation; and use drains only when required, rather than as a routine (10). Supposing these circumstances is constant for surgery, the number and size of skin incisions is certainly related to postoperative pain. The authors have already demonstrated that SPA hysterectomy caused less immediate postoperative pain and better surgical outcome with respect to recovery time than conventional laparoscopic hysterectomy (2).

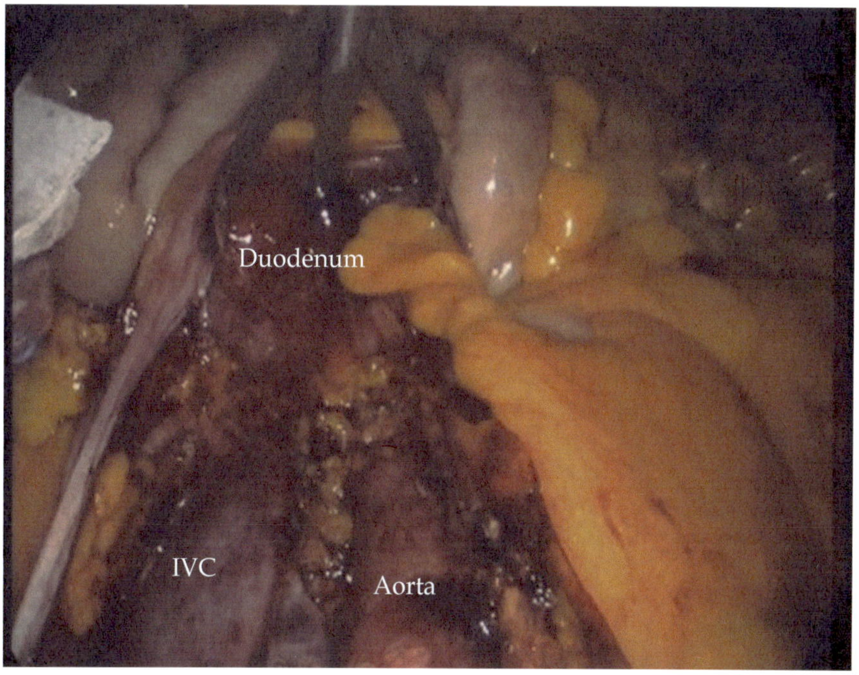

Fig. 8. The use of the 5-mm sized laparoscopic articulating fan retractor for traction of the bowel.

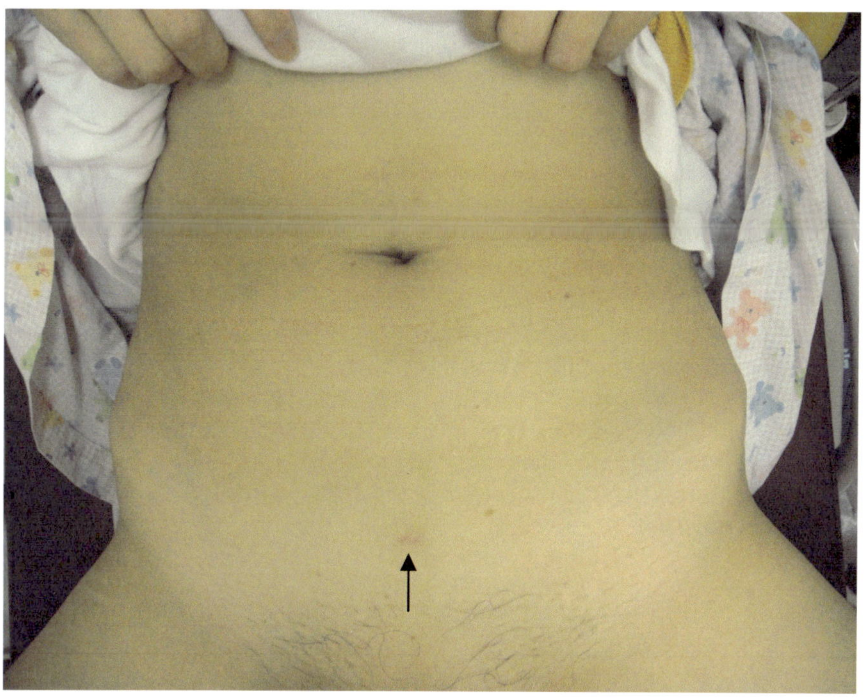

Fig. 9. Postoperative image after 2 months; There is only one small scar on the suprapubic area (arrow).

Putative advantages of the TPA system include enhanced cosmetic results from a hidden umbilical scar and 5-mm suprapubic incision that is covered by pubic hair, a decrease in morbidity related to bowel and vascular injury during trocar placement, and decreased postoperative wound infection and hernia formation (Fig 9).
To clarify the benefits of the TPA system and to complement limitations of this study, a prospective randomized trial is needed. In conclusion, TPA staging laparoscopy using a single multi-channel port and 5-mm ancillary port is a feasible procedure for gynecologic cancer patients and causes only minimal skin incisions.

5. References

[1] Paek J, Nam EJ, Jung YW, Lee SH, Kim JH, Kim YT, et al. Two-port access staging laparoscopy for gynecologic cancers: a pilot study. J Laparoendosc Adv Surg Tech A. 2010 May;20(4):347-53.
[2] Yim GW, Jung YW, Paek J, Lee SH, Kwon HY, Nam EJ, et al. Transumbilical single-port access versus conventional total laparoscopic hysterectomy: surgical outcomes. Am J Obstet Gynecol. 2010 Jul;203(1):26 e1-6.
[3] Escobar PF, Starks DC, Fader AN, Barber M, Rojas-Espalliat L. Single-port risk-reducing salpingo-oophorectomy with and without hysterectomy: surgical outcomes and learning curve analysis. Gynecol Oncol. 2010 Oct;119(1):43-7.
[4] Fader AN, Rojas-Espaillat L, Ibeanu O, Grumbine FC, Escobar PF. Laparoendoscopic single-site surgery (LESS) in gynecology: a multi-institutional evaluation. Am J Obstet Gynecol. 2010 Nov;203(5):501 e1-6.
[5] Fader AN, Escobar PF. Laparoendoscopic single-site surgery (LESS) in gynecologic oncology: technique and initial report. Gynecol Oncol. 2009 Aug;114(2):157-61.
[6] Nougues CP, Harmon CM, Hansen EN, Georgeson KE, Muensterer OJ. Cholecystectomy using single-incision pediatric endosurgery: technique and initial experience in the first 25 cases. J Laparoendosc Adv Surg Tech A. 2010 Jun;20(5):493-6.
[7] Scribner DR, Walker JL, Johnson GA, McMeekin SD, Gold MA, Mannel RS. Laparoscopic pelvic and paraaortic lymph node dissection: analysis of the first 100 cases. Gynecologic Oncology. 2001;82(3):498-503.
[8] Khler C, Klemm P, Schau A, Possover M, Krause N, Tozzi R, et al. Introduction of transperitoneal lymphadenectomy in a gynecologic oncology center: analysis of 650 laparoscopic pelvic and/or paraaortic transperitoneal lymphadenectomies. Gynecologic Oncology. 2004;95(1):52-61.
[9] Holloway RW, Ahmad S, DeNardis SA, Peterson LB, Sultana N, Bigsby GE, et al. Robotic-assisted laparoscopic hysterectomy and lymphadenectomy for endometrial cancer: Analysis of surgical performance. Gynecologic Oncology. 2009;115(3):447-52.
[10] Mouton WG, Bessell JR, Otten KT, Maddern GJ. Pain after laparoscopy. Surg Endosc. 1999 May;13(5):445-8.

Part 10

Laparoscopic Robotic Surgery

14

Do Costs of Robotic Surgery Matter?

Peter van Dam, Jan Hauspy, Luc Verkinderen,
Bich Trinh, Luc Van Looy and Luc Dirix
*Departments of Obstretics and Gynecology, Medical Oncology,
Saint Augustinus Hospital, Wilrijk,
Belgium*

1. Introduction

Although robots began as theoretical constructs devised from science fiction novels, they soon became a reality in the automobile industry in 1958 when general Motors introduced the Unimate to assist production (1). Since then robots have been used in a variety of applications including many industrial tasks, and deep-sea and space exploration (2). The first concept of surgical robotics was developed in the late 1980s at the National Aeronautics and Space Centre (NASA). Together with Stanford Research Institute, virtual reality and surgical robotics were integrated and the first steps toward telepresence surgery were made (3). The original model, known as the PUMA 560, was used for neurosurgical stereotactic maneuvers under computed tomographic guidance (2). Commercialisation of robotic surgery started in the early 1990s with the development of complete robotic systems HERMES (Computer Motion, Goleta, CA, USA) and AESOP (Computer Motion, Goleta, CA, USA) (2,4). These systems used voice recognition to control the laparoscopic camera, light source, insufflation and printer. They were designed to reduce surgeon fatigue and to offer a stable visual field. The ZEUS robotic system (Computer Motion, Goleta, CA, USA) and the Da Vinci robotic system (Intuitive Surgery, Mountain View, CA, USA) were introduced in the late 1990s (5,6). Both systems have remote manupilators that are controlled from a surgical workstation. In 2003, Computer Motion was acquired by Intuitive Surgery (6). Today the Zeus system is no longer commercially available and the Da Vinci system is the only telerobot on the market (6). The Da Vinci robot was approved for general surgery by the US Food and Drug Administration (FDA) in 2000, for the use in urology in 2001 and for gynecology in 2005 (6). The use of robotic assisted surgery has grown exponentially over the last few years as there is a clear trend in surgery, driven by patient demand, to develop less invasive approaches to common procedures (7). By the end of 2010 Intuitive Surgery had sold a total 1752 units. Robotic technology has gained popularity in various surgical specialities such as urology, gynecology, thoracic surgery, general surgery, and currently head and neck surgery.

2. The Da Vinci surgical system

The Da Vinci Surgical system has been described nicely by several authors (2,6,8). In brief it has three major components. The first component is the surgeon console. The surgeon sits ergonomically behind the console and controls the robotic system remotely. The console can be placed anywhere in or even outside the operating room. While operating, the surgeon is viewing a stereoscopic image projected in the console and controls the robotic arms with hand manipulators and foot pedals. The second component is the Insite Vision System. This creates three dimensional view by means of two camera control units and two light sources built in the unit. A 12 mm endoscope is used. The viewer gives a six to ten times magnification of the operating field. Because of the 3D view, the visual feedback is excellent and allows the surgeon to work precisely, even without haptic feedback. The third component is the patient-side cart with the robotic arms. The first series of Da Vinci systems had three robotic arms, and the new series all have four robotic arms. One of the arms holds the laparoscope and the other arms holds the various EndoWrist instruments, which measure either 5-8 mm in diameter. Each grasping instrument has its own preprogrammed maximum pressure and can be used in 10 operations before being obligatory replaced. These laparoscopic instruments have 7 degrees of freedom that replicate the full motion of the surgeon's hand. The external robotic arms provide 3 degrees of freedom (insertion, pitchband yaw) and the EndoWrist mechanism provides 4 additional degrees of freedom (pitch, yaw, rotation and grip). These enable the surgeon to manipulate, coagulate, dissect and suture intuitively. The system also allows variety of scaled motion for precise control while eliminating tremors.

3. Advantages of robotic surgery

Robotic-assisted and laparoscopic surgery eliminates the need for large morbid and less esthetical incisions and often decreases blood loss, post-operative pain, use of pain medication and length of hospital stay (2,6), especially when compared to open surgery. Advantages of robotic surgery compared to laparoscopy and open surgery are: improved dexterity, more precise movements and tremor reduction, and better visualisation of the operating field (magnification and 3D). In addition the robot fingertip hand control mechanism is "intuitive", meaning that the robotic instruments will move just as your hands move, rather than as a mirror image movement as in laparoscopy. This eliminates the fulcrum effect observed in laparoscopy in which a surgeon must move his hand in the opposite direction to the intended location. For example, to have the laparoscopic scissor tips at the patients right ovary, the surgeons hand must move left (8). The robotic digital process allows scaling down the surgeons's hand movements to a level at which microvascular or microscopic procedures are feasible. Difficult, minimal invasive surgery is accesable for surgeons without advanced laparoscopic training as it has a short learning curve (6, 9). Fatigue and frustration become less of a limiting factor for the robotic surgeon compared to the laparoscopic surgeon (10).

4. Limitations of robotic surgery

The major drawback of the Da Vinci system is the loss of tactile and force feedback. This can be surmounted by training and is partially compensated for by the 3-D visual feedback. However it often leads to rupturing of suture material during knot tying by beginning robotic surgeons. In addition placing the trocars is limited in order to avoid collision of the robotic arms. With the current equipment this leads to difficulties to operate in the lower and upper abdomen simultaneously. In gynecologic cancer staging procedures, requiring higher paraaortic lymph node dissection, the robot sometimes must be dedocked after completing the pelvic portion of the surgery, the operating table turned 180 degrees , new ports placed, and the robot redocked facing the upper abdomen (8). This problem can be partially solved by positioning the robot lateral to the patient and not in between the legs, but currently remains a drawback. With laparoscopic surgery, the surgeon tends to place the ports in more 'natural' and anatomical positions. Esthetically, ports of a laparoscopy are much better located (eg the umbilicus and just medial to the anterior superior iliac spine) than the 'forced' trocare placements in an arch, commonly used for robotic assisted procedures. The use of larger trocars (11mm versus 5 mm) is an additional esthetical disadvantage for robotic surgery compared to laparoscopy. The cart with the robotic arms, which is positioned close to the patient, makes access to the patient limited. Particularly in gynecologic surgery it is sometimes difficult to remove the uterus and other specimens from the vagina after the robot has been docked (2). Due to the sophisticated technology a robotic team of specialized surgeons, anaesthesists and dedicated nursing staff is mandatory to make a robotic program function optimally. Particularly the surgeon and nursing staff need specific training. This makes the use of robotic surgery less practical for non-elective cases. Conventional open surgery, laparoscopic surgery and robotic surgery require different skills. As the robot is a high tech complicated instrument to master, adequate training is mandatory before embarking on surgery in patients. It is important to train basic laparoscopic and robotic skills in a box trainer, on a cadaver or on animals (6). However the major disadvantage of robotic surgery are the high cost of purchase, maintenance and instruments of the robotic system.

5. Cost of robotic surgery

5.1 Equipment

There is a major difference in operative costs between open, lapoaroscopic, and robotic surgery resulting from added expense of specialized equipment. Equipment costs associated with laparoscopic surgery have a relatively low per-case cost as it is multipurpose (eg. monitors and cameras can be used for laparoscopy but also for hysteroscopy) and can be used by different specialities for many types of surgery (11). On the contrary, the Da Vinci robot, costsing over 1.500.000 Euro, and requiring a yearly service contract of 150.000 Euro, has a more limited number of applications. The fixed costs depend greatly upon the number of cases being operated over the amortized life span of the robotic system. If utilized for 300 cases per year and amortized over 7 years it adds more then 1000 Euro per case, but if less patients are operated yearly the costs of robotic assisted surgery increase even more. Such costs are not reimbursed by the hospital. The robot also offers a distinct financial disadvantage because each instrument only has a limited preprogrammed (n=10) number of uses, such that the added cost for instruments and drapings per case can be as high as 1700 Euro per case. The major factor affecting the costs of laparoscopic surgery is the price of laparoscopic instruments. This depends on the type and number of instruments which are used. Generally (semi)reusable instruments are cheaper per case compared to disposable instrument (12). Although one would expect equipment costs to decrease with time (analogous to the retail computer market) there has been an increase in costs that exceeds inflation despite an increase in the number of procedures performed nationwide (11,12). There has been no decrease in the costs of robot-related products due to the lack of market competition.

5.2 Operative times

Operative times play an important role in determining the operative costs. They include the time to start up the procedure, to do the surgery and to prepare the surgical theatre for the next operation. These costs are calculated in 15-30 min intervals. Costs of anesthesia also increase over similar time intervals. In general, the set-up and brake-down of the robotic system takes significantly longer compared to the preparation of laparoscopic or open surgery. For many procedures operative times are lower for open surgery, intermediate for robotic surgery and slightly longer for comparable laparoscopic surgery (10). As experience grows with a certain techniques operative time becomes shorter until they stabilize at a certain level. Lenihan et al showed that the the total operative times for robotic hysterectomies stabilized at approximately 95 minutes after 50 cases (9) A study that evaluated the learning curve in a series of robot assisted laparoscopic prostatectomies found that the learning curve may range from a low of 13 cases to a high of 200 cases depending on the surgeon (13). The average initial time to perform this procedure in this cohort was 424 min, with a final operative time of 230 min per case. The costs of the learning curve are high and can vary widely. For robot assisted laparoscopic prostatectomies costs of the initial learning cure varied from 49,613 US Dollars to 554,694 US dollars with an average of 217,034 US dollars (13, 14). As in most centers surgeons already went through their learning curves for open and/or laparoscopic surgery the robotic learning curve is an added cost. To overcome these extra costs, the concept of high volume centers is of great importance. In such units the learning curve can be rapidly traversed and costs minimized. Robotic surgery is specifically suitable for virtual reality training , as the operation itself is computer guided. Different companies are developing virtual reality simulators for robotic surgery. This may reduce the learning curve significantly and is likely to be the training of choice for the surgeons of tomorrow (15).

5.3 Hospital stay

Room and board costs represent an important part of the overall cost of hospitalization. For many procedures, the main financial advantage for the laparoscopic and robotic approach is the decreased hospital stay (11,16). The reduced number of impatient hospital days and earlier return to regular diet allows for cost savings. These savings can compensate for added expenses in the operating room and result in cost superiority of some procedures. It is important to realize that the costs of hospitals beds vary between hospital, especially between community hospitals and academic medical centres (6). Up to now, there have not been any publications demonstrating an advantage of a robotic-assisted laparoscopic approach over 'pure' laparoscopic approach in terms of rooms and board (11).

5.4 Other costs

In general laparoscopic and robotic procedures allow patients to resume their normal family and professional activities sooner (8,10). It is difficult to calculate the savings for society as sick leave, insurance for inability to work, etc… vary enormously on an individual basis. There is no evidence that long term morbidity varies considerably between open, laparoscopic and robot-assisted procedures (16).

An interesting advantage of robotic surgery is the more ergonomic position of the surgeon to perform a procedure. Loss of economic productivity of surgeons related to doing laparoscopic and open surgery (eg cervical hernia) is a severely underestimated factor. A recent survey by Matern et al on this subject shows that 97% of surgeons think improvement of ergonomics in the operating theatre is necessary (17).

6. Cost analysis of robotic procedures

6.1 Gynecologic surgery

Sarlos et al compared the costs of 40 consecutive robot-assisted hysterectomies with 40 matched total laparoscopic hysterectomies. There were no conversions to laparotomy or major morbidity in both groups (18). Operating time was 83 (55-165) versus 109 (50-170) minutes, and hospital stay 3.3 (2-6) versus 3.9 (2-7) days. Average surgical costs were 4067 Euros for the robotic group compared to 2151 Euros in the laparoscopic group.
Using the Premier Hospital Database Paric et al identified women above 18 years of age with a record of minimally invasive hysterectomy performed in 2007 to 2008. Of 361888 patient records analyzed from 358 hospitals, 95% (N=34527) of laparoscopic hysterectomies were performed without robotic assistance (19). Inpatient procedures with and without robotics cost 9640 vs 6973 USD, respectively (difference strongly significant). Similar differences were found for outpatient procedures (7920 vs 5949 USD). There were little clinical differences in perioperative and postoperative events. Only surgical times were significantly longer for robot-assisted procedures.
Barnett et al used decision modeling to compare costs associated with robotic, laparoscopic and open hysterectomy (20). The societal perspective model predicted laparoscopy (10128 USD) as the least expensive approach followed by robotic (11476 USD) and open hysterectomy (12847 USD). In the hospital perspective models laparoscopy was least expensive (6581 USD) followed by open (7009 USD) and robotic hysterectomy (8770 USD).
Rodgers et al made a comparison with open surgery and calculated that robotic surgery increased the costs for tubal anastomosis by 1446 US dollars (21). However Dharia Patel et al found that the cost per delivery was equal (22). Robotic rectopexy proved to be 755 USD more expensive than laparoscopic rectopexy (23). Advicula et al showed that robotic myomectomy had less complications and shorter hospital stay (24). They calculated that mean hospital reimbursement was 30064 USD (SD: 6689) for the robotic procedure vs 13400 USD (SD:7720) for open surgery
Outcomes and costs for endometrial cancer staging via traditional laparotomy (N=40), standard laparoscopy (N=30) and robot assisted surgery (N=40) were compared in one single institution by Bell et all (25). Patients undergoing robotic assisted hysterectomy and staging experienced longer operative times than the laparotomy cohort but with no difference in comparison to the laparoscopic cohort (184 min vs 108 mi vs 171 min, $p> 0.0001$, $p=0.14$). Estimated blood loss was significantly reduced for the robotic cohort in comparison to the laparotomy cohort and comparable to the laparoscopic cohort. The complication rate was lowest in the robotic group (7.5%) relative to laparotomy (27.5%) and laparoscopic group (20%) ($p = 0.015$, $p=0.03$). Average return to normal activity for the robotic patients was significantly shorter then those undergoing laparotomy (24 vs 52 days, $p < 0.001$) and those undergoing laparoscopy (31 days, $p = 0.005$). Lymph node yields were similar in all groups. The total average cost for hysterectomy with staging completed via laparotomy was 12943 USD, for standard laparoscopy 7569 USD and for robotic assistance 8212 USD.

6.2 Urologic surgery

One of the largest cost analyses of robotic surgery, compared to open and laparoscopic surgery, was made by Bolenz et al for radical prostatectomy (26) . The study included 643 consecutive patients who underwent a radical prostatectomy: 262 robotic_assisted laparoscopic radical abdominal prostatectomy (RALP), 220 laparoscopic radical prostatectomy (LRP), and 161 open (retropubic) radical prostatectomy (RRP) Disease characteristics were similar in the three groups. Lymphadenectomy was more commonly performed in RRP (100%), compared to LRP (22%) and RALP (11%) ($p<0.001$). Nerve sparing was performed in 85% of RALP procedures, 96% op LRP procedures and 90% of RRP procedures ($p< 0.001$). Mean length of hospital stay was higher RRP than for LRP and RALP. The median direct costs were higher for RALP compared to LRP or RRP (RALP 6752 USD, LRP 5687 USD, ORP: 4427 USD, $p< 0.001$). The main difference was in surgical supply cost (RALP 2015 USD, LRP 725 USD, RRP 185 USD, $p < 0.001$) and operating room costs (RALP: 2798 USD, LRP: 2453 USD, ORP: 1611 USD, $p < 0.001$). When considering purchase and maintenance costs for the robot, the financial burdon would increase by 2698 USD per patient, given an average of 126 cases a year. The authors conclude that these costs may have significant impact on overall costs of prostate cancer care in the United States.
Smith et al performed a comparative cost analysis of 20 prior cases of robotic and open cystectomy. Mean fixed operating room costs for robotic surgery were 1634 USD higher than for open cases. Operating room variable costs were also higher by a difference of 570 USD directly related to increased operating room time. Hospital costs were nearly identical for the fixed component while variable costs were 564 USD higher for the open approach secondary to higher transfusion costs and longer mean length of stay. Based on these findings robotic assisted laparoscopic cystectomy is associated with a higher financial cost of + 1640 USD than the open approach in the perioperative setting.

6.3 Gastrointestinal surgery

Costs of robotic assisted and laparoscopic cholecystectomy were analyzed in a case-control study by Breitenstein et (28). Fifty consecutive patients undergoing robotic assisted cholcystectomy between December 2004 and February 2006 were matched 1:1 to 50 patients with conventional cholecystectomy. No minor and one major (2%) complication occurred in each group and there were no conversions to open surgery. Operation time (skin to skin: 55 min vs 50 min, $p=0.85$) and hospital stay (2.6 vs 2.8 days) were similar. Overall hospital costs were significantly higher for robotic assisted cholecystectomy: 7985 USD (SD 1760) versus 6255 USD (SD 1956), $p < 0.001$, with a raw difference of 1730 USD (95% CI 991-2468) and a difference adjusted for confounders of 1606 USD (95% CI 1076-2136). This difference was mainly related to the amortization and consumables of the robotic system.
Hubens et al performed a retrospective analysis on 45 patients (mean BMI 44.2) who had a Roux-en-Y gastric bypass procedure (RYGBP) with the aid of the Da Vinci robot system compared to 45 patients (mean MI 43.9) who underwent a laparoscopic RYGBP (29). Although the initial total operating time was shorter for the laparoscopic cases, the last ten robotic cases were performed in a similar time as the laparoscopic cases (136 vs 127 min). There were no differences in postoperative complications between the two groups in terms of anastomotic leakage or stenosis. In the robotic group more conversions to open surgery were noted (five patients) because of laceration of the intestines with the robotic arms. This is probably inherent to the learning curve of the procedure. The costs were higher for robotic surgery than for standard RYGBP, mainly because of the extra equipment used.

6.4 Thoracic surgery

The financial impact of employing minimally invasive techniques for lobectomy compared with traditional open thoracotomy was assessed by Park et al (30). A retrospective review was conducted using ICD9 codes for thoracotomy, video-asisted thoracic surgery (VATS) and robotic VATS lobectomy to determine total average costs associated with the resultant hospital stay in Memorial-Sloan Kettering Cancer Center (USA). Robotic VATs lobectomy had higher associated costs then VATS only, primarily attributed to increased costs of the first hospital day, but was still less costly than thoracotomy. The average cost of VATs is substantially less than thoracotomy primarily because of a decreased length of stay. Casali and Walker could partially confirm these data in a retrospective analysis of 93 patients undergoing a VATS lobectomy and 253 a lobectomy by thoracotomy in the Royal Infermary of Edinburgh (UK) (31). Overall cost for a VATS lobectomy was 8023+/-565 Euro which was less than open lobectomy 8178+/-167 Euro (p=0.0002).

6.5 Cardiac surgery

Jones et al prospectively analyzed two cohorts undergoing off-pump coronary revascularization by minithoracotomy using robotic procedure or by classic sternotomy (32). The patient groups were matched for the number of coronary arteries revascularized and risk factors known to influence perioperative outcome. Patients undergoing robotic minithoractomy had shorter intubation times (4.8 vs 12 hours, $p < 0.001$), intensive care unit stay (22 vs 51 hours, $p < 0.001$)), total hospital stay (3.8 vs 6.4 days, $p< 0.001$) and lower blood transfusion requirements (0.2 vs 1.4 units, $p < 0.001$). Despite increased operative costs for supplies, longer operating room times, and additional radiology services, the total hospital costs were equivalent between groups. However, this analysis did not include the initial acquisition of the robot ! These authors found that the advantages of robotic technology had the greatest impact on postoperative cost for patients with characteristics that places them at high risk for long hospital stays (eg elderly, ejection fraction 20%, poorly controlled diabetes, chronic obstructive pulmonary disease and receiving home oxygen). The incidence of major postoperative cardiac and cerebrovascular events was 26% in the open CABG group compared with 4% after robotic mini-CABG (hazard ratio 3.9; 95% CI: 1.4-7.6; $p = 0.008$). Minimally invasive CABG was associated with significantly shorter time to return to work versus sternotomy (44 vs 93 days, $p = 0.16$). These findings are particularly relevant to low-risk patients, a subgroup who are especially concerned with the adverse effects of a prolonged recovery on early quality of life.

Robotic mitral valve repair (MVR) has been performed in Australia since 2004. Kam et al retrospectively compared 107 robotic and 40 conventional MVRs and performed an ad hoc cost analysis (33). The post-operative degrees of mitral regurgitation were comparable. Total operating time was 18% longer in robotic compared to conventional (239 vs 202 min, $p< 0.001$). In robotic cases intensive care unit stay (37 vs 45 hours, $p= 0.002$) and hospital stay (6.4 vs 8.8 days, $p< 0.001$) was reduced. Mean hospital cost, without including capital costs, was comparable (18503 AUD vs 17880 AUD, p=0.176).

Morgan and colleagues conducted a retrospective review of clinical and financial data of 20 patients undergoing atrial septal defect closure, and 20 patients who underwent mitral valve repair (MVR) using either robotic techniques or a conventional approach by sternotomy (34). Robotics did not significantly increase the total hospital cost for ASD closure or MVR. However when including the initial capital investment for the robot total hospital costs were increased by 3773 USD for robotic ASD closure and 3444 USD for robotic MVR (p = 0.021 an p=0.004).

6.6 Pediatric surgery

Anderberg et al calculated costs using regional hospital prices for their first 14 robot-assisted fundoplications in children, compared to their last ten similar laparoscopic and open procedures (35). The mean costs of the robotic procedure was 9584 EUR, of the laparoscopic surgery 8982 EUR and of the open surgery 10521 EUR. Patients seemed to benefit from the use of robotic surgery having less postoperative pain and a shorter hospital stay.

7. How important are costs

Technologic innovation in health care is an important driver of cost growth. Doctors and patients often embrace new modes of treatment before their merits and weaknesses are fully understood (36). Robotic technology has been readily adopted over the last five years in both Europe and the United States (16). The number of robot-assisted procedures that are performed world wide has nearly tripled since 2007, from 80000 to 250000 in 2009 (36). The present review of the literature shows that currently robot-assisted surgery is consistently more expensive then video-laparoscopy and in many cases to open surgery. Across the full range of 20 types of surgery for which studies exist the average additional variable cost was about 1600 USD per patient, rising to more then 3000 USD when the amortized cost of the robot itself was included. It seems that currently only for very complex surgical procedures, such as cardiac surgery, its costs can be competitive to similar open surgical procedures. Some authors have suggested that robotic technology may have contributed to the substitution of surgical for non-surgical treatment for certain diseases (36). The observed pattern matches evidence from the Surveillance, Epidemiology and End Results Medicare database, and shows that Medicare beneficiaries who received a diagnosis in of prostate cancer in 2005 were about 14% more likely to have undergone surgery by 2007 than their counterparts whose prostate cancer was diagnosed 3 years earlier (37). This is likely affecting costs on the long run as some studies show more adjuvant radiotherapy is used after robotic prostatectomy (38) It has been calculated that if robotic assisted surgery would replace conventional surgeries for the full range of procedures for which cost studies have been done, it would generate nearly 2.5 billion US$ in additional health care costs in the United States (36).

The development of new technology and new medications often has a financial motive and the willingness of hospitals and healthcare systems to acquire these advancements often is an economic consideration (16). Patients only demand the robot because it is marketed to them by hospitals and purchasers of the machines in hopes of a nice return on investment. The health care system in many countries is prepared to cover new technologies at higher rates than older technologies, even when there is no proof that the newer technologies provide an additional benefit. Therefore the crucial question is whether robotic surgery, being more expensive, is better than comparable traditional video-endoscopic and open surgery. Generally most robotic and laparoscopic procedures have less short term morbidity, blood loss, intensive care unit and hospital stay then open surgery (6,11,18-35). Up to now no major differences have been found between robot-assisted and classic video-assisted procedures for these factors. Most experience on cost calculation for robotics has been gathered in urology. In a recent editorial in European Urology Graefen writes "Are these extra costs justified ? Maybe yes, if an advantage for robotic assisted radical prostatectomy over other approaches were documented, but this is currently not the case" (38). Reviewing the literature on this subject this author concludes that it is clear that high surgical volume is crucial to have a good results, but functional outcome (ie continence and erectile function) is not better and in fact significantly more salvage radiotherapy is necessary after robotic surgery. Currently, long term oncologic outcome is not certain after robot-assisted prostatectomy. Similar echos are coming from the other side of the Atlantic. Lotan from Texas wrote in 2010 in Current Opinion in Urology :"These added costs have not been associated with significant improved outcomes over pure laparoscopy or open procedures. In order for the robot to be cost effective, efficacy needs to be improved over alternative approaches and costs of the robot or instruments need to be decreased" (11). Breitenstein goes even further by saying "Costs of robots are high and currently do not justify the use of this technique due to the lack of proven benefit for patients. A reduction of acquisition, maintenance and disposable costs of the robotic system is a prerequisite for large scale adoption and implementation of this technique. The exponential use of robotic surgery is not based on evidence based benefits but mainly patient driven, stimulated by enthusiastic surgeons who love these "high tech toys" and a smart marketing machine driven by the manufactures. In order to stay viable, robotic programs will need to pay for themselves on a per case basis. Although it is likely that there is a great future for robotic surgery its advantages should not be taken for granted and should be further investigated. Multicenter international trials including a health economic section are needed to demonstrate that the higher costs are warranted by superior outcomes. Until then physicians have a responsibility to society and their patients to deliver the best possible care at justifiable cost.

8. Future perspectives

It has been estimated that the introduction of robotic surgery has increased the costs of certain forms of health care significantly with little proven benefit. Attempts can be made by the surgeon to minimize the costs of robotic surgery by reducing the number of instruments used (4 in stead of 5 instruments: use of only one needle driver saves 292 Euro), reducing the operating time of a procedure (get more experience), training dedicated robotic surgeons (not everybody can and should do this surgery in a unit), and stimulating early discharge of the patient when possible (savings will be greater in high cost university hospital vs low cost hospital). The hospital can decrease the costs by increasing the case load by stimulating multidisciplinary use of the robot centralization of robotic surgery. Robotic surgery should only be used for complex surgery. Last but not least: it is of paramount importance that the price of the robot, the maintenance costs, and the price of the drapings and instruments is reduced by the manufacturer in order to keep robotics affordable in most health care systems. Intuitive Surgical virtually has a monopoly in robotic surgery and competition is needed in this field. Manufacturers of laparoscopic devices should be creative to make laparoscopic surgery more accessible to facilitate the use of video-endoscopic surgery, which up to now seems to have a similar efficacy as robotic surgery. However, the future of robotics looks bright as robots will become even smaller and easier to handle, surgeons will get better performing robotic surgery, and eventually robots will become cheaper as almost all electronic devices did when they became more mature with many competitors on the market.

9. References

[1] Hockstein NG, Gourin Cg, Faust RA, terries DJ. A history of robots from science fuction to surgical robots. J Robot Surg 2007;1:113-118.

[2] Advicula AP, Wang K. Evolving role and current state of robotics in minimally invasive gynecologic surgery. J Min Invasiv Surg 2009;16:291-301.

[3] Kwoh YS, Hou J, Jonckheere EA, Hayati S. A robot with improved absolute positioning accuracy for CT guided steraotactic brain surgery. IEEE Trans Biomed Eng 1988; 35:153-60.

[4] Luketich JD, Fernando HC, Buenaventura PO, Christie NA, Grondin SC, SChauer PR. Results of a randomize trial with HERMES assisted versus non Hermes assisted laparoscopic anti-reflux surgery. Surg Endosc 2002;16:1264-1266.

[5] Marescaux J, Rubino F. The ZEUS robotic system: experimental and clinical applications. Surg Clin North Am 2003;83:1305-1315.

[6] Schreuder HW, Verheijen RH. Robotic Surgery. BJOG 2008; 116: 198-213

[7] Bren L. Alternatives to hysterectomy, new technologies, more options. FDA Consum 2001;35:23-28.

[8] Chen CC, Falcone T. Robotic Gynecologic Surgery: Past, present and Future. Clinical Obs and Gyn 2009;52:335-343.

[9] Lenihan JP, Kovanda C, Seshadri-Kreaden U. What is the learning curve for robotic assisted gynecologic surgery. J Minim Invasive Gynecol 200;15: 589-594.

[10] Holloway RW, Patel D, Ahmad S. Robotic surgery in Gynecology. Scan J Surg 2009;98:96-109.

[11] Lotan Y. Economics of robotics in urology. Curr Opni Urol 2010;20:92-97.

[12] Lotan y, cadeddu JA. Financial aspects of laparoscopy. In: Gill I, editor. Textbook of laparoscopic urology. New York: Informa Healthcare USA, Inc, 2006; Chapter 90:1009-1016.

[13] Steinberg Pl, Merguerian PA, Bihrle W, Seigne JD. The cost of learning robotic-assisted prostatectomy. Urology 2008;72:1068-1072.

[14] Steinberg PL, Merguerian PA, Bihrle W, Heaney JA, Seigne JD. A da Vinci robot system can make sense for a mature laparoscopic prostatectomy program. JSLS 2008;12:9-12.

[15] Albani JM, Lee DI,. Virtual reality-assisted robotic surgery simulation. J Enourol 2007;21:285-7.

[16] Leddy LS, Lendvay TS, Satava RM. Robotic surgery: applications and cost effectiveness. Open Access Surgery 2010:3:99-107.

[17] Matern U, Koneczny S. Safety, hazards and ergonomics in the operating room. Surg Enodsc 2007;21:1965-9.

[18] Sarlos D, Kots L, Stevanovic N, Schaer G. Robotic hysterectomy versus convetional laparoscopic hysterectomy: outcome and cost analyses of a matched case control study. Eur J Obstet Gynecol Reprod Biol 2010;150:92-6.

[19] Pasic RP, Rizzo JA, Farig H, Ross S, Moore M, Gunnarsson C. Coparing robotiassisted with conventional laparoscopic hysterectomy: impact on cost and clinical outcomes. J Minim Invasive Gynecol 2010;17:730-8.

[20] Barnett JC, Judd JP, Wu JM, Scales CD, Myers ER, Havrilevsky LJ. Cost coparison among robotic, laparoscopic and open hysterectomy for endometrial cancer. Obstet Gynecol 2010;116:685-93

[21] Rodgers AK, Goldberg JM, Hammel JP, Fancone T. Tubal anastomosis by robotic compared with outpatient minilaparotomy. Obstet Gynecol 2007;109:1375-80.

[22] Dharia Patel SP, Steinkampf MP, Whitten SJ, Malizia BA. Robotic tubal anastomosis: surgical technique and cost effectiveness. Fertile Steil 200:90:1175-9.

[23] Heemskerk J, de Hoog DE, van Gemert WG, Baeten Cg, Greve JW, Bouvy ND. Dis Colon rectum 2007;50:1825-30.

[24] Advincula AP, Xu X, Goudeau S, Ransom SB. Robot-assisted laparoscopic myomectomy versus abdominal myomectomy: a comparison of short-term surgical outcomes and immediate costs. J Minim Invasive Gynecol 2007:14:698-705.

[25] Bell MC, Torgerson J, Seshadri-Kraeden U, Suttle AW, Hunt. Comparison of outcomes and cost for endometrial cancer staging via traditional laparotomy, standard laparoscopy and robotic techniques. Gynecol Oncol 2008;111:407-11.

[26] Bolenz C, Gupta A, Hotze T, Ho R, Cadeddu JA, Roehrbom CG, Lotan Y. Cost Comparison of robotic, laparoscopic and open radical prostatectomy for prostate cancer. Eur Urol 2010;57:453-8.

[27] Smith A, Kurpad R, lal A, Nielsen M, Wallen EM, Pruthi RS. Cost analysis of robotic versus open radical prostatectomy for bladder cancer. J Urol 2010;183:505-9.

[28] Breitenstein S, Nocito A, Puhan M, Held U, weber M, Clavien PA. Robotic assisted versus laparoscopic cholecystectomy: outcome and cost analyses of a matched control study. Ann Surg 2008;247:987-93.

[29] Hubens G, Balliu L, Ruppert M, Gypen B, Van Tu T, vaneerdeweg W. Roux-enY gastric bypass procedure performed with the da Vanci robot system: is it worth it ? Surg Endosc 2008;22:1690-6.

[30] Park BJ, Flores RM. Cost Comparison of robotic, video-asisted thoracic surgery and thoracotomy approaches to pulmonary lobectomy. Thor Surg Clin 2008;18:287-300.

[31] Casali G, Walker WS. Video-assisted thoracic surgery lobectomy: can we afford it ? Eur J Cardiothorac Surg 2009;35:423-8.

[32] Jones B, Desai P, Proston R. Establishing the case for minimally invasive, robotic assisted CABG in the treatment of multivessel coronary artery disease. Heart Surg Forum 2009;12:E147-9.

[33] Kam JK, Cooray SD, Kam JK, Smith JA, Almeida AA. A cost analysis study of robotic versus conventional mitral valve repair. Heart Lung Circ 2010;19:413-8.

[34] Morgan JA, Thornton BA, Peacock JC, Hollingsworth KW, Smith CR, Oz MC, Argenziano M. Does robotic technology make minimally invasive cardiac surgery too expensive ? A hospital cost analysis of robotic and conventional technques. J Card Surg 2005;20:246-51.

[35] Anderberg M, Kockum CC, Arnbjornsson E. Paediatric robotic surgery in clinical practice: a cost analysis. Eur J Pediatr Surg 2009;19:311-5.

[36] Barbash GI, Gilled SA. New technology and health care costs.The case of robot assisted surgery 2010;363:701-4.

[37] Snyder CF, Frick KD, Blackford AL, Herbert RJ, Neville BA, Carducci MA, Earle CC. How does initial treatment choice affect short-term and long term costs for clinically localized prostate cancer ? Cancer 2010;116:5391-9.
[38] Graefen M. Low quality of eveidence for robot-asisted laparoscopic prostatectomy: a problem not only in robotic literature. Eur Urol 2010:57:943-4.

15

Robotic Surgery in Gynecologic Oncology

Behrouz Zand and Pedro T. Ramirez
University of Texas-M.D.
Anderson Cancer Center Department of Gynecologic Oncology
U.S.A

1. Introduction

Approximately 83,000 women were diagnosed in the United States with gynecologic malignancies in 2010 (Jemal et al., 2010). Treatment typically involves major abdominal surgery to remove the primary cancer. In addition to a hysterectomy, staging procedures such as pelvic and para-aortic dissection are often needed. In order to minimize the morbidity of surgery, a minimally invasive approach has been shown to provide numerable benefits to patients. These include shorter hospitalizations, reduced blood loss, faster recovery, and fewer postoperative complications.

The da Vinci Surgical System (Intuitive Surgical, Inc, Sunnyvale, California, USA) was approved by the FDA in 2005 for use in gynecology. This system has several advantages over traditional laparoscopy including 7 degrees of motion, 3-dimensional views, tremor filtration, and improved dexterity. Potential drawbacks of this system include lack of haptic feedback, cost, and the size of the system that often requires special operating rooms. In this chapter, we will focus on the outcomes, safety and feasibility reported on robotic assisted surgery in cervical, endometrial and ovarian cancer.

2. Cervical cancer

Cervical cancer is the second most common malignancy in women worldwide (Schiffman et al., 2007). The number of cancer cases in developed countries has dramatically declined since the advent of frequent screening with "Pap" smears. In 2010, 12,200 cervical cancer cases were diagnosed in the U.S., and 4,210 cervical cancer deaths were reported (Jemal et al., 2010).

2.1 Radical hysterectomy

Historically, patients with stages IA2 to IB1 cervical cancer have been managed with radical hysterectomy performed by laparotomy. The first laparoscopic radical hysterectomy with pelvic and para-aortic lymphadenectomy was published in 1992 (Nezhat et al., 1992). Since that time, laparoscopic radical hysterectomy has been shown to be a safe and feasible alternative for treatment of early-stage cervical cancer. (Ramirez et al., 2006; Frumovitz et al., 2007). However, the use of laparoscopic radical hysterectomy has not been embraced by most gynecologic oncologists due to its technical difficulty.

Sert & Abeler described the first robotic-assisted radical hysterectomy with pelvic lymph node dissection (Sert & Abeler, 2006). The same group went on to publish the first comparative study investigating the feasibility of robotic assisted laparoscopic radical hysterectomy and pelvic lymphadenectomy in patients with early stage cervical cancer compared to conventional laparoscopy. The mean operating time was 241 minutes and 300 minutes in the robotic and laparoscopic group, respectively. However, this difference was not statistically significant. The robotic-assisted group had less blood loss (71 mL vs. 160 mL, p=0.038). There was no difference in the number of lymph nodes, parametrial tissue, and cuff size between the two groups. The robotic-assisted group had a shorter hospital stay (4 days vs. 8 days, p= 0.004) (Sert & Abeler, 2007).

In a case-control cohort study, fifty one patients underwent robotic-assisted type III radical hysterectomy and pelvic lymph node dissection, while forty-nine patients underwent traditional laparotomy radical hysterectomy. The robotic group had significantly less blood loss (96 mL vs. 417 mL), and operative time (211 minutes vs. 248 minutes). The robotic group also had significantly higher lymph node retrieval (33.8 vs. 23.3). The robotic group had a shorter hospital stay (1 day vs. 3.2 days). The laparotomy group had a higher complication rate than the robotic group, 16.3% versus 7.8%; however, this was not statistically significant (Boggess et al., 2008a).

Magrina et al. compared perioperative results of 27 patients undergoing robotic radical hysterectomy from 2003 to 2006. Comparisons were made with laparoscopic and laparotomy patients matched by age, BMI, type of hysterectomy (radical or modified radical), site and type of malignancy, and FIGO staging. The operating times of the robotics and laparotomy groups were similar (189.6 minutes vs. 166.8 minutes), and significantly shorter compared to laparoscopy (220.4 minutes). There were no differences in the number of lymph node retrieval between the three groups. Blood loss (133.1 mL vs. 208.4 mL) was similar between the robotic and laparoscopic group, and highest for laparotomy group (443.6 mL). The length of hospital stay was similar between robotic and laparoscopic group (1.7 vs. 2.4 days, respectively). The laparotomy group had the longest average length of hospital stay (3.6 days). There were no differences in the complication rates between the 3 groups (Magrina et al., 2008).

2.2 Setup & technique

The patient is placed in the dorsal lithotomy position using Allen stirrups (Allen Medical, Acton MA) with arms tucked to the side. The robotic tower and the tower containing the electrosurgical generators and smoke evacuator are positioned lateral to the patient's right foot. A uterine manipulator is often used. The da Vinci column is positioned between the patient's legs.

A 10 mm transumbillical trocar is introduced approximately 20 cm above the pubic symphisis. Another 10 mm trocar is placed approximately 8 cm lateral in the left upper quadrant in the left mid-clavicular line. This trocar is used as an assistant port. The robotic trocars are then placed. These are all 8 mm trocars. The first is placed 8-cm lateral to the assistant port, the second is placed 8 cm lateral and 15 degrees below the midline camera port, and the third trocar is placed 8 cm lateral to the last trocar on the right side (Figure 1). The operating table is placed in Trendelenburg position until the small bowel and sigmoid are displaced out of the pelvis and to a maximum of 30 degrees.

Once the robotic column is advanced to the operating table and placed between the patient's legs, the robotic system is docked and instruments are introduced. There are a number of instruments that may be used and surgeons are encouraged to test several before deciding what is ideal for their practice. We prefer to use an EndoWrist bipolar grasper (Intuitive Surgical, Sunnyvale, CA) on the left upper quadrant port, an EndoWrist monopolar scissor in the right hand through the right sided trocar immediately next to the camera port, and an EndoWrist Cadiere grasper in the most lateral right trocar.

The robotic radical hysterectomy is performed in the same manner as a traditional Piver type III abdominal radical hysterectomy with the use of scissors and monopolar cautery for isolation and ligation of small vessels and bipolar cautery for the ovarian vessels, uterine artery, and vascular branches of the cardinal and uterosacral ligaments. After isolation of the uterine artery and division at its origin on the pelvic sidewall, the artery is dissected free of the ureter, exposing the ureteral tunnel of Wertheim. The ureter is freed from the medial leaf of the broad ligament until it enters the cardinal ligament. The anterior vesical ligament is then coagulated and divided with scissors. Any remaining medial attachments of the ureter to the vagina is then released, and the ureter and bladder is dissected free of the anterior vagina to allow vaginotomy with an adequate margin.

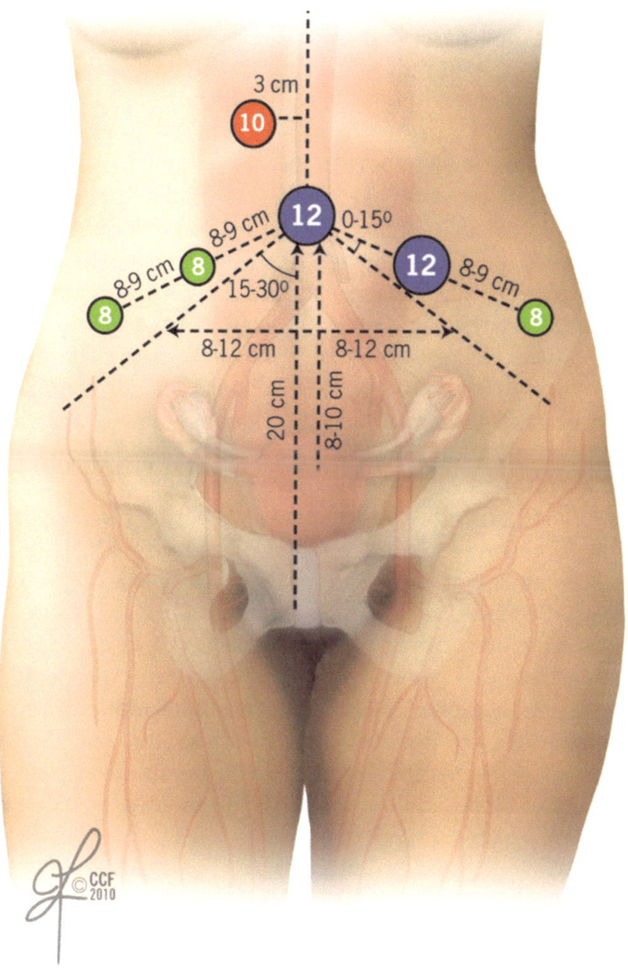

Fig. 1. Trocar placement in radical hysterectomy

The rectovaginal space is developed by an incision of the peritoneum over and between the uterosacral ligaments. The uterosacral ligament is then transected to its insertion into the posterior vaginal wall, and the remainder of the cardinal ligament is resected to the sidewall of the vagina. After the same dissection on the patients left side is completed, vaginotomy is performed. Once the vaginotomy is completed, the specimen is delivered vaginally, and a sponge is placed in the vagina to restore pneumoperitoneum. The specimen is inspected to evaluate the adequacy of the vaginal and parametrial margins. If additional vaginal margin is required, then it is resected easily at this point in the procedure.

Once the radical hysterectomy is completed a complete bilateral pelvic lymphadenectomy is performed from the common iliac artery proximally to the circumflex iliac vein distally. The specimens are placed in an EndoCatch bag (Ethicon Endo-Surgery Inc, Cincinnati, OH) and delivered vaginally. The vaginal cuff is closed using a continuous barbed suture.

2.3 Radical trachelectomy

Radical trachelectomy has been shown to be a safe and feasible option in patients diagnosed with cervical cancer who wish to preserve their fertility (Beiner et al., 2008; Plante et al., 2011). The procedure was first described by Dargent et al. in 1994 (Dargent et al., 1994). Most of the published literature on radical trachelectomy has been on the vaginal approach. However, the vaginal approach can be technically difficult in nulliparous women without pelvic descent and requires a surgeon comfortable with a radical vaginal approach. Alternatively, several studies have reported the safety and feasibility of the abdominal approach (Ungar et al., 2005; Pareja et al., 2008). The robotic approach can offer the same advantages of minimally invasive surgery (decreased blood loss, decreased pain, quicker return of bowel function, etc.) to patients requiring this challenging procedure. The literature on this procedure is limited to isolated case reports and small case series.

A study by Ramirez et al. reported on four patients with stage IA1-1A2 cervical cancer that underwent robotic radical trachelectomy and bilateral pelvic lymphadenectomy. The median operative time was 339.5 minutes. The median blood loss was 62.5 mL. The median number of pelvic lymph nodes removed was 20. There were no conversions to laparotomy and no intraoperative complications. The median length of hospital stay was 1.5 days. One patient experienced a transient left lower extremity sensory neuropathy postoperatively (Ramirez et al., 2010). Another study by Burnett et al. reported their experience with robotic radical trachelectomy. Six women underwent this procedure with stage IBI squamous cell carcinoma or adenocarcinoma of the cervix. Median age was 27 years old. The mean duration of surgery was 360 minutes. Mean blood loss was 108 mL. None of the women had positive lymph nodes. Five out of the six women had negative margins. All patients were discharged on postoperative day one or two. There were two postoperative complications. One patient developed a herniation of small bowel through 8 mm port site on day 4 and one patient had ecchymosis of anterior abdominal wall to the left flank consistent with hemorrhage from the inferior epigastric vessels which required no intervention except for transfusion with 2 units of blood. Follow up from 9-13 months revealed no recurrences or pregnancies (Burnett et al., 2009).

2.3.1 Setup & technique

The patient is placed in the dorsal lithotomy position. A V-Care manipulator (Utica, NY) is placed in the uterus for manipulation. Once the manipulator is placed, attention is focused on the abdominal part of the procedure. A 12 mm bladeless trocar (Ethicon Endosurgery,

Cincinnati, OH) is introduced in the left upper quadrant approximately 2 cm below the left costal margin at the midclavicular line and the abdomen is insufflated. This trocar is used during the procedure by the patient-side assistant. The patient is then placed in the steep Trendelenburg position. The abdomen is explored for evidence of metastatic disease. Another 12 mm bladeless trocar is placed in the umbilicus under direct visualization. Alternatively, this trocar may be placed 2 cm above the umbilicus to gain better visualization of the pelvis. This second trocar is used for the robotic camera. The robotic trocars are then placed. The first robotic trocar is placed 8 cm lateral to and 15 degrees below the patient-side assistant's trocar. The second robotic trocar is placed 8 cm to the right of and 15 degrees below the trocar at the umbilicus. The third robotic trocar is placed 8 cm lateral to the second robotic trocar (Fig. 2).

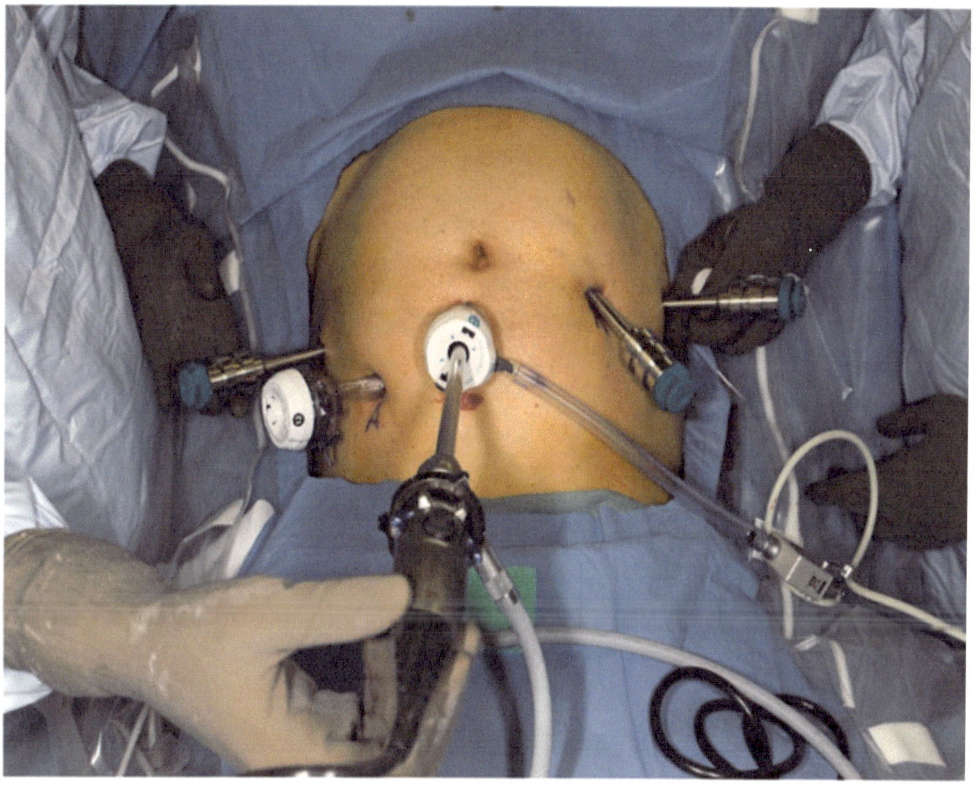

Fig. 2. Trocar placement for robotic radical trachelectomy

The robotic instruments are then placed. These include an EndoWrist bipolar grasper (Intuitive Surgical, Sunnyvale, CA) through the first robotic trocar, an EndoWrist monopolar scissor through the second robotic trocar, and an EndoWrist Cardiere grasper through the third robotic trocar. The da Vinci System is then docked. The radical trachelectomy is performed as follows: An incision is made over the round ligament and the peritoneum lateral to the infundibulopelvic ligaments is opened bilaterally. The paravesical and pararectal spaces are then developed. The ureters are then separated from the peritoneum down to where they enter the lateral parametrial tissue. The level of resection of the parametria is as follows: the ureters are dissected from the parametria and mobilized completely to the bladder after division of the anterior and posterior vesicouterine ligaments. The peritoneum over the bladder is then incised, and the bladder is mobilized inferiorly over the anterior vaginal wall. The uterine vessels are transected bilaterally at their origin and dissected over the ureters bilaterally. The anterior vesicouterine ligaments are then divided. The peritoneum over the rectovaginal space is then incised, and the uterosacral ligaments are divided bilaterally. While upward traction is placed on the vaginal cuff, a circumferential incision is made in the vagina to assure an adequate 2 cm margin. The V-Care manipulator is then removed.

The specimen is then held by the parametria bilaterally using graspers. A monopolar scissor or Harmonic scalpel (Ethicon Endo-Surgery, Cincinnati, OH) is used to amputate the cervix, leaving approximately 1 cm of residual cervical stump. The specimen—including cervix, bilateral parametria, and upper vaginal margin—is then removed through the vagina. The specimen is then sent for frozen section evaluation. The endocervical margin should be tumor-free at least 5mm from the level of the tumor. A Smit sleeve cannula (Nucletron, Columbia, MD) is then introduced vaginally and placed into the uterus by using the robotic graspers. We use the Smit sleeve cannula (See figure 3) to decrease the potential for scarring of the residual cervix. It is usually left in the uterus for approximately 2–4 weeks. A cerclage is placed using 0-Ethibond suture (Ethicon, Inc.), and the uterus is sutured to the upper vagina using interrupted 0-Vicryl sutures placed using the EndoWrist Mega Needle driver. Alternatively, a single continuous barbed suture may be used to anastomose the uterus to the vagina. The cerclage is placed abdominally using the robotic system. The pelvic lymphadenectomy is performed bilaterally from the level of the mid-common iliac vessels to the circumflex iliac vein distally.

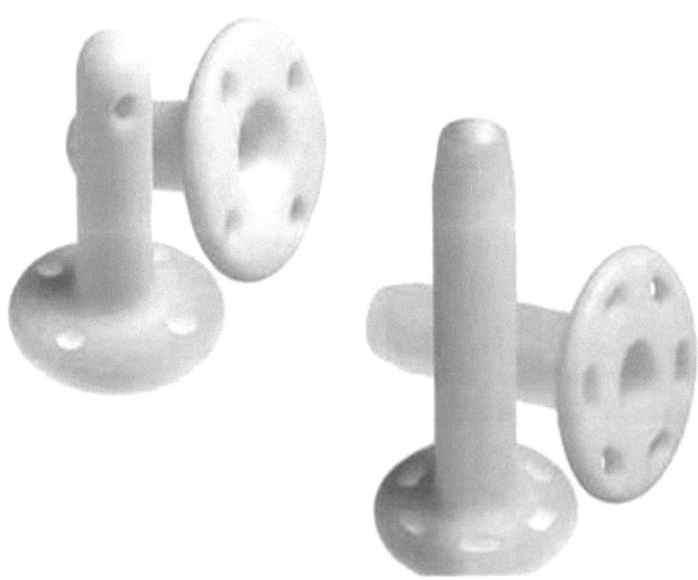

Fig. 3. Smit sleeve cannula used in radical trachelectomy

3. Endometrial cancer

Endometrial cancer is the most common gynecologic malignancy in developed countries. The American Cancer Society estimates that 43,470 American women were diagnosed in

2010 and approximately 7,950 women died of the disease during that time. (Jemal et al., 2010). The majority of patients are diagnosed with early stage disease. Endometrial cancer is staged surgically. Historically, surgical staging in endometrial cancer has been done by open laparotomy which includes hysterectomy, bilateral salpingo-oophorectomy, and bilateral pelvic and para-aortic lymphadenectomy in select patients with specific risk factors. In the 1990s, small single institution studies showed the safety and feasibility of laparoscopic surgical staging in endometrial cancer (Querleu et al., 1991; Childers et al., 1994; Spirtos et al., 1995). In 2009, a prospective, multi-institutional, randomized trial showed the feasibility and safety of laparoscopic comprehensive surgical staging for endometrial cancer. Of the 1,682 patients, 74.2% were completed without conversion to laparotomy. The laparotomy group did have a shorter operative time despite no difference in intraoperative complications. No difference in overall detection of advanced stage (stage IIIA, IIIC, or IVB) was seen. The laparoscopy group had fewer postoperative adverse events and significantly shorter hospital stay than the laparotomy group (Walker et al., 2009). Therefore, minimally invasive surgery is a safe and feasible option for surgical staging in endometrial cancer.

3.1 Robotic assisted hysterectomy and staging

Robotic surgery has several advantages over laparotomy in the management of endometrial cancer. It has been shown to be potentially equivalent to laparoscopy in this setting. In a study by Boggess et al., the authors compared the outcomes in women who underwent hysterectomy and staging by robotic, laparoscopy or laparotomy. The number of cases was 138 for the laparotomy group, 81 for the laparoscopy group, and 103 for the robotic group. The robotic cohort had a statistically significant higher BMI ($p= 0.0008$). Operative time was longest for the laparoscopy group at 213.4 minutes followed by robotic group at 191.2 minutes and laparotomy group at 146.5 minutes. The estimated blood loss was lowest for the robotic technique ($p<0.0001$). Lymph node retrieval was highest for robotic group. Length of hospital stay was lowest for the robotic group ($p<0.0001$). The postoperative complications rates were lower for the robotic group versus laparotomy group, 5.8% versus 29.7% respectively. The complication rate between laparoscopy and robotic group were not statistically different (Boggess et al., 2008b). Similar results were seen in other studies (Veljovich et al., 2008; Bell et al., 2008, Seamon et al., 2009).

Comparison of clinical outcomes of robotic cases versus laparoscopic or laparotomy for endometrial cancer was evaluated in a meta-analysis by Gaia et al. in 2010. The analysis included 1,591 patients from eight comparative studies. Operative time was similar between robotic and laparoscopic cases, but longer than laparotomy group. The estimated blood loss was lower in the robotic hysterectomy group compared to the laparotomy and laparoscopy group. There were no differences in the pooled analysis on the number of pelvic and para-aortic lymph nodes in all three groups. The length of hospital stay was shorter for both robotic and laparoscopic groups compared to the laparotomy group. Differences in complication rates were not seen between the three groups. Therefore, clinical outcomes between laparoscopy and robotic surgery for endometrial cancer seem similar with the exception of less blood loss in robotic surgery (Gaia et al., 2010).

3.1.1 Setup & technique

The trocar placement for the robotic-assisted hysterectomy for endometrial cancer is the same as that described above for robotic-assisted radical hysterectomy. To initiate the hysterectomy, the bipolar device grasps the right round ligament. This is then coagulated and transected. An incision is made lateral to the infundibulopelvic ligaments. The right ureter is identified, and the ovarian vessels are coagulated and transected. The broad ligament is then skeletonized with monopolar scissors as the bipolar graspers are used to apply medial traction of the right adnexa. Dissection is continued along the broad ligament to the vesicouterine peritoneum. The assistant places upward traction on the uterine manipulator while the surgeon advances the dissection, and the bladder flap is created. The uterine vessels are coagulated with the bipolar forceps and transected with the monopolar scissors. The same procedure is performed on the left side of the uterus.

The vaginal incision is made anteriorly with the monopolar scissors just below the cervix. This incision is extended lateral to the right and left fornix. Exposure is further facilitated by upward traction in the anterior vaginal fornix. The vaginal assistant places counter tension in the posterior fornix and the posterior vaginal incision follows the scored peritoneum to meet the anterior incision and the uterus is removed through the vagina. Once hemostasis of the vaginal cuff is confirmed, the assistant exchanges the monopolar scissors for robotic needle drivers. The recto sigmoid colon is retracted with the suction irrigator or bipolar grasper, and the blunt grasper displaces the bladder away from the vagina. The cuff may be closed with a single running or multiple interrupted sutures.

For the pelvic lymphadenectomy, the bipolar grasper and monopolar scissors are used to perform the dissection. The pararectal and paravesical spaces are developed, and the ureter and superior vesicle artery is identified. The bipolar grasper then provides gentle retraction at the bifurcation and displaces the ureter medially. After the landmarks are established, the pelvic lymphadenectomy is performed adhering to the following boundaries: mid-psoas muscle laterally, above the bifurcation of the common iliac proximally, the deep circumflex iliac vein distally, and the obturator nerve inferiorly. During the obturator dissection, the assistant provides gentle traction on the external iliac vein with the blunt grasper, and the suction irrigator is used to retract the superior vesicle artery. Each side of the pelvic lymph node dissection results in 1 or 2 large node bundles that are placed in 1 bag for each side.

To begin the right aortic lymphadenectomy, the peritoneum over the right common iliac artery is grasped and incised with the monopolar scissors. The Cadiere grasper is used to place lateral traction on the peritoneum on the right side and the assistant grasps the peritoneum overlying the aorta, also placing lateral traction to the left side. The incision is extended along the right side of the aorta mobilizing the duodenum.

The ureter is identified by retroperitoneal dissection under the lateral peritoneal reflection between the right common and ovarian vessels. The right psoas muscle, genitofemoral nerve, ovarian vessels, and ureter are visualized. The assistant reflects the ureter laterally. The node dissection is performed by skeletonizing the nodal bundle over the inferior vena cava from the bifurcation of the common iliac vessels to just below the right renal vein. A wide field of dissection is essential for optimal exposure. Once the planes are created, the assistant may provide lateral ureteral retraction with the blunt grasper allowing the suction-irrigator to remain free to facilitate a dry operative field and to retract small bowel. The lymph node bundle is skeletonized from the right common iliac artery and aorta. Further dissection is performed just under the lymph node bundle and away from the inferior vena cava, creating small pedicles so that lymphatics or small venous perforators can be safely coagulated and sealed before the transection. The surgeon must be visually aware of the amount of tension that is placed on the lymph nodes. After the medial aspect of the dissection is completed, the superior boundary of the bundle is coagulated and cut; the bundle is freed from its loose lateral attachments down to the inferior boundary. Once the en-bloc dissection is complete, the lymph nodes are placed in an Endo Catch Gold bag (Auto Suture Division, Tyco Healthcare, and Norwalk, CT) and removed.

For the left aortic lymphadenectomy, the peritoneal incision is extended over the left common iliac artery and above the inferior mesenteric artery (IMA). The ideal dissection plane is created by sharply opening the retroperitoneal areolar tissue close to the aorta and left common iliac artery in the direction of the psoas muscle. The bedside assistant places gentle counter tension on the aorta and the blunt grasper retracts the distal ureter and mesentery out of the field of dissection. Next, the bipolar grasper gently retracts the superior aspect of the peritoneal window created a few centimeters distal to the IMA insertion into the aorta. The lymph nodes on the left side lie lateral and often posterior to the great vessels and are first dissected away from the aorta, and pedicles are created and ligated close to the node bundle. Occasionally, the assistant is able to grasp the nodal bundle and provide counter tension during dissection. The lymph node bundle lateral to the aorta is removed en-bloc from just above the bifurcation of the common iliac vessels to the IMA. Dissection above this level may be performed at the discretion of the surgeon.

The pelvis is irrigated, and the abdomen/pelvis including all vascular pedicles are inspected. The midline port is closed at the fascial level with interrupted suture. Depending on surgeon preference, the 5- to 12-mm port is either left open or sutured with the Inlet Carter-Thomason CloseSure System (Ascent Healthcare Solutions, Phoenix, AZ).

4. Ovarian cancer

The studies for ovarian cancer staging in minimally invasive surgery are very limited. There is a paucity of data on the feasibility and safety of robotic surgery in patients with ovarian cancer. In a recent study by Magrina et al., a retrospective analysis case-control analysis of 25 patients who underwent robotic surgical treatment were compared to similar patients who underwent standard laparoscopy and laparotomy. The rate of intraoperative complications was similar for the 3 groups. Laparoscopy and robotics were preferable in patients with primary tumor excision (hysterectomy, adnexectomy, omentectomy, pelvic and para-aortic lymphadenectomy, appendectomy, and removal of metastatic peritoneal disease). However, with advanced ovarian cancer, laparotomy was the preferred method as robotic outcomes were not improved because operative times were 138 minutes longer, and length of stay were similar between the two groups. There was no difference in overall survival among the 3 groups. The median length of follow up was 2.2 years for the robotic group, 4.4 years for the laparoscopy group, and 2.9 years for the laparotomy group. Progression free survival was significantly higher for the robotic and laparoscopy group compared to laparotomy group. This difference in progression free survival was most likely due to selection bias as patients with more disseminated disease underwent laparotomy. Furthermore, the robotic and laparoscopy groups had an overall higher rate of neoadjuvant or intra-peritoneal chemotherapy as compared to the laparotomy group, which likely, further contributed to the improved progression free survival (Magrina et al., 2010). Although robotic assisted surgery in treatment and staging of ovarian cancer seems promising especially in early stage cancer, further long term outcome data are needed. At this time, we do not find robotic assisted surgery to be a safe and feasible option for surgical staging in advanced ovarian cancer.

5. Conclusion

Robotic surgery in gynecologic oncology provides the benefits of minimally invasive surgery (shorter hospital stay, decreased blood loss, faster recovery, and fewer postoperative complications with the added benefits of 7 degrees of motion, 3-dimensional views, tremor reduction, improved dexterity and decreased surgeon fatigue). The main drawbacks are the expense, absence of haptic feedback, and longer term outcome data are needed since it is a new technology.

Robotic surgery in gynecologic oncology holds great promise. If long term and large population data show its efficacy and safety to be comparable or superior to conventional laparoscopy and laparotomy, then robotic surgery will play a pivotal role in gynecologic oncology surgery. Short term data and small case series, comparing robotic surgery with laparoscopy in cervical and endometrial cancer, show comparable or superior outcomes for robotic surgery. With regard to ovarian cancer, although the data is scant, robotic surgery may hold promise in surgical staging for treatment of ovarian cancer, especially in the early stages of ovarian cancer.

6. References

Beiner ME, Hauspy J, Rosen B, Murphy J, Laframboises, Nofech-Mozes S, Ismiil N, Rasty G, Khalifa MA, Covens A. Radical vaginal trachelectomy vs. radical hysterectomy for small early stage cervical cancer: a match case control study. *Gynecol Oncol*, Vol. 110, Issue 2 (August 2008), pp 168-171.

Bell MC, Torgerson J, Seshadri-Kreaden U, Suttle AW, Hunt S. Comparison of outcomes and cost of endometrial cancer staging via traditional laparotomy, standard laparoscopy, and robotic techniques. *Gynecol Oncol*, Volume 111, Issue 3 (December 2008), pp. 407-411.

a. Boggess JF, Gehrig PA, Cantrell L, Shafer A, Ridgway M, Skinner E, Folwer WC. A case control study of robot-assisted type III radical hysterectomy with pelvic lymph node dissection compared with open radical hysterectomy. *Am J Obstet Gynecol*, Vol. 199, Issue 4 (October 2008), pp 357.e1-357.e7.

b. Boggess JF, Gehrig PA, Cantrell L, Shafer A, Ridgway M, Skiiner E, Fowler WC. A comparative study of 3 surgical methods for hysterectomy with staging for endometrial cancer: robotic assistance, laparoscopy, laparotomy. *Am J Obstet Gynecol*, Vol. 1999, Issue 4 (October 2008), pp. 360e1-360.e9.

Burnett AF, Stone PJ, Duckworth MD, Roman JJ. Robotic radical trachelectomy for preservation of fertility in early cervical cancer: Case series and description of technique. *J of Min Inv Gynecol*, Vol. 16, Issue 5, (September/October 2009), pp. 569-572.

Childers JM, Spirtos NM, Brainard P, Surwit EA. Laparoscopic staging of the patient with incompletely staged early adenocarcinoma of the endometrium. *Obstet Gynecol*, Vol. 83, Issue 4 (April 1994), pp 597-600.

Dargent D. Laparoscopic surgery and gynecologic cancer. *Curr Opin Obstet Gynecol*, Vol. 5, Issue 3 (June 1993), pp 294-300.

Gaia G, Holloway RW, Santoro L, Ahmad S, Silverio ED, Spinillo A. Robotic-assisted hysterectomy for endometrial cancer compared with traditional laparoscopic and laparotomy approaches. *Obstet Gynecol*, Vol. 116, Issue 6 (December 2010), pp 1422-1431.

Frumovitz M, Dos Reis R, Sun CC, Milam MR, Bevers MW, Brown J, Slomovitz BM, Ramirez PT. Comparison of total laparoscopic and abdominal radical hysterectomy for patients with early stage cervical cancer. *Obstet Gynecol*, Vol. 110, Issue 1 (July 2007), pp 96-102.

Jemal A, Siegel R, Xu J, Ward E. Cancer statistics, 2010. *CA Cancer J Clin*, Vol. 60, Issue 5 (September-October 2010), pp 277-300.

Magrina JF, Kho RM, Weaver AL, Montero RP, Magtibay PM. Robotic radical hysterectomy: comparison with laparoscopy and laparotomy. *Gynecol Oncol*, Vol 109, Issue 1 (April 2008), pp 86-91.

Magrina JF, Zanagnolo V, Noble BN, Kho RM, Magtibay P. Robotic approach for ovarian cancer: Perioperative and survival results and comparison with laparoscopy and laparotomy. *Gynecol Oncol*, Article in Press, Available online December 2010.

Nezhat CR, Burrell MO, Nezhat FR, Benigno BB, Welander CE. Laparoscopic radical hysterectomy with paraaortic and pelvic node dissection. *Am J Obstet Gynecol*, Vol. 166, Issue 3 (March 1992), pp 864-865.

Pareja RF, Ramirez PT, Borrero MF, Angel CG. Abdominal radical trachelectomy: a case series and literature review. *Gynecol Oncol*, Vol. 111, Issue 3 (December 2008), pp 555-560.

Plante M, Gregoire J, Renaud MC, Rov M. The vaginal radical trachelectomy: An update of a series of 125 cases and 106 pregnancies. . *Gynecol Oncol*, (Jan 2011) Article in Press(November 2008), pp s105-s110.

Querleu D, Leblanc E, Castelain B. Laparoscopic pelvic lymphadenectomy in the staging of early carcinoma of the cervix. *Am J Obstet Gynecol*, Vol. 164, Issue 2 (February 1991), pp 579-581.

Ramirez PT, Schmeler KM, Malpica A, Soliman PT. Safety and feasibility of robotic radical trachelectomy in patients with early-stage cervical cancer. *Gynecol Oncol*, Vol. 116, Issue 3, (March 2010), pp. 512-515.

Ramirez PT, Slomovitz BM, Soliman PT, Coleman RL, Levenback C. Total laparoscopic radical hysterectomy and lymphadenectomy: the M.D. Anderson Cancer Center experience. *Gynecol Oncol*, Vol. 102, Issue 2 (August 2006), pp. 252-255.

Schiffman M, Castle PE, Jeronimo J, Rodriguez AC, Wacholder S. Human papillomavirus and cervical cancer. *Lancet*, Vol. 370, Issue 9590 (September 2007), pp. 890-907.

Seamon, LG, Cohn DE, Henretta MS, Kim KH, Carlson MJ, Phillips GS, Fowler JM. Minimally invasive comprehensive surgical staging for endometrial cancer: Robotics or laparoscopy? *Gynecol Oncol*, Vol. 113, Issue 1 (April 2009), pp. 36-41.

Sert BM, Abeler VM. Robotic-assisted laparoscopic radical hysterectomy (Piver type III) with pelvic node dissection—case report. *Eur J Gynaecol Oncol*, Vol 27, Issue 5 (2006), pp 531-533, ISSN 0392-2936

Sert B, Abeler V. Robotic radical hysterectomy in early-stage cervical carcinoma patients, comparing results with total laparoscopic radical hysterectomy cases. The future is now? *Int J Med Robot*, Vol 3, Issue 3 (Sep 2007), pp. 224-228.

Spirtos NM, Schlaerth JB, Spirtos TW, Schlaerth AC, Indman PD, Kimball RE. Laparoscopic bilateral pelvic and paraaortic lymph node sampling: An evolving technique. *Am J Obstet Gynecol,* Vol. 173, Issue 1(July 1995), pp 105-111.

Ungar L, Palfalvi L, Hogg R, Siklos R, Boyle DC, Del Priore G, Smith JR. Abdominal radical trachelectomy: a fertility preserving option for women with early cervical cancer. *Br J Obstet Gynaecol,* Vol. 112, Issue 3 (March 2005), pp 366-369.

Veljovich DS, Paley PJ, Drescher CW, Everett EN, Shah C, Peters WA III. Robotic surgery in gynecologic oncology: program initiation and outcomes after the first year with comparison with laparotomy for endometrial cancer staging. *Am J Obstet Gynecol,* Vol. 198, Issue 6 (June 2008), pp. 679.e1-e9.

Walker JL, Piedmonte MR, Spirtos NM, Eisenkop SM, Schlaerth JB, Mannel RS, Spiegel G, Barakat R, Pearl ML, Sharma SK. Laparoscopy compared with laparotomy for comprehensive surgical staging of uterine cancer: Gynecologic Oncology Group Study LAP2. *J Clin Oncol,* Vol. 27, Issue 32 (November 2009), pp 5331-5336.

Part 11

Laparoscopic Hysterectomy

16

Laparoscopic Hysterectomy

Cezary Dejewski
Center of minimally invasive gynecological surgery
Amper Kliniken AG, 85221 Dachau
Germany

1. Introduction

The first hysterectomy was performed by Charles Clay in November 1843. It was performed due to a large myomatosus uterus. The operation was successful, however, the patient died on the fifteenth postoperative day. The first patient who survived a hysterectomy was in 1853 and it was performed by Walter Burnham. Out of his subsequent 15 patients, three patients did not survive. These early hysterectomies were all subtotal hysterectomies.

The complete abdominal hysterectomy was recommended in 1929 by Richardson to the prevention of the cervical cancer. Supracervical hysterectomies were preferred for prevention of peritoneal contamination with vaginal bacterial flora and for prevention of peritonitis. However, in the 1950's, when penicillin and other antibiotics became available, Dr. Richardson's technique of total abdominal hysterectomy started to become popular.

Since the first in 1989 from Reich described laparoscopic hysterectomy (LH) the laparoscopic assisted vaginal hysterectomy had spread first in the medical centres (LAVH).

In 1991 Kurt Semm was first who reported about first laparoscopic subtotal hysterectomy. He called his version "CASH" (Classic Abdominal Semm Hysterectomy) and combined the Morcellement of the uterus with the coring out of the cervix. The Semm hysterectomy never became popular due to technical difficulties.

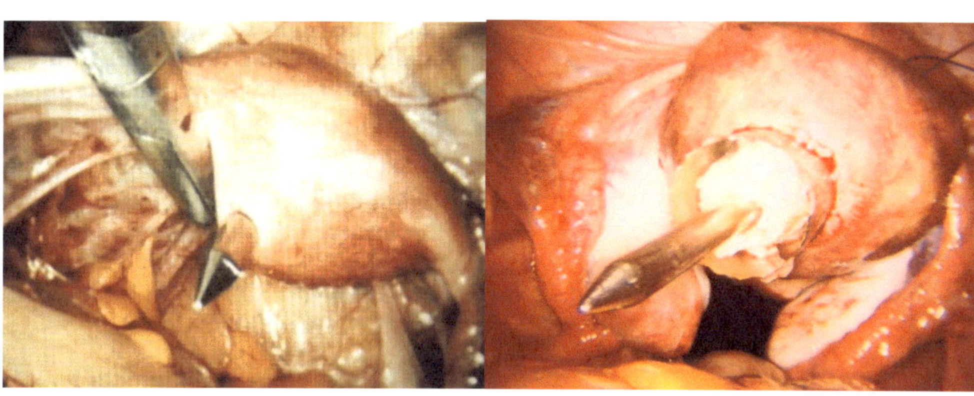

Fig. 1.

2. Indications and contraindications

The indications for laparoscopic hysterectomy are the same, as those which are count to the abdominal hysterectomy - symptomatic uterine fibroids, in the treatment of genital prolaps, endometriosis and adenomyosis, dysmenorrhoe, hypermenorrhoe or dysfunctional uterine bleeding.

After 23 years of development of laparoscopic approach for hysterectomy we haven't any major contraindications to the LH. The removal of very large uterus has become possible by technical development. With clear benefits of LH versus AH, the time-consuming morcellation isn't also a contraindication any more. Patients benefit from less complications and faster convalescence. The author takes the laparoscopic hysterectomy (TLH or LASH) routine even with large uterus (1603 G, the largest uterus until now).

Slightly different is the indication position for supracervikal hysterectomy (LASH), because of preservation of the Cervix. As main indications for the LASH are the symptomatic uterus myomatosus, the adenomyosis uteri with discomfort and dysfunctionally bleeding disturbances which are resistant to therapy. Missing premalignant or malignant changes of the cervix or the body uteri are counted as essential conditions for the realisation of a LASH. Cervixmyoma and recto-vaginal endometriosis show relative contraindications.

For women after LASH lies the risk to fall ill with an invasive cervical cancer, in countries with early diagnosis programs for the cervical cancer, between 0.1 and 0.2%. It is comparable with the risk, reported in the literature of 0.17 %, to develop a carcinoma of the vaginal butt after abdominal hysterectomy. Early lesions can be removed without problems by a specific biopsy or cervixconisation.

The LASH isn't suitable as a standard operation or as a randomly alternative to the hysterectomy in countries without existing early diagnosis programs because of the lack of guaranteed screening examinations before and after a LASH.

3. Operating room setup

The preparing for the laparoscopic case is the most important factor to get a successful laparoscopic procedure. This includes; the ergonomic position of the lights, video screens, and the power supply tower. In order to proceed with the procedure, there should be given functioning monitors/screens for the surgeon and all assistants.

The patient is placed in the dorsolithotomy position on the operating table. A nosogastric tube have to be placed to decompress the stomach. The patient should be moved downwards on the table so that the uterine manipulator can be moved in all directions. The patient`s arms must be tucked alongside the body to allow the surgeon a moving ability without restrictions. The shoulder bolster are very important. They are centred on the acromnion process, over a gel pad, and clipped to the sidebar of the table to prevent upward slippage during Trendelenburg position. A foley catheter should be placed in the bladder to allow to drainage before trocars are inserted. Both; a disposable and reusable uterine manipulator can be used.

The surgeon is positioned on the left side of the patient while the first assistant is placed at the right side and the second assistant stands between the legs. Each surgeon must have a monitor/screen in front of him which he can adjust to his needs. The power supply tower should be positioned close to the patient.

A very important aspect by the acquisition of instruments for the laparoscopic surgery is the choice of the coagulation and preparation technique. The industry courts with little smoke production and OP shortening (LigaSure, Harmonic scalpel).

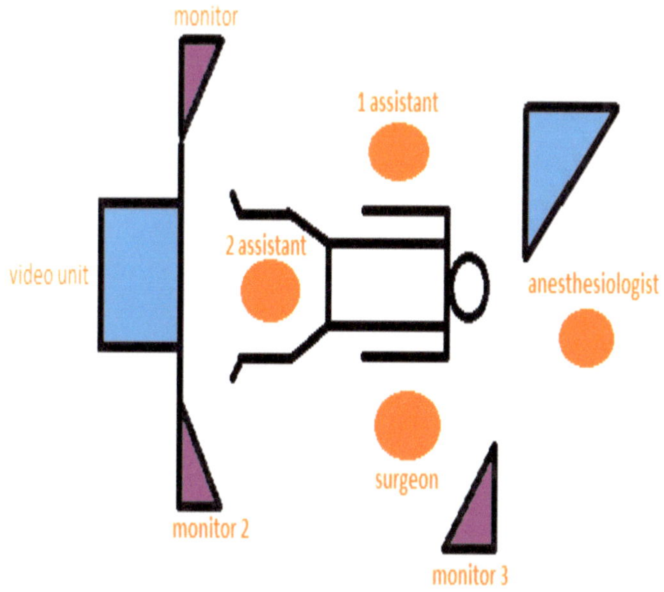

Fig. 2. Operating room setup.

The influence of different operation technologies within the long enduring operation is low. However, the operation duration is significantly influenced by the size of the uterus and not by the used instruments.

A work of the Hessler and al (13) examines and compares the application of different instruments.

172 patients obtained from the same surgeon a total laparoscopic hysterectomy. 60 patients were operated with SonoSurg™, 60 with Ultracision™, 34 with BiClamp™, 11 with BiSect™ and 7 with classical bipolar instruments. Every hysterectomy were executed with standardised Op steps. There were no determining differences between the several technologies considering of the whole operation duration and the pure hysterectomy duration.

The advantages of the classical bipolar instruments with the coagulation of bigger vessels are qualified through the obligatory instrument change to the scissors and the worse preparation qualities, in particular in the area of the cervix, bladder and bowel.

The disadvantages of the ultrasonic technology with the coagulation of the bigger vessels are compensated by the good preparations qualities in this area again. Therefore, the economic aspects, in particular the costs per operation, remain decisively for the equipment purchasing choice.

4. Positioning the trocars

The typical placement of the laparoscope is umbilical (Figure 3). Most surgeons use 10mm instruments with 0 degree. At a large uterus (16 weeks and exceeding) a 30 degree optic is often helpful to present uterine vessels and ureters. If the the uterine fundus reached the umbilicus or beyond, the umbilical optic insertion is impossible. In such cases we used the left subcostal access. We place the trocar on the left below the ribs with two fingers-width and medially 1-2 cm to the epigastric line. The preparation is carried out openly.

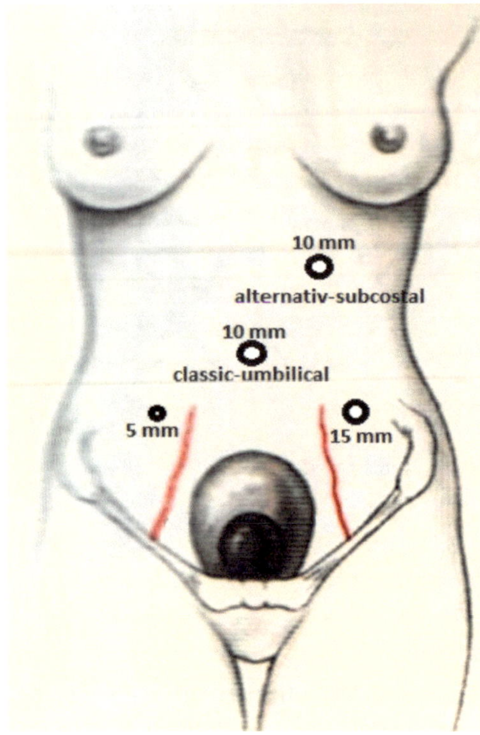

Fig. 3.

We perform all hysterectomies with two ports. On the right lower abdomen is always a 5 mm port placed and on the left lower abdomen, a 12 mm port. The left access will be extended to 15 mm for the morcellation. When peritoneal Adhesions is suspected primary, we choose a left subcostal access also.

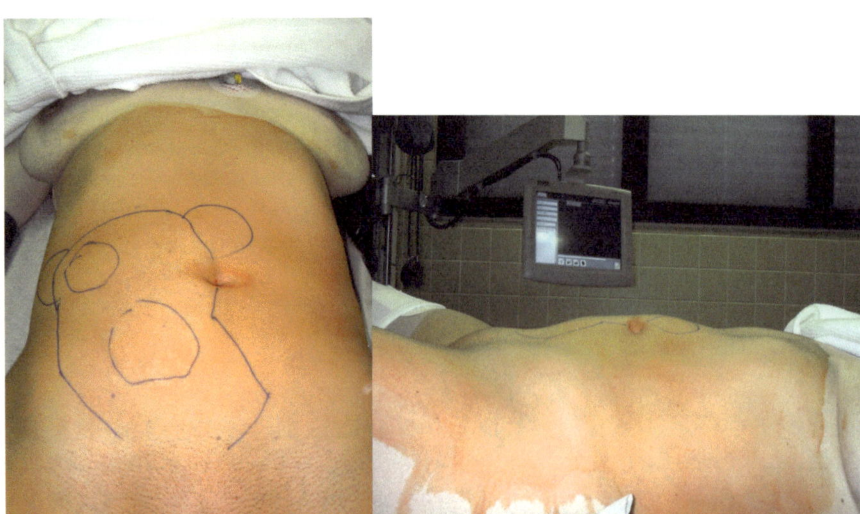

Fig. 4. Very large uterus makes the use of navel trokar-optics impossible.

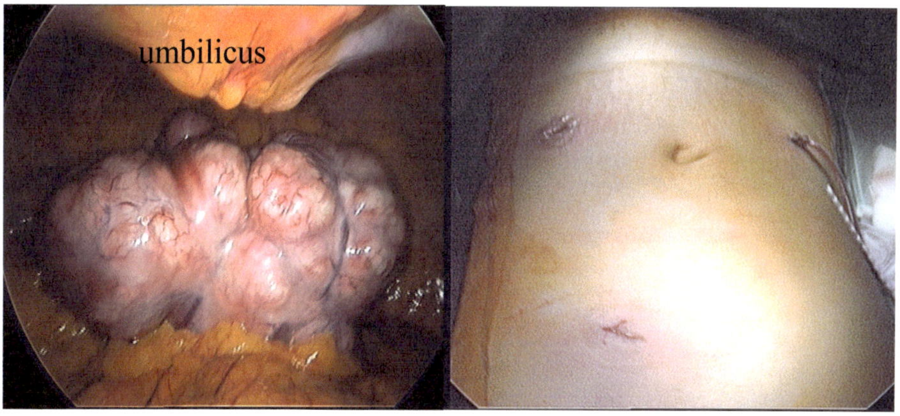

Fig. 5. The same patient. Subcostal access on the left for the optic and very big uterus.

5. Classic laparoscopic hysterectomy (LH)

- LAVH - laparoscopic-assisted vaginal hysterectomy
- LASH - laparoscopic supracervical hysterectomy
- TLH - total laparoscopic hysterectomy
- TLIH - total laparoscopic intrafascial hysterectomy

All hysterectomies made by us are proceeded with standardised methods. Depending on the chosen technique, the operations conduct to a certain point always same.

We always use a uterine manipulator. We are convinced that this is a very important component of surgical technique. By the manipulator, the uterus is pushed anteriorly and laterally. This saves us one laparoscopic port. Additionally, the distance between the uterine vessels and the ureter is amplified. The distance to the ureter allows low-risk vessel coagulation.

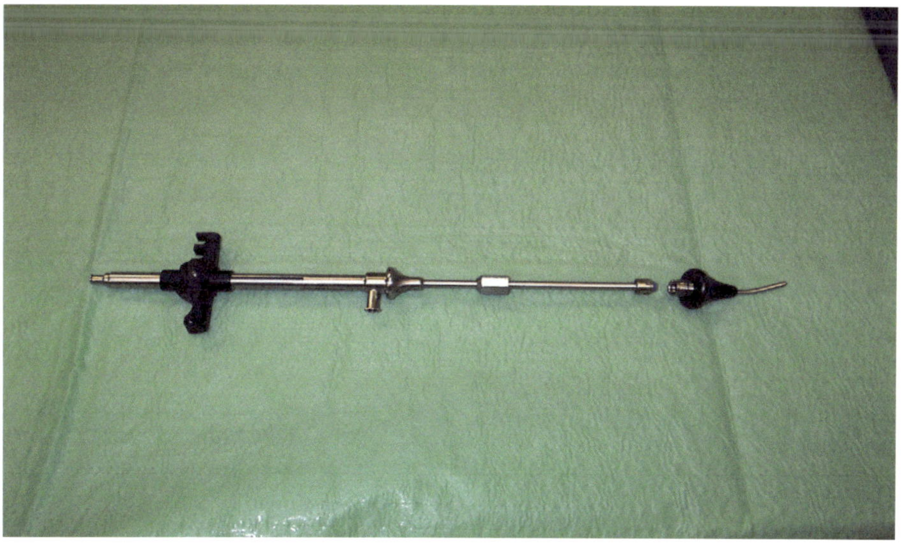

Fig. 5. Uterine Cohen manipulator which we use for LASH, LAVH, TLIH.

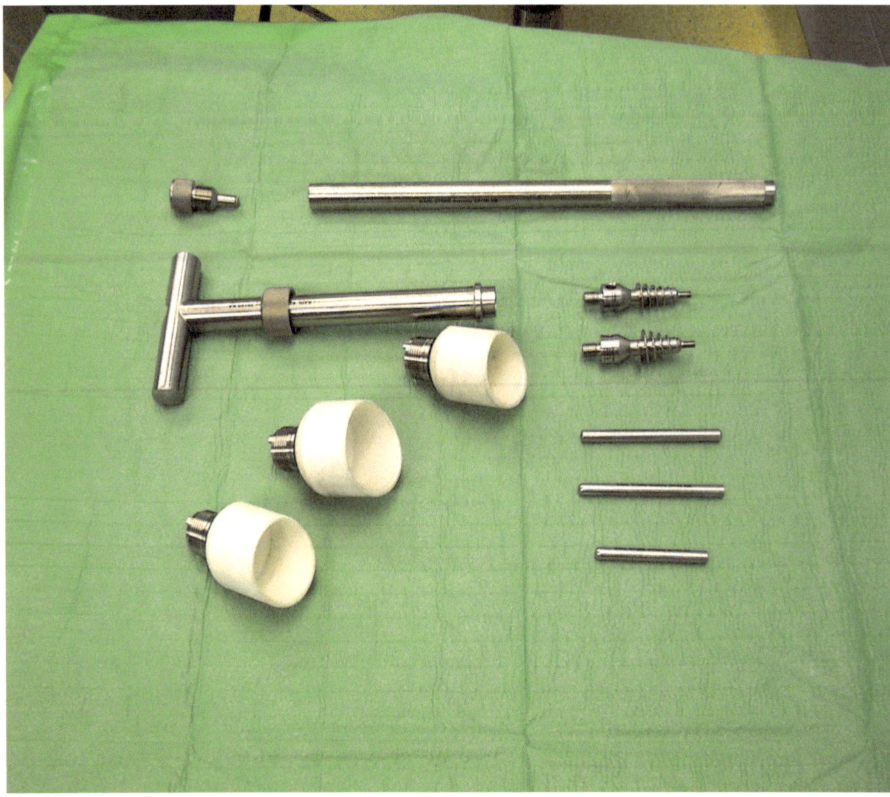

Fig. 6. Uterine Hohl manipulator for TLH, TLIH.

Single standardised surgical technique steps of the LH in our clinic are:

1. Cauterization and transection of the round ligament ("liga sure" or bipolar).

After cutting the round ligament the retroperitoneal space is opened. Now the ovarian ligament can be presented with ovarian vessels and it can be better targeted to achieve a coagulation. At large uterus, depending on the situation, we cut sometimes the fallopian tube or ovarian ligament first.

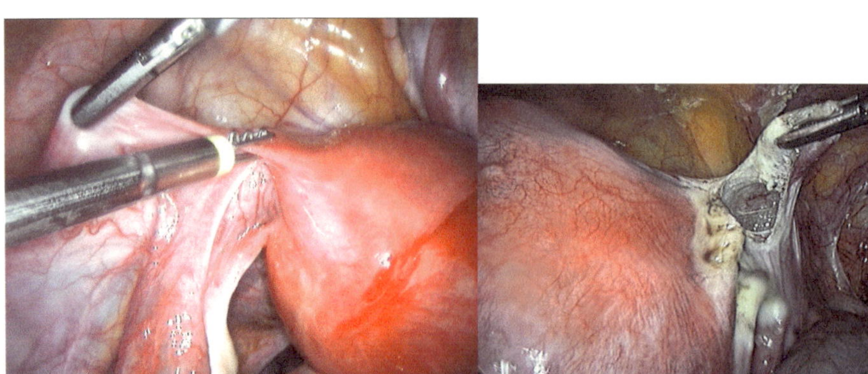

1.a. Small uterus. 1.b. Big uterus.

2. Ligation of the tube and of the ovarian ligament with the vessels.

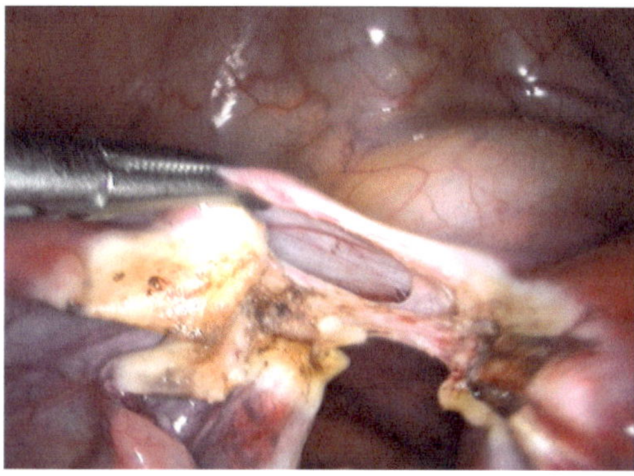

2.a. Small uterus.

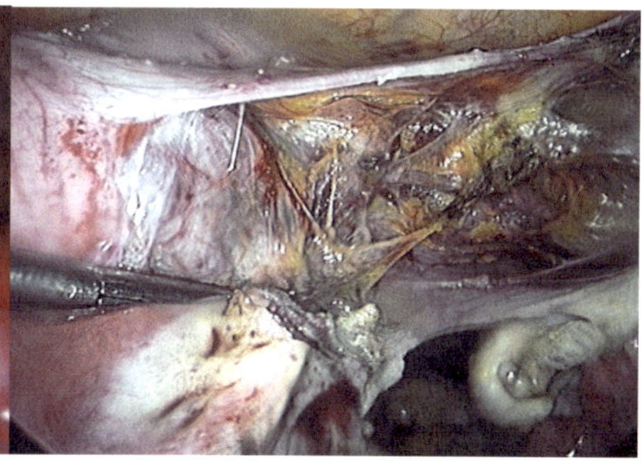

2.b. Big uterus

The retroperitoneal space is wide open by the blunt preparation. All anatomical structures are clearly visible. If necessary, the ureter can already be now grounded and identified on the back page of the broad ligament.

3. Dissection of the anterior broad ligament peritoneum to cervix level.

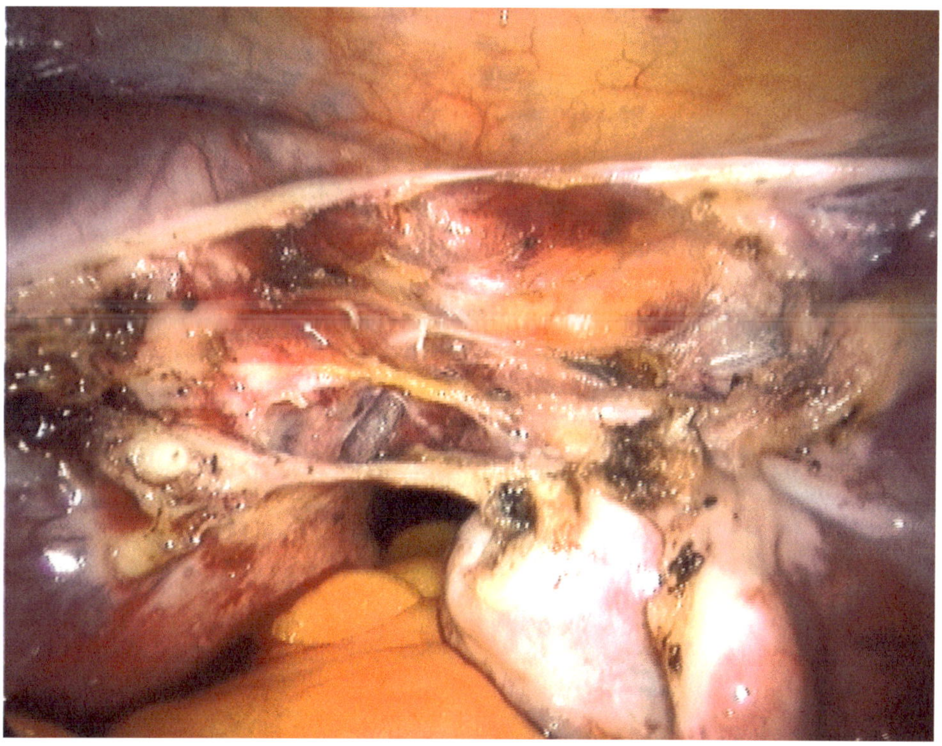

4. Search and localisation of the ureters.
5. Dissection of the posterior broad ligament peritoneum to uterosacral ligament. The broad ligament peritoneum is skeletonized to expose the uterine vessels.

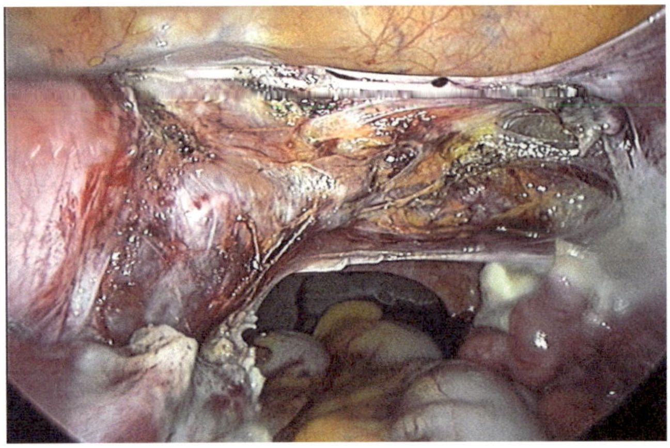

6. Ligation and incision of the uterine vessels with „bi-clamp“ or bipolar coagulation.

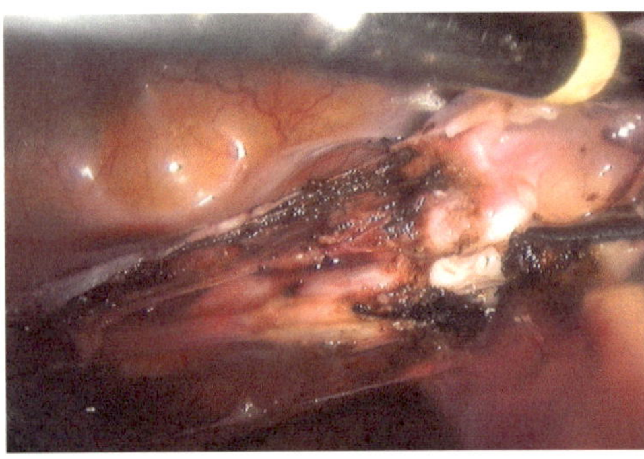
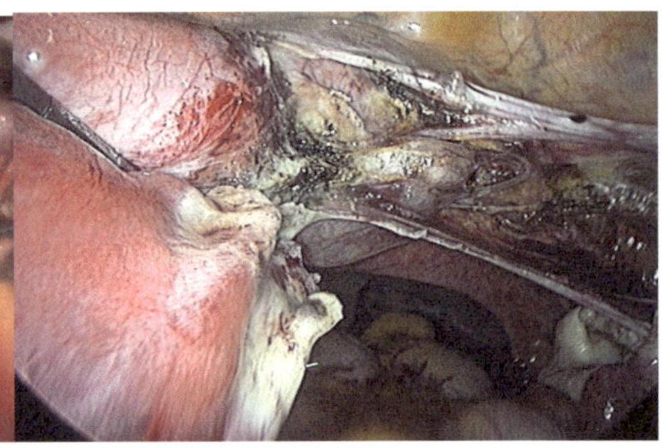

It is extremely important that the uterus will be strongly positioned anteriorly and laterally to the opposite direction with the uterine manipulator.
Alternatively, the uterine vessels can be torn down after a titan clip supply or a suturing. The Bi-clamp or bipolar coagulation is the safest and fastest option.

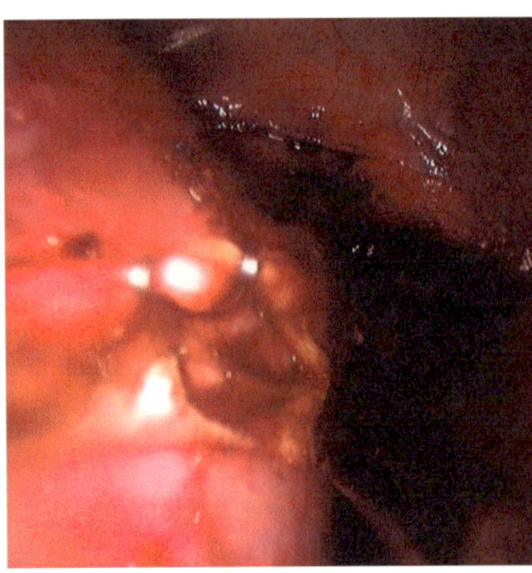
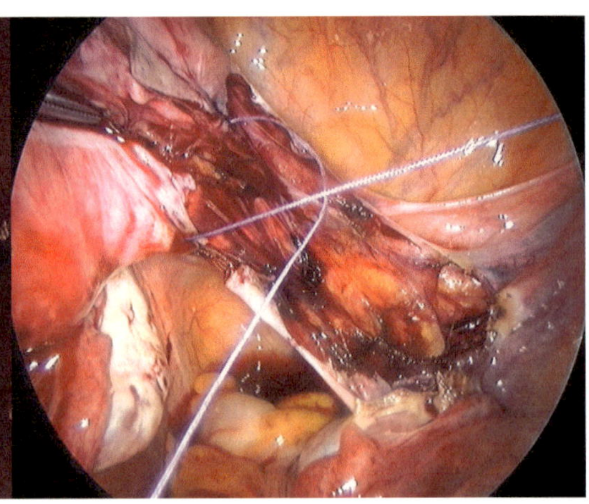

7. Dissection of the bladder.

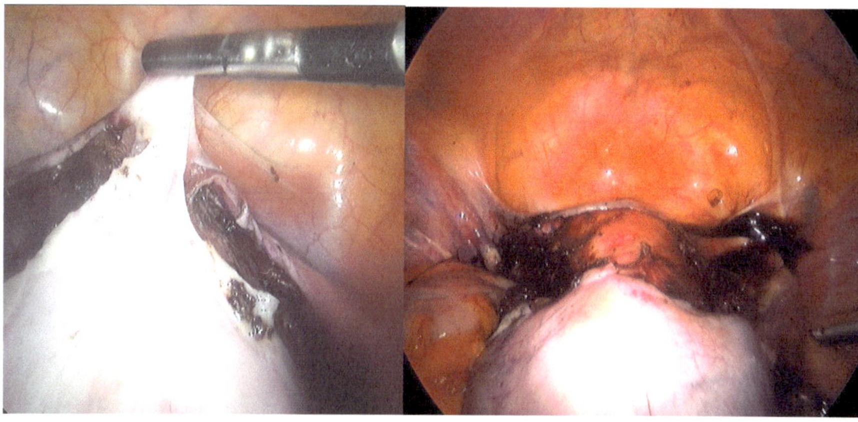

First the vesicouterine fold must be identified, afterwards elevated prior to incise it. This space must be dissected carefully, especially in the case at surgery, in particular previous caeserean section.

8. The skeletonized uterus.

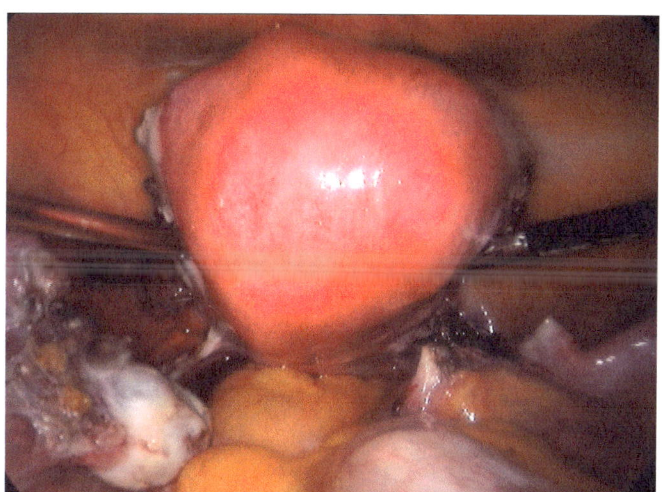

All surgical steps of these hysterectomy techniques (LAVH, LASH, TLH, TLIH) were until now identical.

If the LAVH technique is chosen, you have to start the vaginal part of the operation. The uterus body will be removed from the cervix within the LASH operation.

Further preparations shall be conducted within the TLH and TLIH (total laparoscopic intrafascial hysterectomy) technique (14).

9. The excision of the cervix (LASH) or the uterus from the vagina can be made laparoscopically (TLH) , as well as the dissection of the vagina through a vaginal route (LAVH).

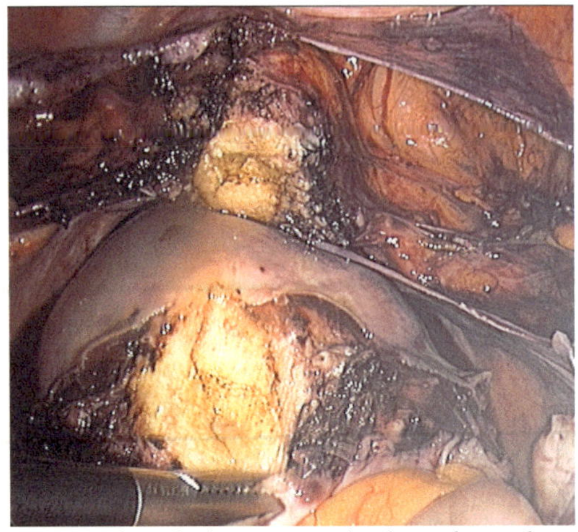

9.a. The uterine body is removed with the monopolar loop from the cervix.
The cervix stump and the cervical canal are now bipolar coagulated. This is made to avoid the cyclical residual bleeding after surgery.

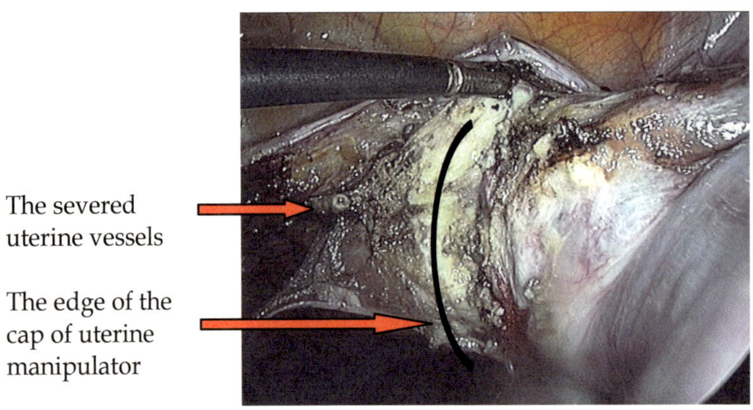

9.b. The uterine vessels are divided. The cap of uterine manipulator shows the edge where the cut must be made. We use for this mono-polar power.

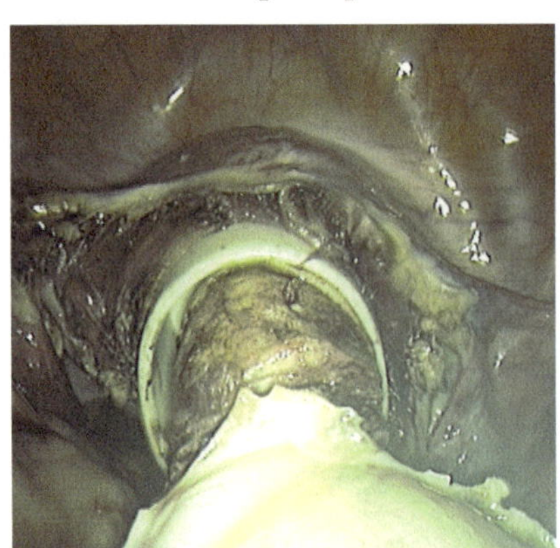

9.c. The uterus is removed from the vagina. In the vagina the cap from the manipulator is visible.

10. Vaginal closure with PDS suture (ethicon). When possible remove the uterus through the vagina.

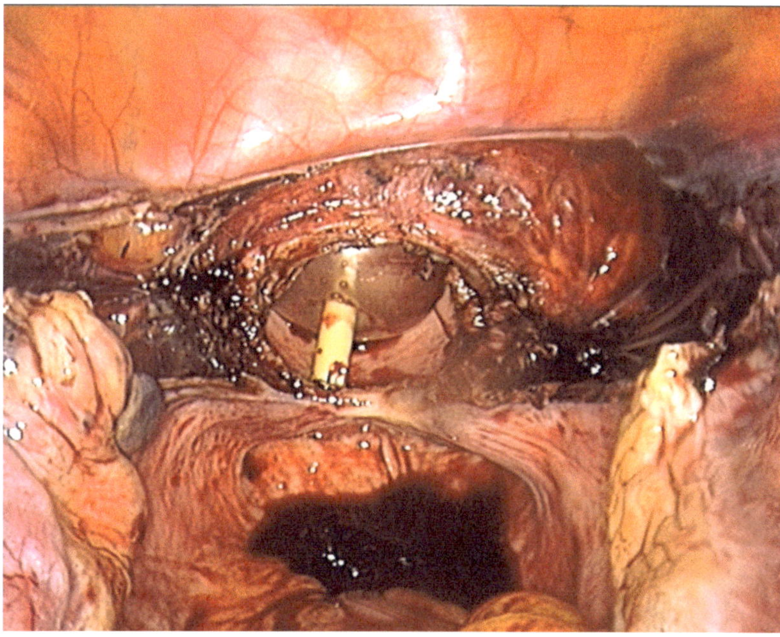

10.a. In the vagina a thick Foley catheter is placed for CO2 sealing.

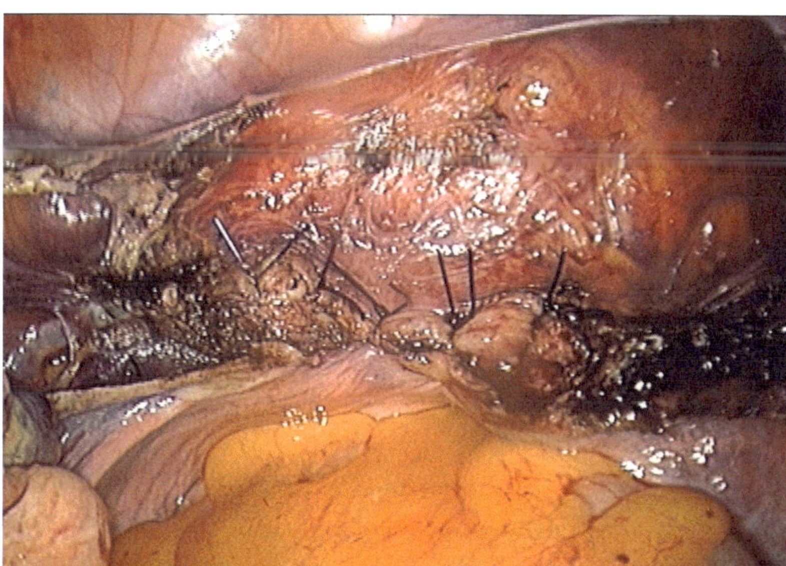

10.b. The vaginal stump is closed with sutures.

11. Closure of the peritoneum over cervix or over vaginal cuff with PDS - "Lahodny - Clip" suture or PDS - "Endosuture" (both-Ethicon).

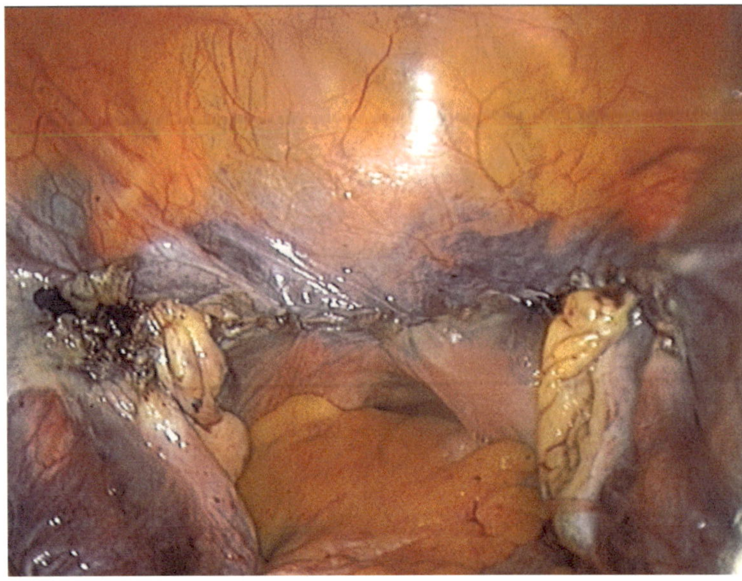

12. Morcellation of uterus.

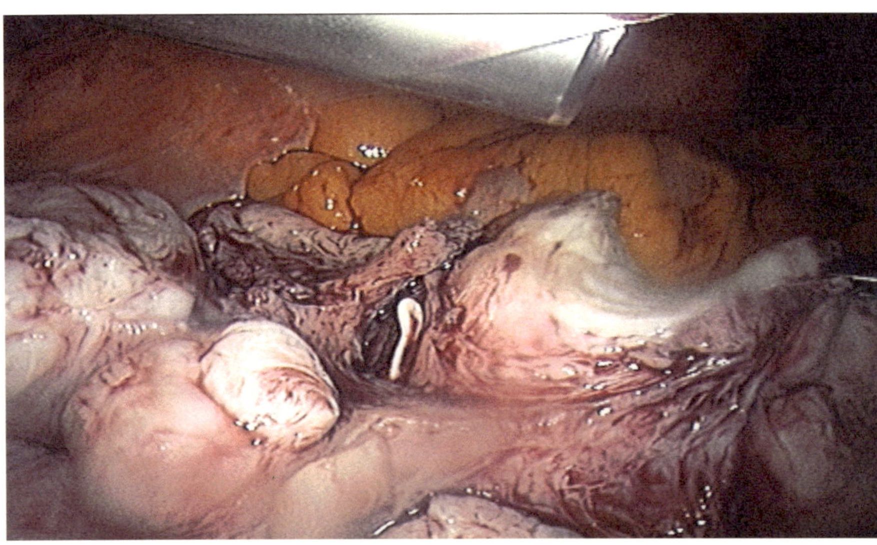

6. Comparison of abdominal, vaginal and laparoscopic hysterectomies

There are not so many prospective, randomized studies to compare the different technique of hysterectomy. A recent meta-analysis of 27 randomized trials showed that patients after laparoscopic hysterectomy (LH) compared to the abdominal (AH) has less blood loss, had suffered less perioperative infections and had a significantly shorter recovery time (15). In contrast, was the AH operation duration shorter and the injuries to the urinary tract (bladder and ureter) significantly higher after LH. The LH has comparing to the VH significantly longer operating durations. It is noted that most studies compare various modifications of LAVH to the VH. The operating endurances depend in the LH significantly more from the operational skills of the surgeon-dependent than in the VH. In english-speaking countries, the vaginal surgery is less operated, and the percentage of vaginal hysterectomies in all uteri removed due to benign indications is accordingly lower. In the USA amounts the percentage 25% (16) and in UK one-third (17).

A major advantage of the VH over the LH is its feasibility in the spinal anaesthesia and the lower costs.

The LH implicates perfect anatomical overview and the image magnification of the video camera. This is for example in the diagnosis and treatment of endometriosis of prime importance. It delivers also enormously further development of nerve-sparing surgical techniques.

After the LH the hospitalization was at the shortest. In Germany, the TLH and LASH is an outpatient procedure. Outpatient means that the patients are able to leave the clinic after approximately 6 hours. All patients were cared for at the operating evening by telephone. The results are similar to the process in the hospital (6).

Meta analyse: vaginal hysterectomy (VH) vs. abdominal hysterectomy, (AH), vs. laparoscopic hysterectomy (LH/LAVH) delivered in 2009 in a Cochrane overview Nieboer et al (18).

Hospitalisation:

VH vs. AH	-1,1 Days [0,92-1,92]
LH vs. AH	-2,0 Days [1,86-2,17]
VH vs. **LH**	No difference

Febrile episodes or unclear infections:

VH vs. AH	OR :0,42
LH vs. AH	OR: 0,65
VH vs. **LH**	No difference

Operative middle blood loss:

LH vs. AH	MD: -45 ml
LH vs. VH	OR: 2,76 (significant blood loos)

Resumption of normal activities:

VH vs. AH	9,5 Tage (95% CI: 6,4-12,6)
LH vs. AH	13,6 Tage (95% CI: 11,8-15,4)

Wound infections:

LH vs. AH	OR: 0,31

Injury of the urinary ways:

LH vs. AH	OR: 2,41
LH vs. **VH**	No difference

Operating time:

LH vs. AH	20,3 minutes
LH vs. VH	39,3 minutes

7. Laparoscopic radical hysterectomy

A pioneer of laparoscopic oncologic gynaecology was Daniel Dargent. Laparoscopic lymphadenectomy was described by him in 1989. His greatest achievement however, was the involvement of Schauta radical vaginal hysterectomy according to laparoscopy. Developed by Dargent laparoscopically assisted radical hysterectomy (LAVRH) was successfully used in the treatment of cervical cancer. The work of Querleu on pelvic lymph node dissection were very important as well (22).

The LAVH was more frequently performed with lymph node dissection in the endometrial carcinoma. Thanks to technological developments, the TLH displaced the LAVH not only as hysterectomy management, but also as part of the surgical treatment of endometrial cancer. Today it is a standard therapy of endometrial carcinoma and not too large uterus. Afterwards the laparoscopic way was performed entirely by the radical hysterectomies - the laparoscopic Wertheim operations (TLRH - total laparoscopic radical hysterectomy)(23,24).

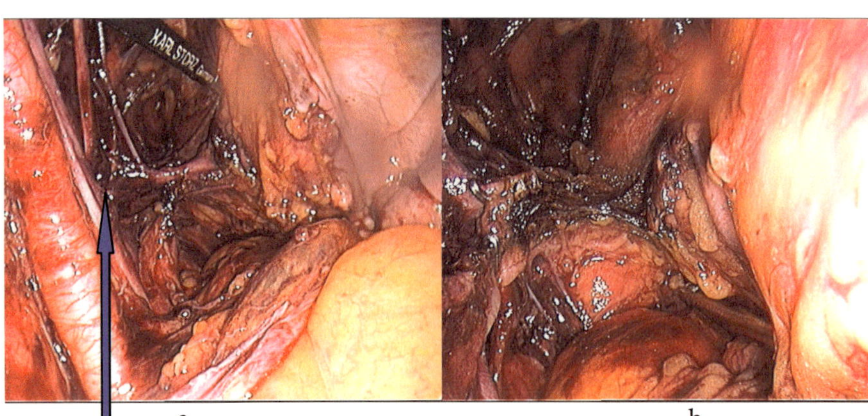

a. b.

Fig. 7. a. Dissected cardinal ligament left after pelvic lymph node dissection - laparoscopic Wertheim operation. b. Cardinal ligament left after the division of the pars vaskularis. The pars nervosa of the ligament is spared.

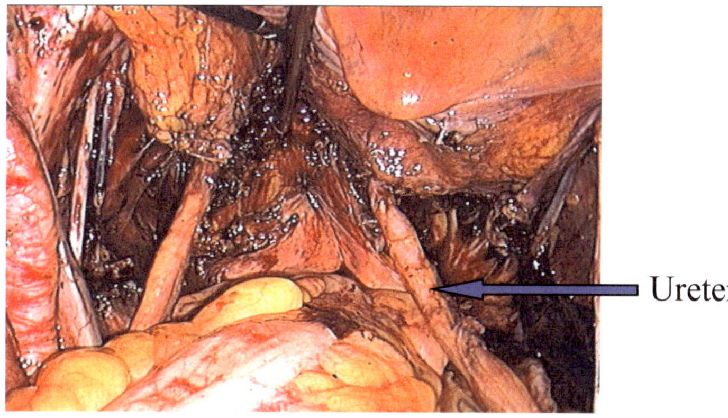

Fig. 8. Situs after TLRH (laparoscopic Wertheim operation).

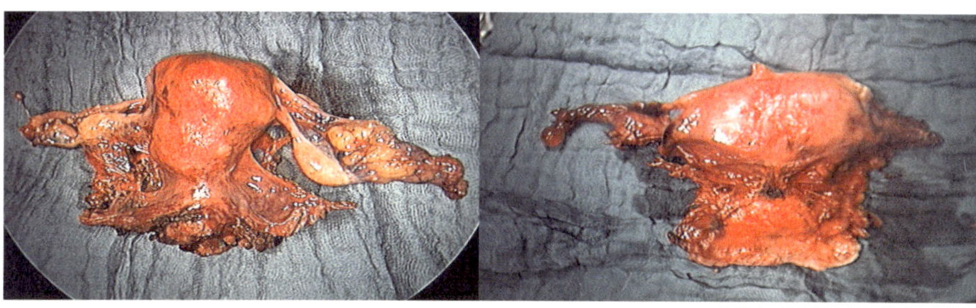

a. b.

Fig. 9. a. Wertheim preparation (Piver III radicalness). b. Schauta preparation.

1992 Netzhat refereed to the para-aortic lymphadenectomy (23). The feasibility of lymphadenectomy by laparoscope were combined with the trachelectomy when the wish to conceive existed beside an early cervical cancer. The process can be carried out vaginal, abdominal or laparoscopically assisted. Between 40% and 70% patients after trachelectomy were pregnant (26).

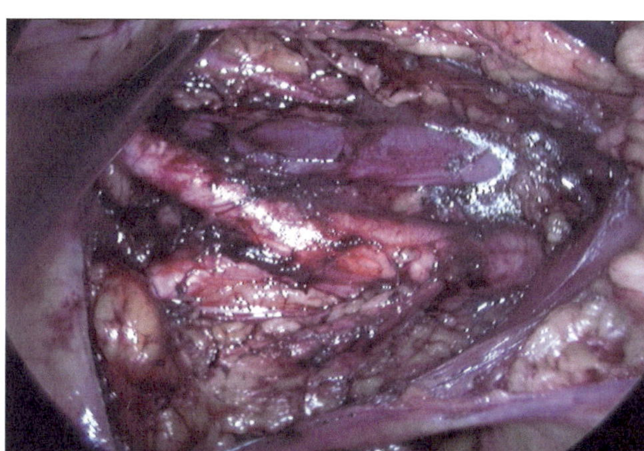

Fig. 10. Para aortic lymph nodes dissection.

Laparoscopy in comparison to open surgery:
- Perfect anatomical overview. Magnifying glass enlargement permits nerves-spare surgery.
  Patients with high BMI and endometrium carcinoma profited from the laparoscopy by the reduction of perioperativ complications like incisional hernia, ileus and due to quicker mobilisation - thrombosis and embolism.

Early endometrial cancer: the comparison of laparotomy and laparoscopy (27):

Procedure	Patient (n)	Middle Op-duration (min)	Middle blood loss (ml)	Removed lymph nodes (n)	Hospitalisation (Days)	Complications all together (%)
Laparotomy	1458	123	402	17,7	7,5	31,3
Laparoscopy	1023	176	236	18,3	4,1	14,9

Result:
- Laparoscopic onkosurgery offers the same oncological security like the open surgery.
- Laparoscopy is associated with less blood loss and less complications. There was less need of blood transfusions.
- The post surgical morbidity can be reduced.
- High-price equipment and a long training curve are facing reduced hospitalization costs and a lower morbidity.

Similar results were shown by other studies (28). Laparoscopic therapy for early cervical and endometrial cancer is the open approach in oncological point of view equivalent. There are nearly identical numbers of lymph nodes obtained via laparotomy (pelvic 18, 7 paraaortal inframesenterial) or laparoscopy (pelvic 17, 7 paraaortal inframesenterial) (27).

8. New laparoscopic device – transumbilical endoscopy (TUE)

In 2004 is the origin year of the N.O.T.E.S. - Treatment (Natural Orifice Transluminal Endoscopic Surgery) of the study group around Anthony Kallo. The technology uses as access roads the so-called natural body openings like stomach, large intestine, bladder or the vagina. From that movement also comes the surgery through the navel – e . N.O.T.E.S. (Embryonic Natural Orifice Transluminal Endoskopic Surgery). All ports required by the surgeon are positioned in the navel pit. In addition are mostly used so-called "single ports". The best well known technologies are the SILS - technology (single Incision Laparoscopic Surgery) of the company Covidien and the LESS – technology (Laparo-Endoscopic single site Surgery) from the company Olympus as disposable ports.
Endoscopic umbilical techniques (Embryonic – N.O.T.E.S.) get in the gynaecology more common. The LAVH, LTH, LASH and the colposacropexie are among, beside the adnexal surgery, this treatment. Some years previously a rapid development could have been followed in the visceral surgery which came along with a wide range of operations opportunities within this technique. In 1995 the first cholecystectomy were accomplished in Ferrara. Today nephrectomy, gastric sleeve – resections, inguinal hernia operations, sigmaresection, colectomy, fundoplication, RY – gastric bypass and pancreas head resections are carried out.

The first e.N.O.T.E.S. Hysterectomy was reported in Juli 2007, in the USA by Dr. Kate O'Hanlan (20). In Europe the first TLH, with SILS - port on 08.05.2009 and the first SILS - LASH on 30.06.2009 by Dr. Cezary Dejewski in Bremerhaven, Germany (19).
Synonyms of the transumbilical laparoscopic surgery:

- Transumbilical single port surgery - TUSPS
- Transumbilical multi port surgery - TUMPS
- Embryonic NOTES - e.N.O.T.E.S.
- Transumbilical Endoscopic Surgery - TUES
- One Port Umbilical Surgery - OPUS
- Natural orifice trans-umbilical surgery - NOTUS
- Single Port Access (SPA) surgery
- Single-Access-Site (SAS) laparoscopic surgery
- Single-Site-Access (SSA) laparoscopic surgery
- Trans-Umbilical Laparoscopic Assisted (TULA) surgery
- Single Incision Laparoscopic Surgery - SILS™
- Laparo-Endoscopic Single-site Surgery - LESS™

The minimization of the access trauma results in less postoperative pain, reduced postoperative intestinal atony, less strain on the lung function and provides a better cosmetic scar results. Patients benefit from quicker recovery and improved quality of life. All the benefits of laparoscopy compared with conventional open surgery are embraced by the e.N.O.T.E.S. technology.
The less postoperative wound pain results from that navel access in which no abdominal muscle were injured. The reduction of two or three trokars on the lower abdomen reduces the intraoperative risk of injury to epigastric vessels (Figur 6).

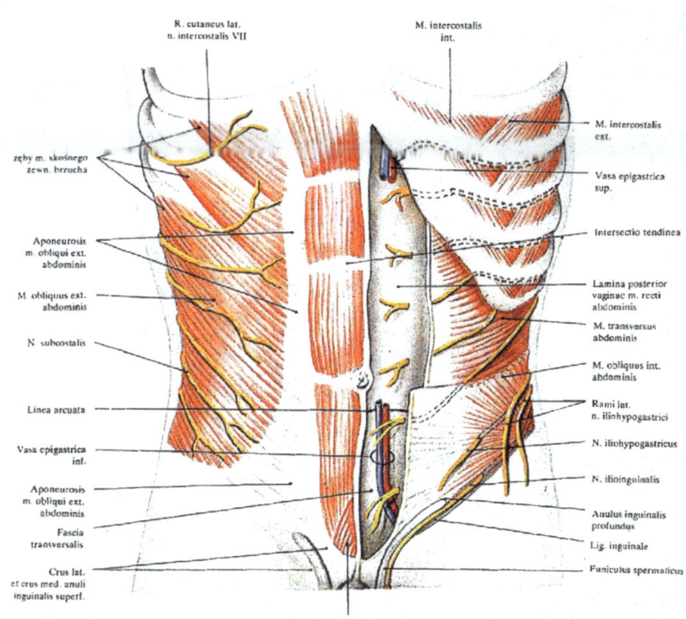

Fig. 6. Abdomen anatomy.

The size of the umbilical scar after the "single port" is from 2 to 3.5 cm.

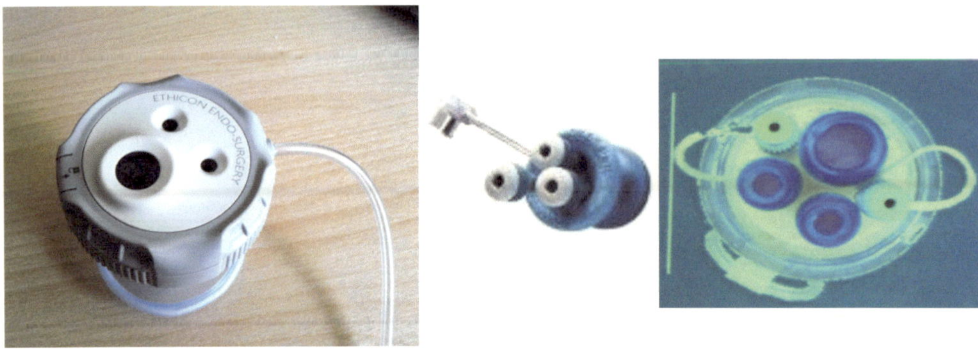

Fig. 7. Various disposable ports (Ethicon, Covidien, Olympus).

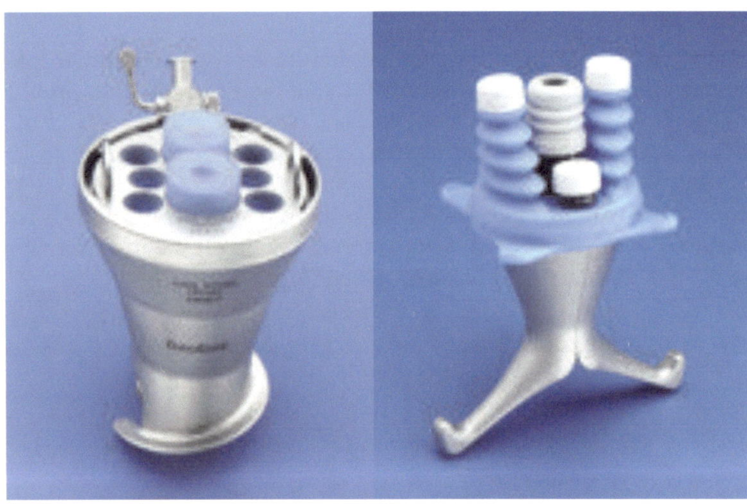

Fig. 8. Single ports from Storz (reusable).

The author had performed about 60 e.N.O.T.E.S. operations between the 1st june 2008 and the 30th april 2010. Including 18 total and 22 supracervical hysterectomies, 1 appendectomy, 11 ovarial surgery, 5 adnexectomy and 6 laparoscopic sacrocolpopexy.

The technique has significant advantages over N.O.T.E.S. surgery. First it is clinically proven and allow on any time to switch to conventional laparoscopy, and many procedures can be performed without quality loss.

Our position is that the ovarial surgery (cystenenukleation with suture ovarian reconstruction) cannot be regarded as an entry in the transumbilical endoscopy because present technology doesn`t allow us a non tissue sparing surgery as a result of confined space conditions and optic collisions. Loss of substance on the ovary at awkward surgery exercises are the result. The transumbilical surgical technique inflicts the surgeon a greater challenge than the conventional technique. The prerequisite for the application of the TUE presume the training and experience in traditional endoscopy. Everything else would discredit the entire development.

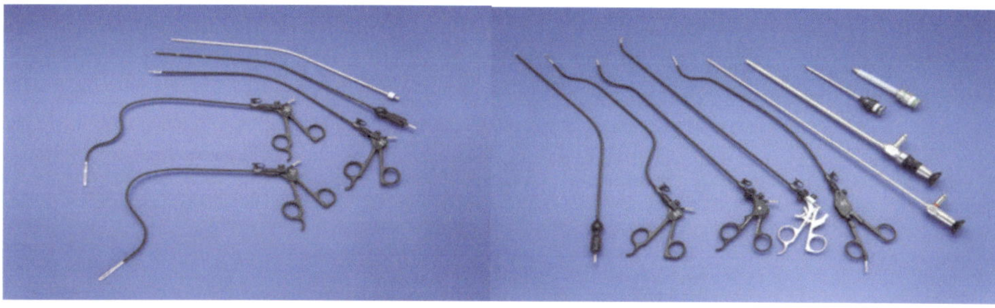

Fig. 9. Several curved endoscopic instruments for transumbilical endoscopy.

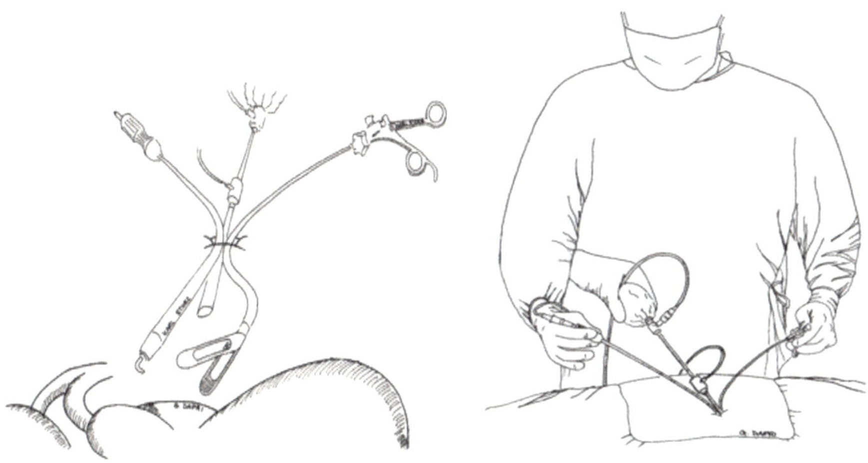

Fig. 10. Problem of limited space and instruments collision.

A further development of instruments and optics for establishing the transumbilical endoscopy are urgently needed. The industry attract currently their biggest attention on the "single port" technology (SPA - single port access). The previously developed SILS (single incision laparoscopic surgery - Covidien) and LESS (Laparo Endoscopic Single Site Surgery - Olympus) are followed by reusable items such as "Endocone" and "X-Cone" ports from Storz. The Wolf and the Esculap company announced now their own ports.
The scar after the cut for the insertion of singel-ports is 2.5 to 3 cm.

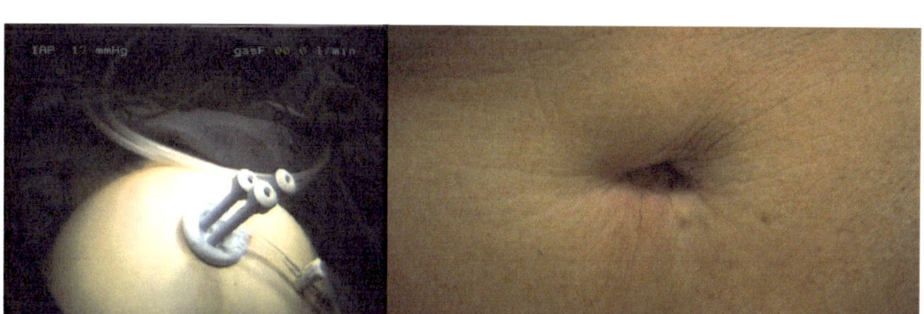

Fig. 11. SILS Single-Port (Covidien) and the umbilical scar 8 weeks after.

We have next to the TUSPS also the "multi-port" technology (TUMPS – transumbilical multi port surgery) applied. We place in the navel instead of a single port three 5 mm trocars (flexible, reusable - from Wolf).

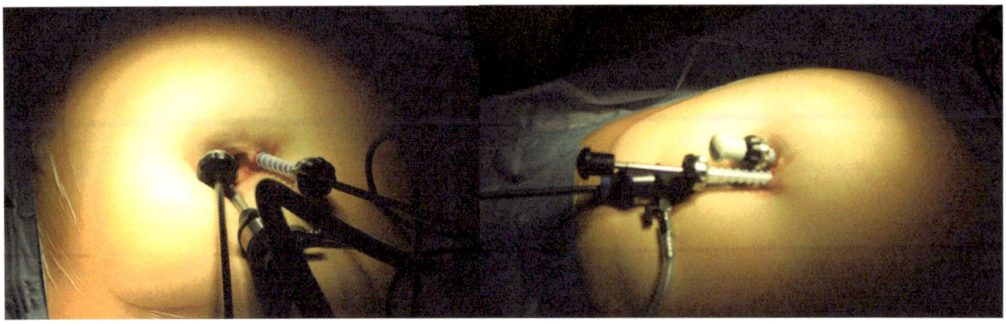

Fig. 12. Transumbilical multi-port endoscopic surgery (TUMPS) - three 5,5 mm ports umbilical.

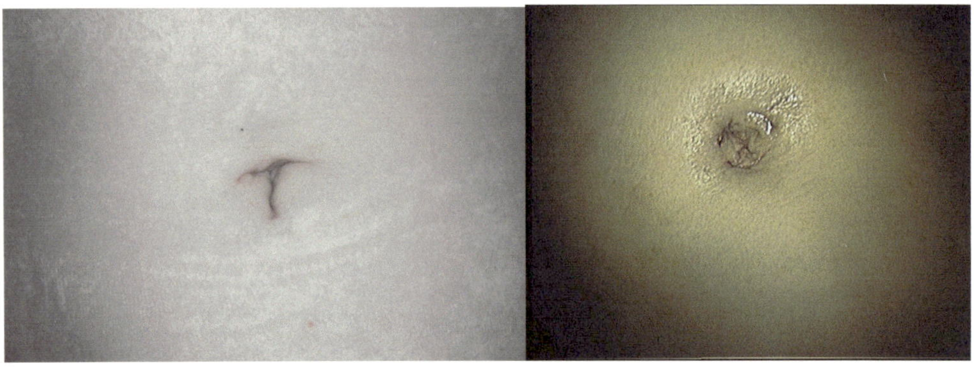

a. 4 weeks after b. 4 days after (another patient)

Fig. 13. Umbilical scars after TUMPS.

Our operating experience has not shown any advantage of "Single Port" (TUSPS - transumbilical single port surgery) technique against the "multi-port" method (TUMPS - transumbilical multi port surgery). Because of placing more ports through the navel, you achieve a wider operating radius so that optic and instruments collisions are much rarer in contrary to the single port technique. In addition with curved instruments it is easily to use the the conventional laparoscopic instruments. The operation is not as cost intensive, and leaves only three 5.5 mm wide scars. The grooves are with the "skin bridge" separated, so a lower risk of hernia can be expected. The pain is being investigated by us, but appears to be lower.

It is possible for the morcellator to expand a 5,5 mm tip to 15 mm and to morcellate it parallel to the camera. The transvaginal morcellation must be used with "single-port", but working with a mirror inverted camera, operations appear much more difficult and assume a longer training curve.

The tumoraseptic extraction of ovarian masses by the rear colpotomy is more convenient for large-adnexal findings, so we use this management in TUSPS and TUMPS technique.

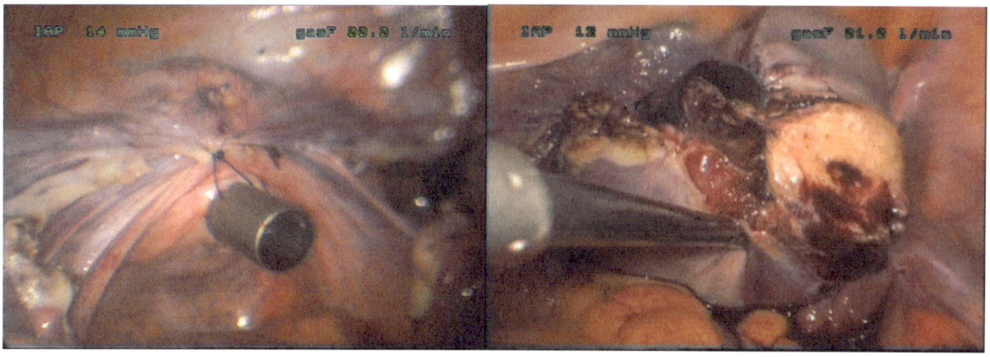

Fig. 14. Morcelation with the rear colpotomy.

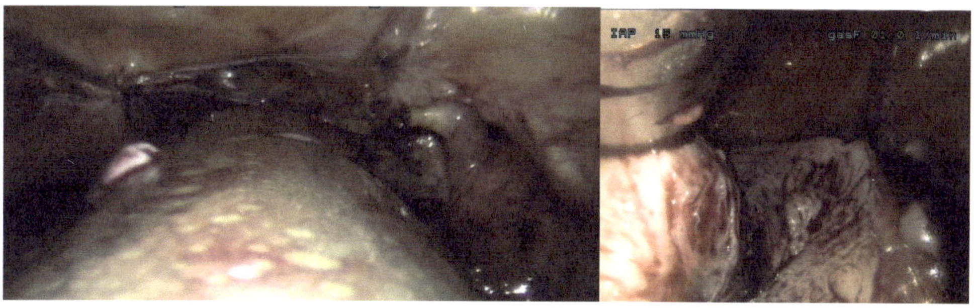

Fig. 15. The umbilical morcelation, multi-port umbilical surgery.

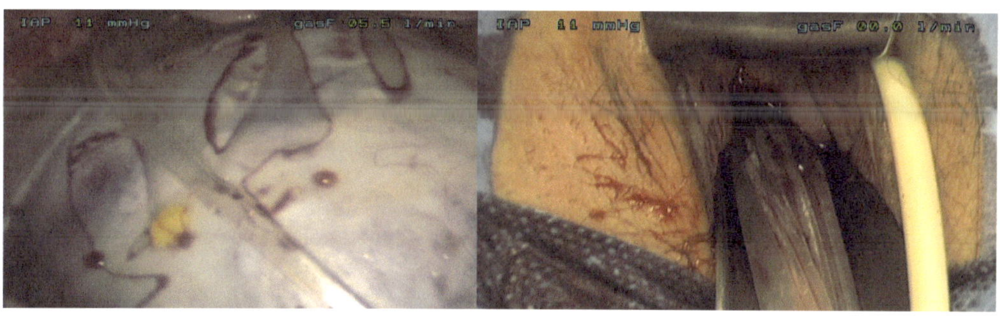

Fig. 16. Recovery of 16 cm big cystoma through the vagina with endo bag.

The total or supracervical hysterectomy by transumbilical access was made, according to the standards of the laparoscopic hysterectomy (LH), with conventional technique. All the individual steps of those procedures remained identical.

9. Complications

In review of Hurd (15), which includes over 1.5 million gynaecological patients, is reported that complications in 0.1 to 10 percent of procedures and 20 to 25 percent of complications were not recognized until the postoperative period.

Between 1980 and 1999 the incidence of entry access injury was 5 to 30 per 10,000 procedures. Bowel and retroperitoneal vascular injuries comprised 76 percent of all injuries and almost 50 percent of small and large bowel injuries were unrecognised for at least 24 hours. The type and proportion of organ injury during entry was: small bowel (25 percent), iliac artery (19 percent), colon (12 percent), iliac or other retroperitoneal vein (9 percent), secondary branches of a mesenteric vessel (7 percent), aorta (6 percent), inferior vena cava (4 percent), abdominal wall vessels (4 percent), bladder (3 percent), liver (2 percent), other (less than 2 percent).
A literature review of procedures performed from 1975 to 2002 reported entry-related visceral lesions occurred in 0.3 to 1.3 per 1000 procedures and entry-related vascular lesions occurred in 0.07 to 4.7 per 1000 procedures. The open technique was not associated with fewer complications than the closed technique; however, this result likely reflects the high risk status of patients undergoing the open procedure.

9.1 Patient risk factors

A very important patient risk factors displays obesity. Increased weight takes on a special significance for laparoscopy. Placement of laparoscopic instruments becomes much more difficult. Bleeding from abdominal wall vessels may be more common because these vessels become difficult to locate. Many intra-abdominal procedures become increasingly difficult because of a restricted operative field secondary to retroperitoneal fat deposits in the pelvic side walls and increased bowel excursion into the operative field. This second problem is probably related to increased volume of bowel, decreased elevation of a heavier anterior abdominal wall by the pneumoperitoneum, and the inability to place many patients who are obese in steep Trendelenburg position because of ventilation considerations.
Another well-described surgical risk factor is age. As the population ages, more women of increased age will have indications for laparoscopy. Older patients are at increased risk of having concomitant disease processes that affect their perioperative morbidity and mortality. Probably the single most important consideration is age-associated increase in cardiovascular disease. Of special importance is the increased susceptibility of elderly persons to hypothermia. In older patients, even mild degrees of hypothermia may increase the risk of cardiac arrhythmia.
As far as laparoscopic complications are concerned, one of the most important risk factors is a history of previous abdominal surgery. The risk of adhesions of omentum and/or bowel to the anterior abdominal wall after previous abdominal surgery is greater than 20%. The most common of these strategies is the use of an open technique for laparoscopic trocar placement, as first advocated by Hasson.
In patients with previous laparotomy in which the scar is located at the umbilicus, use of an alternative location for trocar insertion is usually located in the left subcostal quadrant. The closest organ to the left upper quadrant is the stomach. Therefore, an oral gastric tube is recommended before.

9.2 Anaesthetic risk factors

One of the most critical time-dependent aspects of preparation is the degree to which the patient's stomach is empty because both general anaesthesia and increased intra-abdominal pressure may increase the risk of regurgitation and resultant aspiration.
Preoperative evaluation should include a search for evidence of underlying cardiac disease. With a positive history or physical examination findings suggestive of cardiac disease, preoperative evaluation by both a cardiologist and an anaesthesiologist is extremely important.

Finally, patients at risk for congestive heart failure should be evaluated carefully prior to laparoscopy because a decrease in cardiac output may be related to decreased venous return and increased peripheral vascular resistance.
Any patient with a significant history of pulmonary problems should be evaluated by both a pulmonologist and an anaesthesiologist prior to laparoscopy. Hypercarbia and decreased ventilation associated with laparoscopy may be especially deleterious in pulmonary patients with chronic respiratory acidosis.

By example of bladder and ureter injuries by l total aparoscopic hysterectomy (TLH):

Number:	830 (1)	512 (2)	567 (3)
Uterus weight:	239 g	241 g	242 g
OP time:	132 min	133 min	104 min
Blood loss:	130 ml	309 ml	1,45 g/dl
Hospitalisation:	1,4 Tage	2,7 Tage	5,6 Tage
Conversion to LAP:	0,60%	1,80%	0,20%
Complications rate:	4,70%	4,80%	1,40%
Bladder injury:	12 (1,4%)	2 (0,4%)	4 (0,7%)
Ureter injury:	10 (1,3%)	1 (0,2%)	1 (0,2%)
Bowel injury:	3 (0,4%)	5 (0,97%)	1 (0,2%)

10. References

[1] O`Hantan et al „Total laparoscopic hysterectomy", JSLS 2007
[2] Ng et al „Total laparoscopic hysterectomy", Arch Gynecol Obstet 2007
[3] Mueller et al „Total laparoscopic hysterectomy" ....submitted
[4] Lim et al „Lower urinary tract injurys" J Obstet Gynaecol Res 2010
[5] Donnez et al „A serieas of 3190 laparoscopic hysterectomies", BJOG 2008
[6] Salfelder A. et al „Hysterektiomie als Standarteingriff in der Tagesklinik - ein Wagnis?", Frauenarzt 48 (2007),954-958, 10.
[7] Müller A. et al „ Hysterektomie - ein Vergleich verschiedener Operationsverfahren", Dtsch Arztebl Int 2010; 107(20): 353-9
[8] Reich H. „Laparoscopic hysterectomy", Surgical Laparoscopy & Endoscopy. Raven Press, New York. 1992 ; 2: 85-88.
[9] Mettler L, Lutzewitch N, Dewitz T, Remmert K, Semm K. „From laparotomy to pelviscopic intrafascial hysterectomy". Gyn Endoscopy 1996; 5 : 203-209.
[10] Liu CY, Reich H. „Complications of Total Laparoscopic Hysterectomy in 518 Cases". Gynaecological Endoscopy 1994 ; 3 : 203-208.
[11] Stovall Th. Et al „Complications of gynecologic laparoscopic surgery",UpToDate 18.3, 2011.
[12] Hurd W.W. „Gynecologic Laparoscopy", eMedicine online 2009.
[13] Hessler P.-A., „Comparative Assesment of the Impact of Different Instruments in Total Laparoscopic Hysterectomies" Geburtsh Frauenheilk in 2008; 68: 77-82.

[14] Lee PJ; Total Laparoscopic Intrafascial Hysterectomy, J Am Assoc Gynecol Laparosc. 1996 Aug;3(4, Supplement):S25.
[15] Johnson N et al. Cochrane Database Syst Rev 2005; (2): CD 00 36 77.
[16] Farquhar CM et al Obstet Gynecol 2002, 99 (2). 229-34.
[17] Magos J Obstet Gynaecol AD et al 2001, 21 (2). 166-170
[18] Surgical approach to hysterectomy for benign gynaecological disease (Review), Nieboer TE, Johason N, Lethaby A, Tavender E, Curr E, Garry R, van Voorst S., Mol BWJ, Kluivers KB.
[19] Dejewski C et al „New Technique for Laparoscopic Hysterectomy - SILS (Single Incision Laparoscopic Surgery) Hysterectomy", Geburtsh Frauenheilk 2010; 70: 123-126.
[20] Pope Kerry, President and CEO Novare Surgical System Inc., Cupertino, CA 95014 United States, Calif., July 25 2007 /PRNewswire/; 408/873-3161, kpope@novaresurgical.com
[21] Steed H, Rosen B, Murphy J et al „A comparison of laparoscopic-assisted radical vaginal hysterectomy and radikal abdominal hysterectomy in the treatment of cervical cancer", Gynecol Oncol. 2004;93(3):588-593.
[22] Querleu D, Leblanc E, Castelain B „Laparoscopic pelvic lyphadenectomy in the stging of early carcinoma of the cervix", Am J Obstet Gynecol. 1991;164(2):579-581.
[23] Netzhat CR, Mahdavi A, Nagarseth NP et al „Laparoscopic radical hysterectomy with paraaortic and pelvic node dissection", Am J Obstet Gynecol. 1992;166(3):864-865.
[24] Canis M, Mage G, Wattiez A et al „Does endoscopic surgery have a role in radical surgery of cancer of the cervix uteri?", J Gynecol Biol Reprod (Paris).1990;19:921.
[25] Altgassen C et al „Trachelektomie - Indikationen und Operationsmetoden", Gynäkologe 2009.42:925-931.
[26] Solomayer E, Juhasz-Bösz I et al „Laparoskopische Therapie des frühen Endometrium- und Zervixkarzinom", Frauenarzt 50(2009)1:24-27.
[27] Walker Jl, Piedmonte MR et al „Laparoscopy compared with laparotomy for comprehensive surgical staging of uterine cancer", Gynecologic Oncology Group Study LAP2.J Clin Oncol 27(32):5331-5336.
[28] Meinhold-Heerlein I et al „Endoskopie in der gynäkologischen Onkologie - Chancen und Grenzen", Gynäkologe 2010.43:441-444.

17

Total Laparoscopic Hysterectomy: Surgical Technique and Results

William Kondo, Monica Tessmann Zomer, Lorne Charles, Nicolas Bourdel, Gérard Mage and Michel Canis
[1]*Centro Médico-Hospitalar Sugisawa, Curitiba, Paraná,*
[2]*CHU Estaing, Clermont-Ferrand,*
[1]*Brazil*
[2]*France*

1. Introduction

Hysterectomy is the most commonly performed major gynecologic procedure around the world. Benign diseases are responsible for more than 70% of the indications for hysterectomy and include menstrual disorders, fibroids, pelvic pain and uterine prolapse (Whiteman et al., 2008).

Traditionally, hysterectomy is performed by laparotomy or by vaginal access (Clayton, 2006). In 1989, Reich et al. (1989) described the first totally laparoscopic hysterectomy, which is currently considered an alternative means of access to traditional techniques for hysterectomy.

Despite the advantages of the laparoscopic and vaginal routes compared with laparotomy, this remains the most widely used access route for performing hysterectomy worldwide. In Denmark, 80% of hysterectomies for benign disease between 1988 and 1998 were performed by laparotomy (Gimbel et al., 2001). In the period between 1988 and 1990, approximately 1.7 million hysterectomies were performed in the United States and 75% were by the abdominal route (Wilcox et al., 1994). In 2003, 538,722 hysterectomies were performed for benign disease in the United States and the abdominal route was still the most common (66.1%), followed by vaginal (21.8%) and laparoscopic (11.8%). This study demonstrated that there was a statistically significant difference in the average hospital stay among the three types of surgical access (3 ± 0.03 days, 2 ± 0.03 days and 1.7 ± 0.03 days, respectively, $p < 0.001$), for abdominal, vaginal and laparoscopic approaches (Wu et al., 2007). In a multicenter cross-sectional study including 23 French university hospitals (Chapron et al, 1999), the rates of laparoscopic, vaginal and laparotomic hysterectomy were 9.6%, 47% and 43.4% respectively. In another study conducted between June and December 2004, including 634 women undergoing hysterectomy for benign disease in 12 French university hospitals, total laparoscopic hysterectomy was performed in 19.1%, laparoscopic assisted vaginal hysterectomy in 8.2%, total abdominal hysterectomy in 24.4% and vaginal hysterectomy in 48.3% (David-Montefiore et al., 2007), showing a significant reduction in the rate of laparotomies for performing hysterectomies. This trend indicates an adaptation to the modern concept of minimally invasive surgery. In some referral centers for gynecological laparoscopy in France, such as Clermont-Ferrand, the rate of total laparoscopic hysterectomy is up to more than 90%.

The advantages of the laparoscopic approach compared to open surgery include less intraoperative bleeding, shorter hospital stay, faster recovery and lower rates of wound and / or abdominal wall infections, at the expense of a longer surgery (Johnson et al., 2006). Although several authors have demonstrated an increased rate of ureteral and bladder injuries with the laparoscopic access (Johnson et al., 2006; Mäkinen et al., 2001), a recently published series including 4505 women undergoing hysterectomy using different routes of access (laparoscopy, laparotomy and vaginal) showed no statistically significant difference in the rate of major complications when the 3 groups were compared (Donnez et al., 2009).

In this chapter we discussed the technical details of laparoscopic hysterectomy and clinical outcomes of this surgical technique.

2. Overview of the previous studies

2.1 Laparoscopic vs. laparotomic vs. vaginal hysterectomy

There are several studies in the literature comparing the different routes of access to perform hysterectomy. A meta-analysis comparing women undergoing total abdominal hysterectomy (n = 103) and total laparoscopic hysterectomy (n = 98) observed a reduction in the rate of intraoperative and postoperative complications (30.1% vs. 9.2%) and in the intraoperative blood loss (Walsh et al., 2009). There was no statistically significant difference in the rate of major complications (2.9% vs. 4.1%), which included bladder injury, ureteral injury, bowel injury, vaginal vault dehiscence and pulmonary thromboembolism. Surgical time was significantly longer in the laparoscopic surgery, exceeding the laparotomy group by 22 minutes. A systematic review by Kluivers et al. (2008) which included seven randomized controlled studies comparing the quality of life for women after laparoscopic (n = 874) and abdominal hysterectomy (n = 576), observed that the laparoscopic procedure had a quality of life equal to or above the laparotomic procedure. In two studies in which statistically significant differences between the two groups were found, they occurred in the short term, ie. the first 6 weeks after surgery. Vaisbuch et al. (2006) compared 167 women who underwent total laparoscopic hysterectomy and 119 women who underwent total abdominal hysterectomy. A longer surgical time was noted in laparoscopic group (156 vs. 91.2 minutes; $p<0.001$), but a shorter hospital stay (3.9. vs. 6.5 days; $p<0.001$). The rate of conversion to laparotomy was 1.8%.

A Cochrane review (Nieboer et al., 2009) which compared the access routes for hysterectomy included 34 studies with a total of 4495 women. The benefits of vaginal hysterectomy compared with abdominal were quicker return to normal activities (mean difference of 9.5 days), fewer episodes of fever or nonspecific infection (OR 0.42) and shorter hospitalization (mean difference of 1.1 days). The benefits of laparoscopic surgery compared with open surgery were early return to usual activities (mean difference of 13.6 days), lower intraoperative blood loss (mean difference of 45ml), smaller drop in hemoglobin (mean difference of 0.55g/dl), shorter hospital stay (mean difference of 2 days) and lower incidence of fever and abdominal wall infections (OR 0.31), at the expense of a higher incidence of lesions of the urinary tract (bladder and ureter) (OR 2.41) and prolonged operative time (mean difference of 20.3 minutes). The benefits of laparoscopically assisted vaginal hysterectomy compared with total laparoscopic hysterectomy were lower rate of episodes of fever or nonspecific infection (OR 3.77) and shorter operative time (mean difference of 25.3 minutes). There was no evidence of benefit when comparing the laparoscopic and vaginal hysterectomy; the surgical time (mean difference of 39.3 minutes) and substantial bleeding (OR 2.76) were higher in the laparoscopic group.

Schindlbeck et al. (2008) compared the hysterectomy performed by laparoscopy (n = 43), vaginal (n = 87) and abdominal routes (n = 103), noting that the vaginal route had the shortest operative time (130 vs. 90 vs. 115 minutes; respectively; $p<0.01$), but the greater intraoperative blood loss (200 vs. 300 vs. 250ml, respectively; $p=0.07$). The laparoscopic group had less need for analgesics (1.5 vs. 2 vs. 4 days, respectively; $p<0.01$) and shorter hospital stay (7 vs. 8 vs. 9 days, respectively; $p<0.01$). The major complications included three bladder injuries at laparoscopic hysterectomy, 2 lesions of the rectum at vaginal hysterectomy, and 2 cases of postoperative ileus and one case of vesico-vaginal fistula at total abdominal hysterectomy.

Evaluating the clinical and economic outcomes of laparoscopic (n = 3520), vaginal (n = 3130) and open abdominal hysterectomy (n = 8754), Warren et al. (2009) observed that the rate of postoperative infection was higher in the group undergoing abdominal surgery (15% vs. 14% vs. 18%, respectively; $p<0.05$), length of hospital stay was shorter in the laparoscopic group (1.6 vs. 2.2 vs. 3.7 days; $p<0.001$) and the cost of the procedure was higher in the group undergoing surgery by open approach ($10,868.00 vs. $9544.00 vs. $12,086.00, respectively; $p<0.05$).

2.2 Total laparoscopic vs. laparoscopic supracervical hysterectomy

Some authors have preferred to conserve the cervix at the time of hysterectomy. Urinary and sexual function after surgery, were the clinical parameters for comparison between the total and supracervical techniques. Early studies reported better sexual and urinary function after supracervical hysterectomy, however randomized controlled trials have not confirmed these findings. In a Cochrane review in 2006 (Johnson et al., 2006), a group of randomized controlled trials were evaluated with respect to the results of supracervical and total hysterectomy. Three studies which included 733 patients were analyzed and no difference in urinary incontinence, constipation and sexual function was noted. Sexual function was measured by satisfaction with sex life, the prevalence of dyspareunia and rate of general sexual problems. The supracervical group had lower febrile morbidity and higher cyclic bleeding 1 year after surgery (OR 11.31, 95% CI 5.1 to 31.2). The surgery time (mean difference of 11.41 minutes, 95% CI 6.6 to 16.3) and blood loss (mean difference of 85.1 ml, 95% CI 27.4 to 142.9) were lower in the supracervical group, but there was no difference in the need for blood transfusion. These studies included in the Cochrane review compared the supracervical hysterectomy and total hysterectomy performed through laparotomy, but have been extrapolated to the laparoscopy. A randomized study comparing sexual changes and psychological well-being of patients undergoing subtotal hysterectomy (n = 66) and total hysterectomy (n = 66) (Ellström Engh et al., 2010), noted that women in the subtotal hysterectomy group reported positive changes in the frequency of orgasms and greater sexual pleasure than in the total hysterectomy group. Despite the findings of that study, there was no clear difference in terms of sexual or urinary function in the long term when comparing the two surgical techniques (Sokol & Green, 2009). Preoperative sexual activity is predictive factor of postoperative sexual

activity. However, independently, supracervical hysterectomy may lead to an earlier resumption of sexual activity (Helström, 1994).
In a retrospective series of 1000 supracervical laparoscopic hysterectomies (Bojahr et al., 2009), the median duration of surgery was 70.9 minutes (95% CI 69.2 to 72.5 minutes) and mean uterine weight was 212.5g (95% CI 201 - 223.6g). Surgical time decreased from 85.4 minutes in 2002 to 72.4 minutes in 2006, associated with the increasing in the uterine weight from 192.3 g to 228.7g. There was one case of bladder injury (0.1%) and 4 cases of conversion to laparotomy (0.4%). Milad et al. (2001) compared 27 women undergoing laparoscopic supracervical hysterectomy and 105 undergoing laparoscopically assisted vaginal hysterectomy, noting a shorter surgical time (181 vs. 220min; p=0.007), shorter hospital stay (1 vs. 2 days; p<0.001) and less blood loss (125 vs. 400ml; p<0.001) in the supracervical hysterectomy. No complications occurred in group supracervical hysterectomy. In the group of laparoscopically assisted vaginal hysterectomies there was a complication rate of 13% (p = 0.04), which included bladder injury (n = 3), blood loss exceeding 1000ml (n = 7), and vaginal vault hematoma (n = 4). In 2009 (Cipullo et al., 2009), the postoperative results of total laparoscopic hysterectomy (n = 157) were compared with supracervical laparoscopic hysterectomy (n = 157). The women who underwent supracervical hysterectomy had shorter operative time (100 vs. 110 minutes) and lower rate of major complications (1.3% vs. 4.5%) compared with those who underwent total hysterectomy. The reduction in cancer risk has been cited as an indication for removal of the cervix, however, the risk is low, with a 0.1% risk of cancer when the cervix is retained and a risk of 0.17 % of vaginal cancer. The median time to diagnosis was 26 years after surgery, and survival data were similar to those of patients without prior hysterectomy. Although cancer risk is low, the presence of dysplasia would be a contraindication for cervical preservation (Sokol & Green, 2009). Moreover, the risk of cyclical bleeding after surgery should be considered when discussing the removal of the cervix during a hysterectomy. The bleeding rates are between 5% and 20%, based on data obtained in randomized controlled studies of hysterectomies done by laparotomy and 19% in a prospective observational study of cases done by laparoscopy (Ghomi et al., 2005). The rate of reoperation for cyclic bleeding is 1-2% (Falcone & Walters, 2008; Ghomi et al., 2005). The endocervical fulguration has been shown to decrease the rate of future bleeding, although the efficacy of this modality has not been proven (Ghomi et al., 2005). Another option is excision of the endocervical component, but there is a paucity of literature or data on this technique.

3. Preoperative preparation

3.1 Particulars of laparoscopic hysterectomy

The indications for laparoscopic hysterectomy are similar to those for hysterectomy in general. Specific indications for the laparoscopic approach are the cases where there is contraindication for vaginal hysterectomy (Falcone & Walters, 2008). The Cochrane review of 27 studies with 3643 participants, comparing the results of abdominal, vaginal and laparoscopic hysterectomy concluded that the vaginal route of access should be preferred to abdominal access route, based on the best results. The authors also concluded that when vaginal hysterectomy is not possible, laparoscopic hysterectomy can obviate the need for an abdominal hysterectomy, but require a longer surgical time (mean difference of 25.3

minutes), without imposing any additional benefit to the vaginal route of access (Johnson et al., 2006).

Compared with vaginal surgery, laparoscopy allows the performance of concomitant procedures (appendectomy, adnexal surgery, excision of endometriosis) and inspection of the peritoneal cavity. In 2005, the American College of Obstetricians and Gynecologists Committee Opinion (2005) has listed the following information as appropriate for the use of laparoscopically assisted vaginal hysterectomy: lysis of adhesions, treatment of endometriosis, management of leiomyomas which hinder vaginal hysterectomy, ligation of the infundibulopelvic ligaments to facilitate removal of difficult ovaries, and evaluation of the abdomino-pelvic cavity before hysterectomy. The best diagnostic accuracy of the laparoscopic procedure with a clear view of the entire abdomen and pelvis was confirmed by the eVALuate study (Garry et al., 2004b), which consisted of two randomized controlled trials comparing abdominal (laparoscopy or laparotomy) and vaginal hysterectomy. Laparoscopy was associated with a higher detection rate of unexpected pathologies such as fibroids, endometriosis and adhesions, compared with the vaginal (16.4% vs. 4.8%; $p<0.01$) and the abdominal route of access (22.6% vs. 12.7%; $p<0.01$). However, no data shows that these additional findings influenced the performance of additional procedures by the surgeons or results in the long term.

3.2 Contraindications

The contraindications for laparoscopic hysterectomy are as follows (Sokol & Green, 2009):

- Medical conditions that contraindicate the establishment and maintenance of the pneumoperitoneum.
- Inexperience and / or inadequate training of surgeons.
- Malignancy that may require removal of the intact specimen or special procedures that can not be done due to skill, access or other circumstances.
- Lack of proper equipment.
- Contraindication to a possible laparotomy or non-acceptance of the patient. The consent form must include the potential need for conversion to laparotomy.

3.3 Preoperative details

Randomized studies have shown a decrease in surgical site infection with the use of prophylactic antibiotics in potentially contaminated procedures and it is recommended in cases of laparoscopic hysterectomy (Falcone & Walters, 2008). The prophylactic antibiotics should be administered within one hour of incision in the skin and should not be continued beyond 24 hours.

Several randomized studies have also shown a decreased risk of thromboembolism with enoxaparin prophylaxis.

4. Decision-making, anatomy, and key steps in the operations (Bourdel et al., 2009; Velemir et al., 2009)

4.1 Positioning

The patient is placed in the dorsal decubitus position, under general anesthesia with tracheal intubation. The legs are positioned at 30 degrees flexion, the arms along the body and buttocks slightly exceeding the operating table (Figure 1). The bladder is probed.

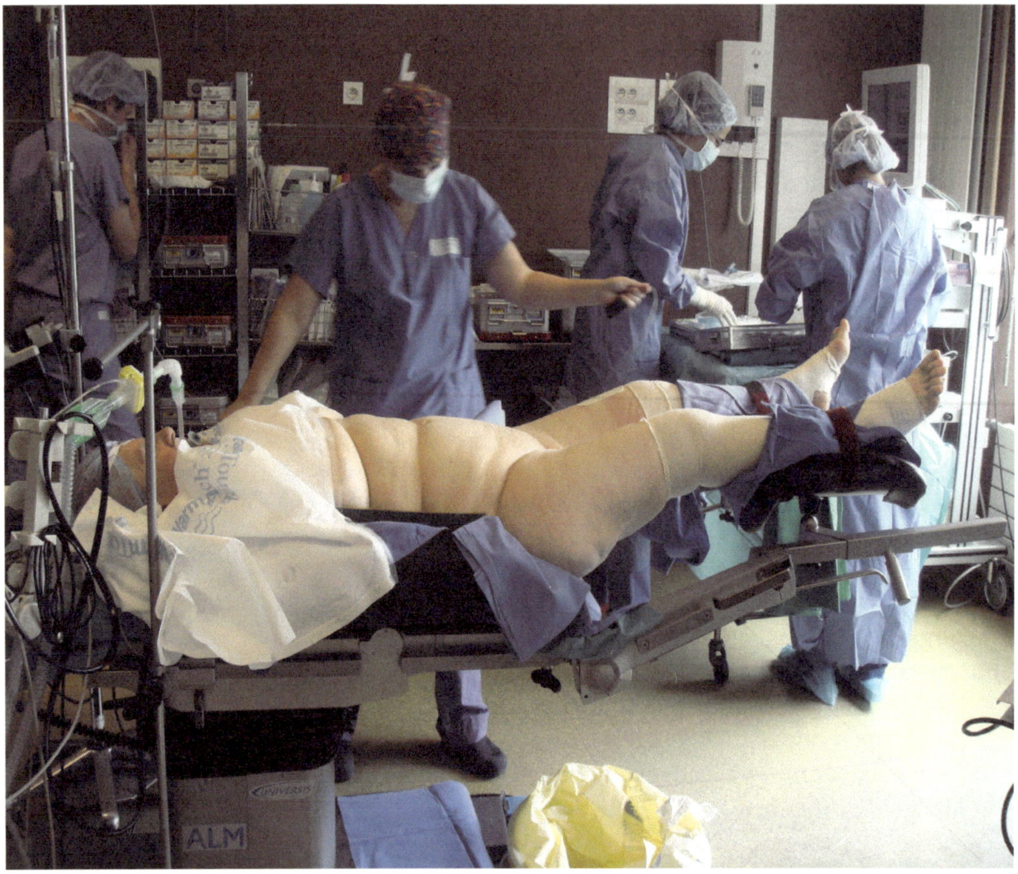

Fig. 1. Positioning of the patient for hysterectomy.

The surgeon is positioned to the left of the patient, the first assistant to the right and the second assistant is responsible for the uterine manipulator.

4.2 Uterine cannulation

Uterine cannulation is performed with a specific instrument: the uterine manipulator Karl Storz type Clermont-Ferrand (Figure 2). The cervix is visualized via speculum and dilated to Hegar number 9. The tip of the manipulator is then inserted into the cervix under direct vision. The size of the tip to be used varies with the size of the uterus.

4.3 Positioning of trocars

Four trocars are placed:

- One 10mm umbilical trocar.
- Three 5mm trocars: one 2cm medial to the right anterior superior iliac spine, another 2cm medial to the left anterior superior iliac spine, and a third in the midline, 8 to 10cm below the umbilicus (Figure 3). The latter 5mm trocar can be replaced by a 10 or 12mm trocar during surgery for the introduction of needles to suture the vaginal vault. In cases of bulkier uteri, the trocars can be positioned more cranially.

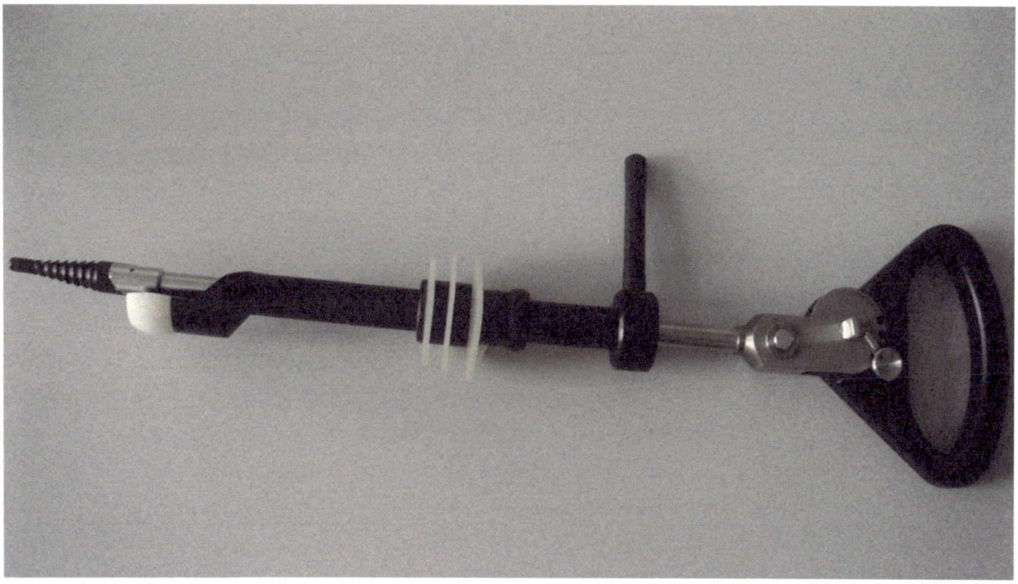

Fig. 2. Uterine manipulator type Clermont-Ferrand (Karl Storz).

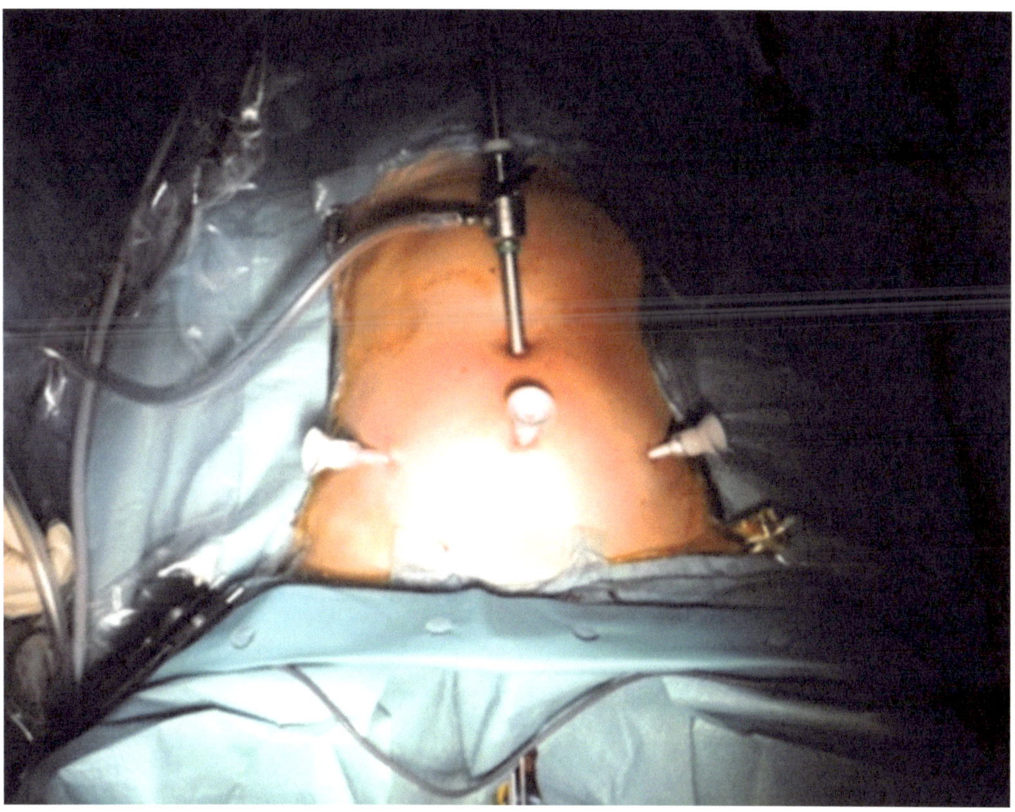

Fig. 3. Positioning of trocars for laparoscopic hysterectomy.

After placing the first trocar, the patient is placed in Trendelenburg position. The small bowel is retracted in cranial direction until the sacral promontory and pouch of Douglas are clearly visible.

The surgeon uses a bipolar cautery in the left hand and scissors in the right hand. The first assistant manipulates the zero degree laparoscope with the left hand and uses an Allis forceps or a grasper in the right hand.

4.4 Presentation of round ligaments

On the left, the release of adhesions between the sigmoid colon and infundibulopelvic ligament allows proper exposure of the round ligament (Figure 4). The uterus is mobilized by the second assistant and maintained in a cranial and anterior position. The round ligament is then grasped and pulled by the first assistant, which facilitates surgical access to the opposite side and thus the beginning of the surgery (Figure 5).

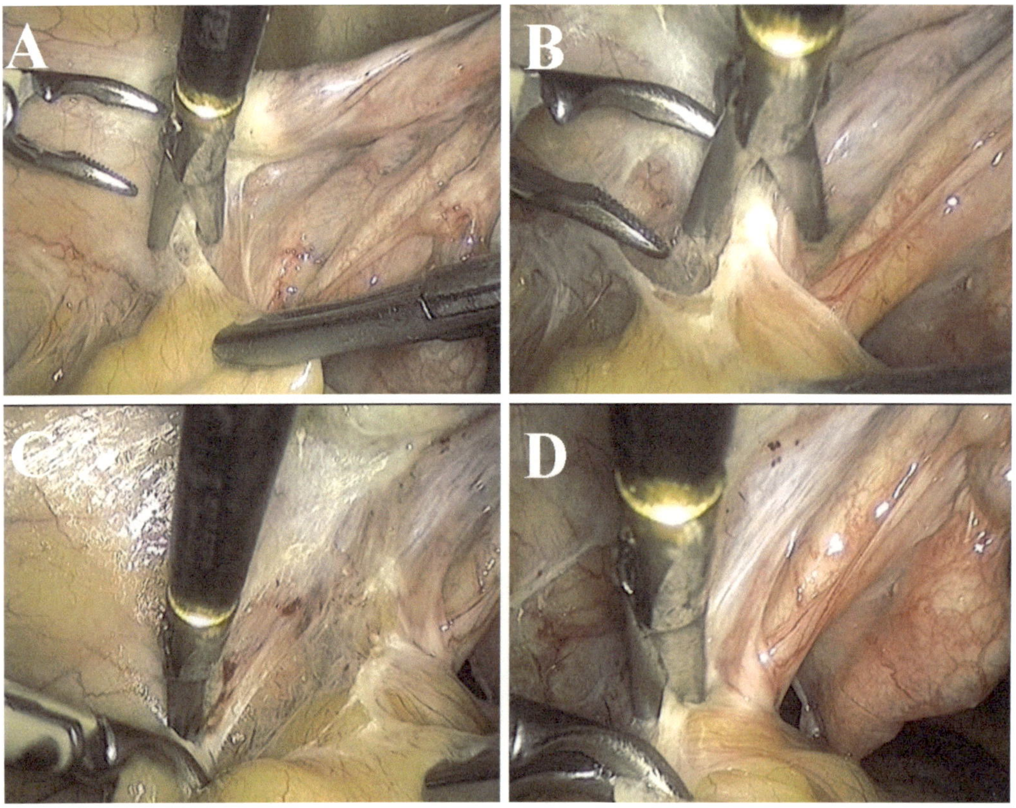

Fig. 4. Releasing the adhesions between the sigmoid colon and the left infundibulopelvic ligament.

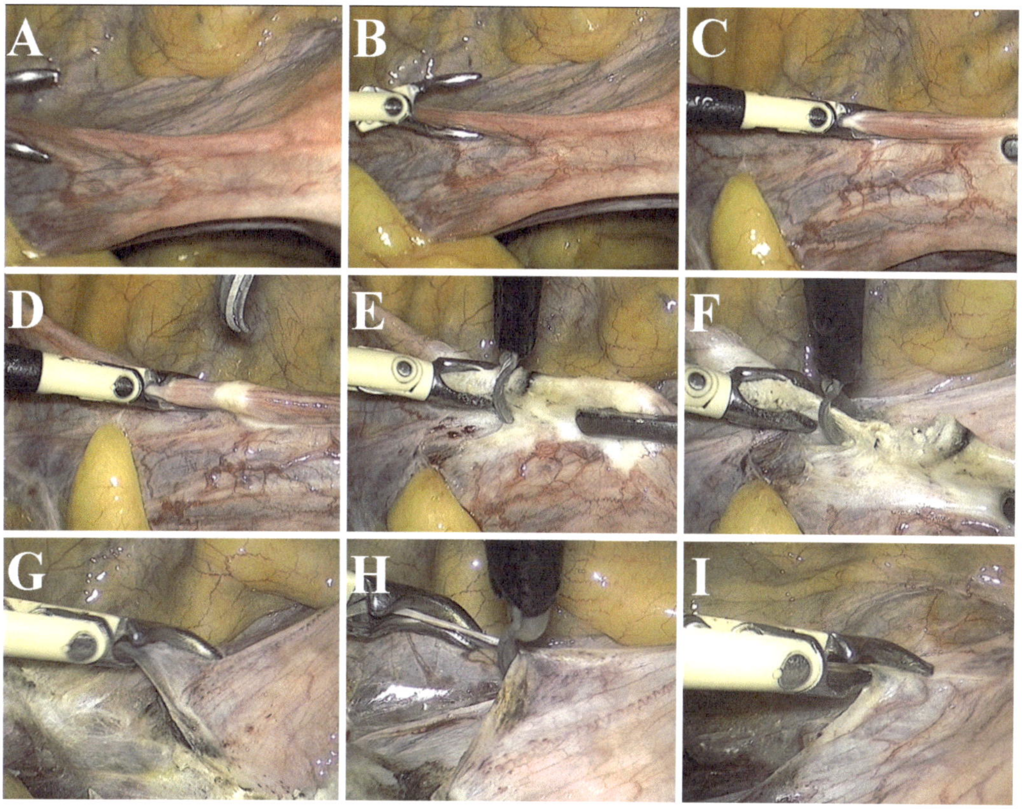

Fig. 5. (A and B) Uterine manipulation using the uterine manipulator of Clermont-Ferrand, exposing the left round ligament. (C) The first assistant pulls the left round ligament and the surgeon starts the coagulation with bipolar cautery. (D to F) Coagulation and section of the round ligament with laparoscopic scissors. (G to I) Opening the anterior leaf of the broad ligament from the round ligament up to the anterior peritoneal reflection.

4.5 Coagulation and division of the round ligaments

The round ligament is held about 2 to 3cm medial to lateral pelvic sidewall. It is then coagulated using bipolar cautery and the transection is performed with laparoscopic scissors (Figure 5).

4.6 Opening the anterior fold of the broad ligament up to the peritoneal vesicouterine fold

The uterus is maintained in a horizontal orientation by the second assistant. The anterior leaf of the broad ligament is coagulated with bipolar forceps and sectioned, from the round ligament up to the vesicouterine peritoneal reflection (Figure 5).

4.7 Fenestration of the broad ligament

The capillaries of the posterior leaf of the broad ligament are coagulated. The blue-gray appearance of the peritoneal leaf indicates that there are no underlying structures which can be inadvertently damaged. The posterior leaf of the broad ligament is cut and the opening is enlarged using divergent traction between the bipolar forceps and scissors (Figure 6). The ureter is then displaced laterally and inferiorly along with the peritoneum where it is less susceptible to injury.

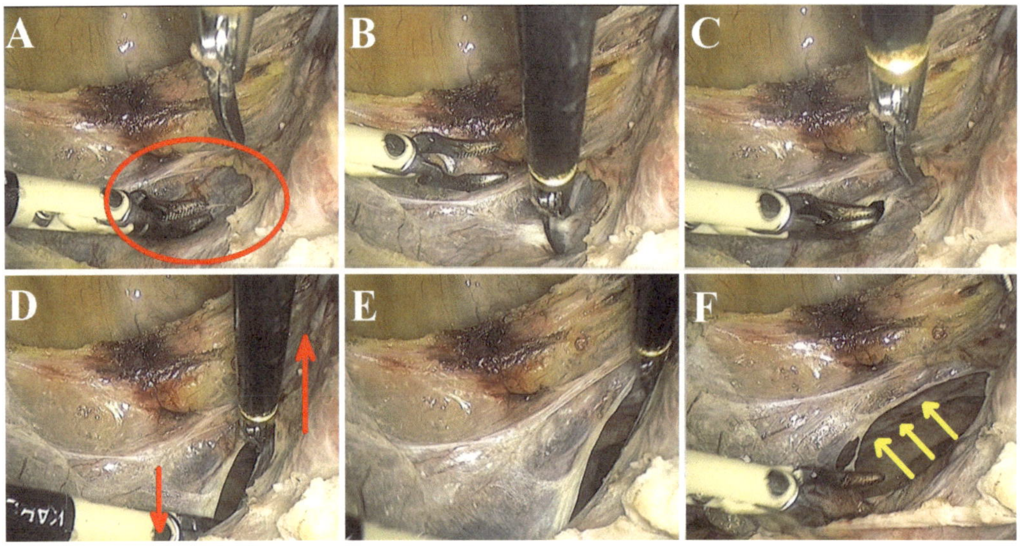

Fig. 6. (A) Coagulation of the capillaries of the posterior leaf of the broad ligament (red circle). (B and C) Opening of the blue region of the posterior leaf of the left broad ligament. (D and E) Fenestration of the broad ligament and the anteroposterior divergent pull of two instruments (scissors and bipolar forceps). (F) The ureter stays laterally along the left pelvic sidewall (yeloow arrows).

4.8 Coagulation and section of the infundibulopelvic ligament (total hysterectomy with bilateral adnexectomy) or the utero-ovarian ligament and the tube (interadnexal hysterectomy)

The first assistant should grasp the round ligament pedicle and apply traction towards the contralateral side of the infundibulopelvic ligament. The coagulation-section of the ligament should be progressive, plane by plane (peritoneum, followed by the vessels and the connective tissue) (Figure 7). When ovarian conservation is desired, the coagulation-section is performed on the tube and the utero-ovarian ligament (Figure 8).

4.9 Opening the posterior leaf of the broad ligament up to the uterosacral ligament

The dissection continues on the posterior peritoneum of the broad ligament, avoiding inadvertent injury of the uterine vessels (Figure 9). The peritoneum is stretched and dissected, coagulated and cut toward the uterosacral ligaments. Thus the uterine pedicle is isolated. All steps, from the coagulation-section of the round ligaments to the opening of the posterior leaf of the broad ligament, are performed in the same way on both sides.

4.10 Opening of the vesicovaginal space

The uterus should be mobilized cranially and slightly posterior, to expose the base of the vesicouterine space. The assistant uses an atraumatic forceps to grasp the peritoneum and bladder in the midline, applying cranial and superior traction. The peritoneum and the adjacent connective tissue are coagulated and sectioned, thus accessing the vesicovaginal plane. The dissection continues in the caudal direction, initially in the midline and then laterally. Coagulation-section of the vesico-uterine ligaments is performed (Figure 10). The second assistant advances the uterine manipulator valve into the vaginal fornix to reveal the plane and facilitate dissection.

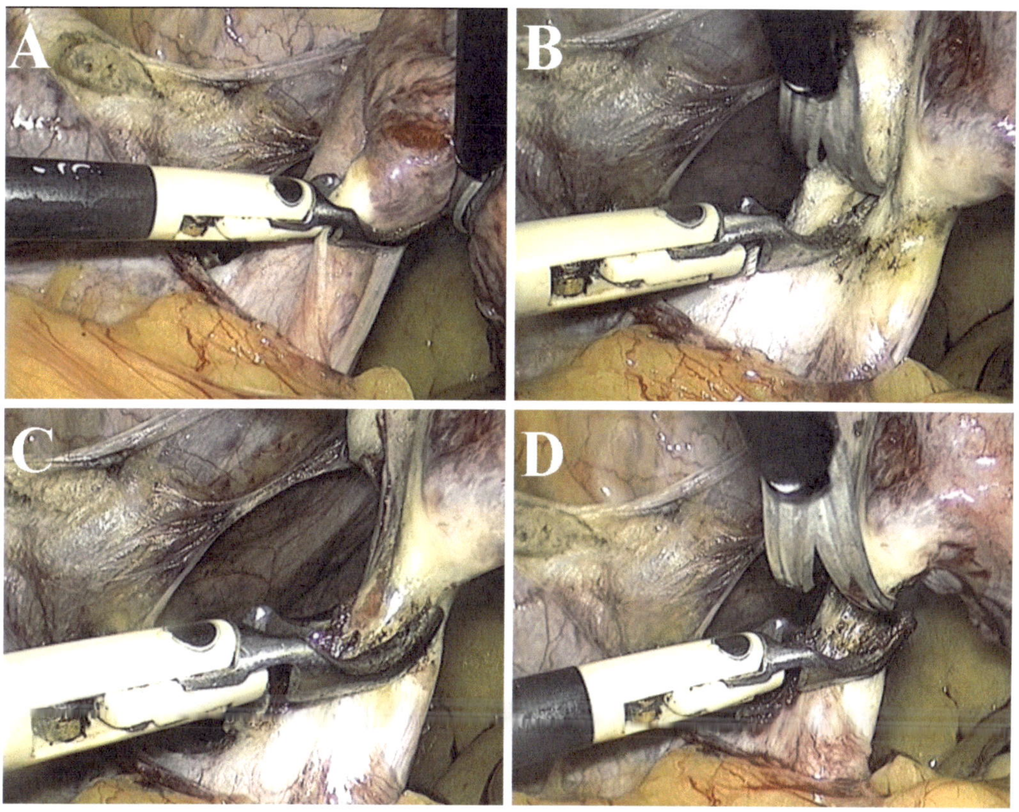

Fig. 7. Traction of the left adnexa by the assistant, followed by progressive bipolar coagulation of the infundibulopelvic ligament.

4.11 Coagulation and section of the uterine pedicles

The uterus is again directed cranially and laterally by the second assistant. The first assistant pulls the adnexa or the round ligament cranially and laterally. The pedicles must be very well isolated to allow an effective bipolar coagulation. The coagulation-section of the uterine pedicles, performed at the ascending uterine artery, should be carried in a progressive manner. The bipolar forceps is introduced by the lateral trocar, on the same side of the pedicle to be coagulated (Figure 11).

After coagulation of the uterine vessels, the pericervical fascia is incised at the same level of the coagulated uterine pedicles in order to enter the intra-fascial plane. The cervicovaginal vessels and the insertion of the uterosacral ligament are coagulated and sectioned (Figure 11).

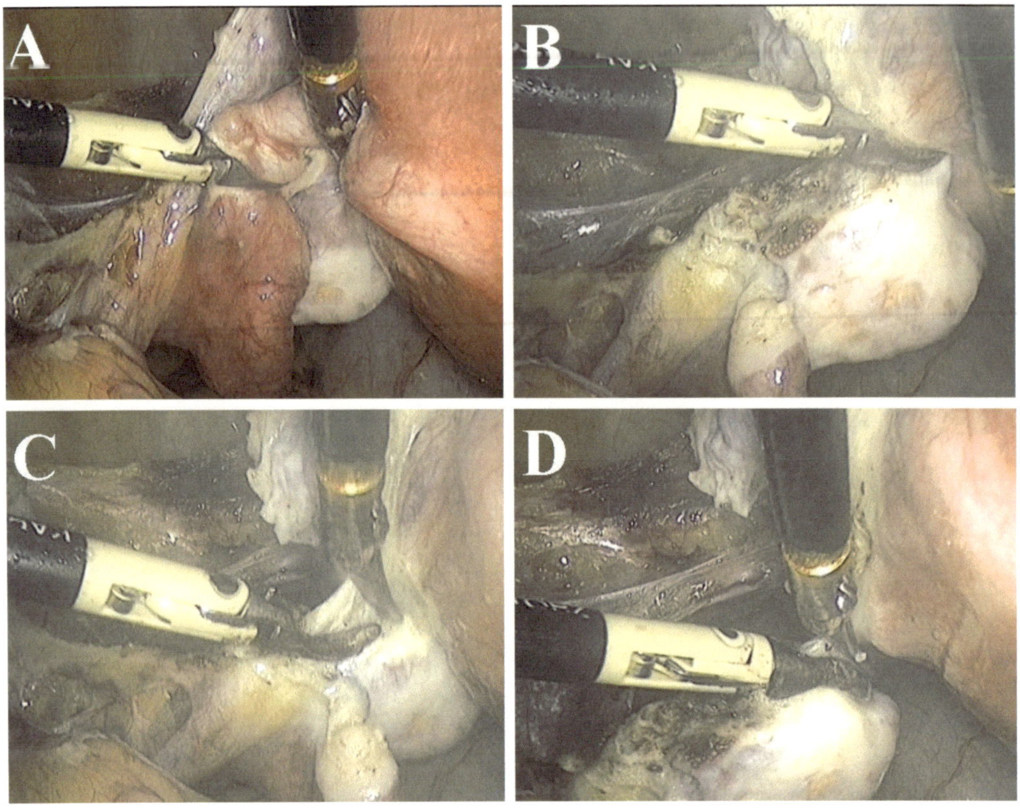

Fig. 8. Coagulation and section of the left fallopian tube and utero-ovarian ligament in case of left adnexal preservation.

4.12 Vaginal opening

The silicone ring system for prevention of loss of pneumoperitoneum is inserted into the vagina and the valve handle is pushed towards head. The monopolar section is performed on the valve starting at the anterior vaginal wall in the midline. It is continued laterally to the left, then posterior. The second assistant systematically exposes each part of the vaginal fornix rotating the valve. The opening of the vaginal vault continues towards the right side and ends posterior. The first assistant aspirates cautery smoke from the operative field. Sometimes additional hemostasis of the vaginal vault with a bipolar forceps is needed (Figure 12).

4.13 Surgical extraction of the uterine specimen

The extraction is performed vaginally in most cases (Figure 12). On some occasions it may be necessary to morcellate the uterus which can be performed laparoscopically, by cold knife or electric morcellator (Figure 13) or vaginally using the classic technique with a cold knife.

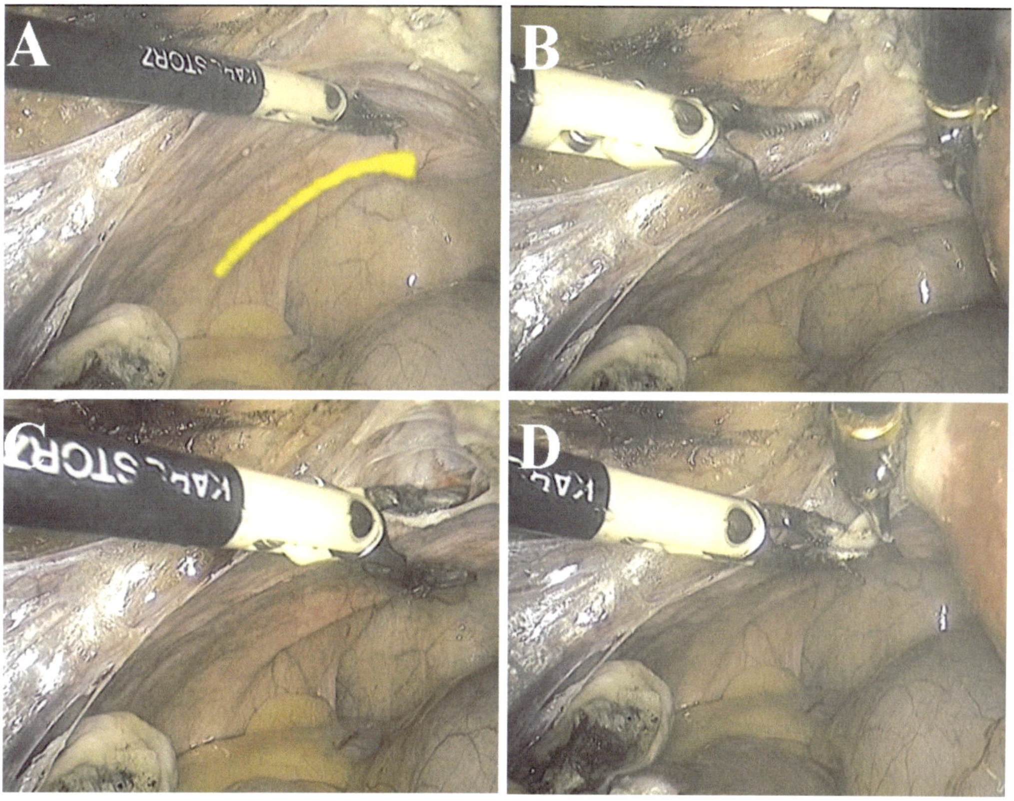

Fig. 9. Opening of the posterior leaf of the broad ligament up to the uterosacral ligament (in yellow).

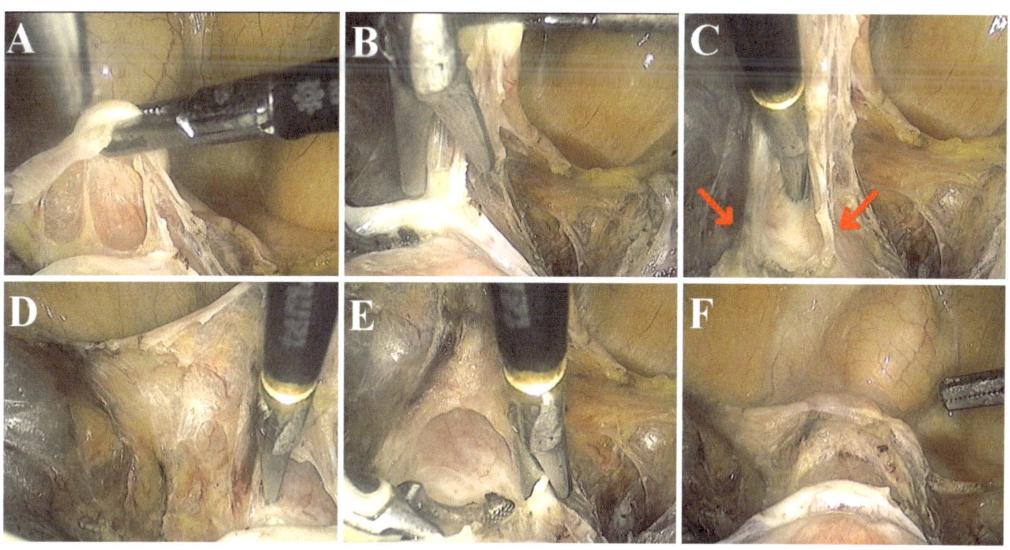

Fig. 10. Dissection of the vesicovaginal space. The green arrows indicate the area to be coagulated (vesico-uterine ligaments).

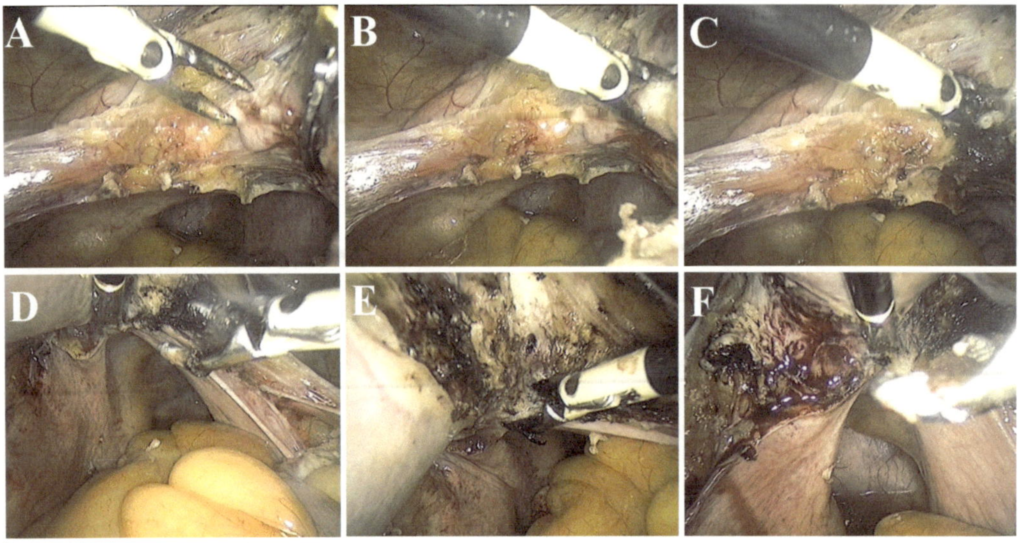

Fig. 11. (A to C) Progressive coagulation of the left uterine vessels using bipolar forceps. (D to F) Intra-fascial plane on right side.

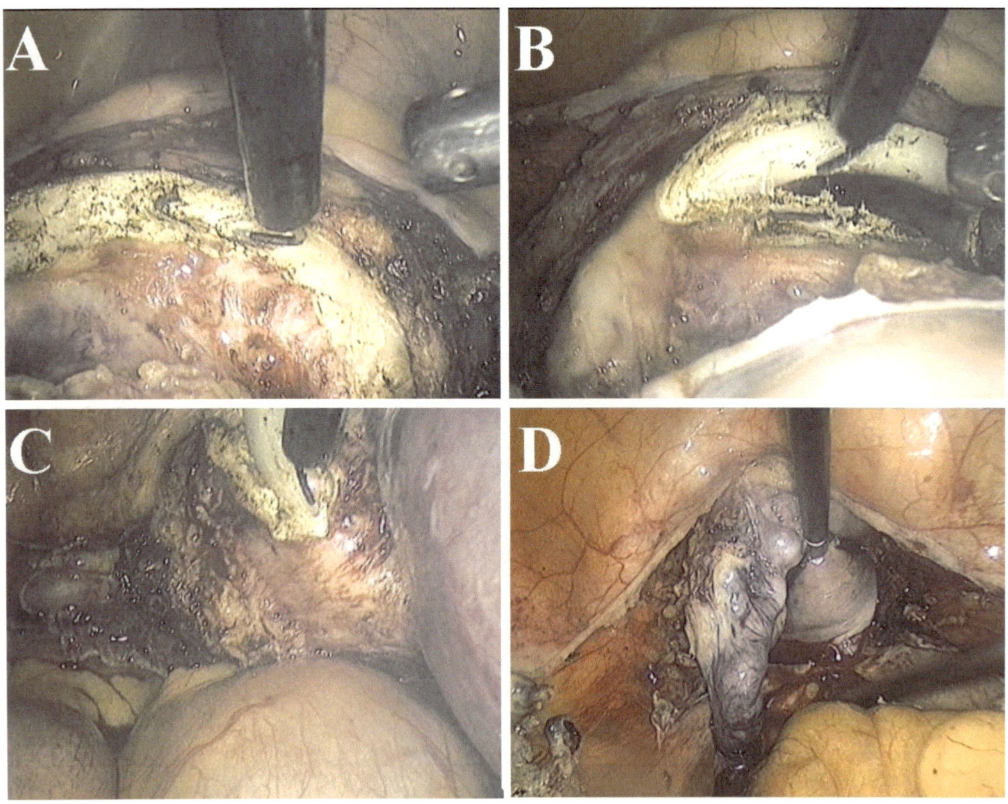

Fig. 12. (A to C) Opening of the vaginal vault with monopolar cautery. (D) Extraction of the uterine specimen without morcellation.

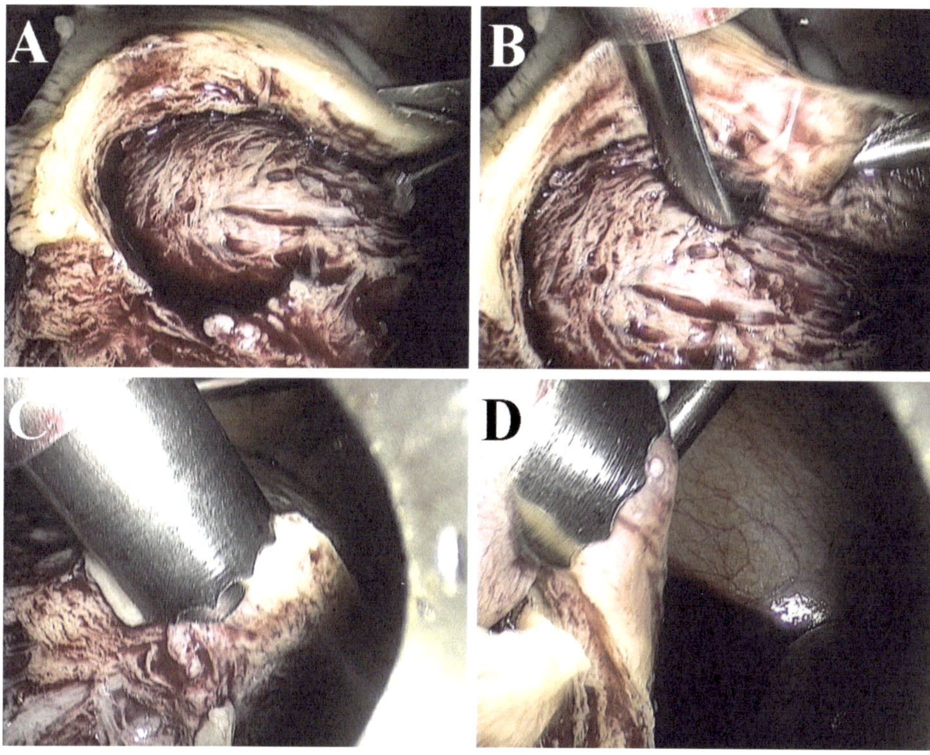

Fig. 13. Extraction of the uterine specimen using an electric morcellator.

4.14 Closure of the vaginal vault

The vaginal vault is sutured at three points using zero monofilament absorbable sutures (Poliglecaprone, Caprofyl ®, Ethicon Inc) (Figure 14).

4.15 Adnexal pexy

In cases of laparoscopic interadnexal hysterectomy we perform the adnexal pexy (fixation of the ovary and tube to the ipsilateral round ligament) using 2-0 polyester (Ethibond®, Ethicon Inc), to avoid adnexal torsion in the postoperative course (Figure 15).
Hemostasis is checked (Figure 15). The fascial defect of the 10mm trocar in the midline is sutured. The pneumoperitoneum is deflated and the skin is sutured with 3-0 monofilament absorbable suture (Poliglecaprone 25, Monocryl ®, Ethicon Inc).

4.16 Alternative techniques to the use of bipolar energy

There are some technical alternatives to the use of bipolar energy for total laparoscopic hysterectomy. Bipolar energy seems to be a safe cost-effective method with good control and accuracy during dissection and sectioning of the uterine vessels and other structures. However, the use of disposable laparoscopic instruments can afford the surgeon a slightly shorter surgical time. Options include endoscopic linear cutting staplers (Figure 16), the LigaSure® Vessel Sealing system (Valleylab) (Figure 17), the EnSeal® tissue sealing system (Advanced Tissue Sealing Technology) (Figure 18), and the Ultracision® harmonic scalpel (Figure 19).

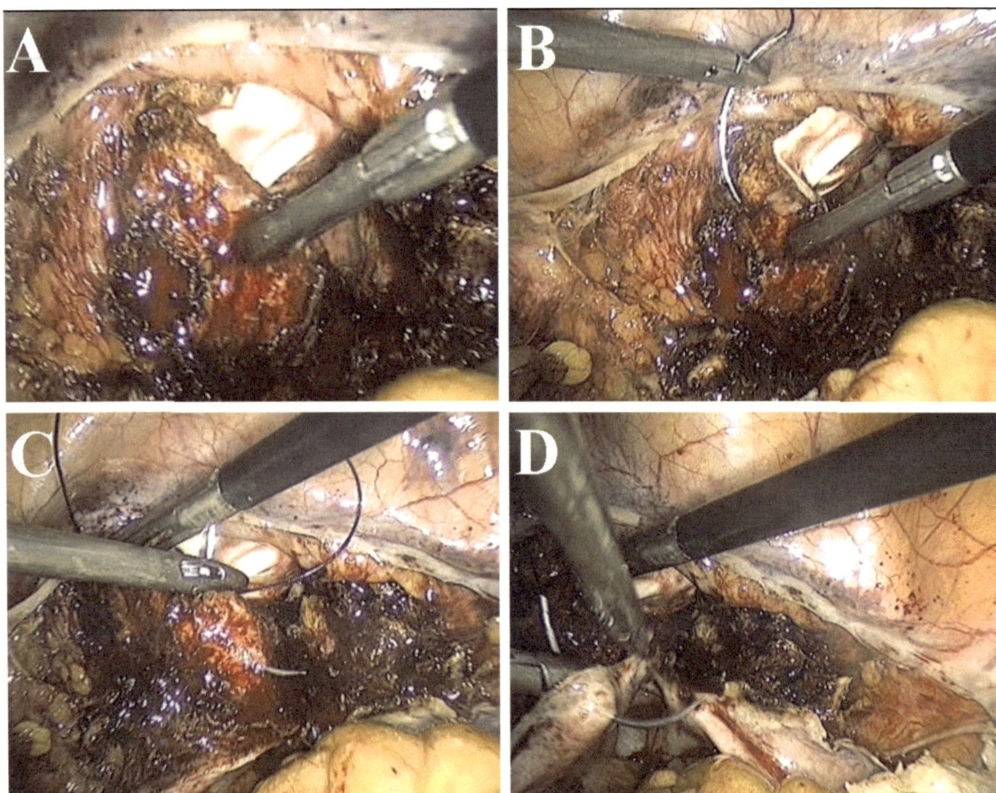

Fig. 14. Suturing the vaginal vault. The first assistant pulls the vagina and three interrupted X-shaped sutures are placed using zero Caprofyl®. The picture illustrates the suture at the left corner of the vagina, which must include the left uterosacral ligament (D).

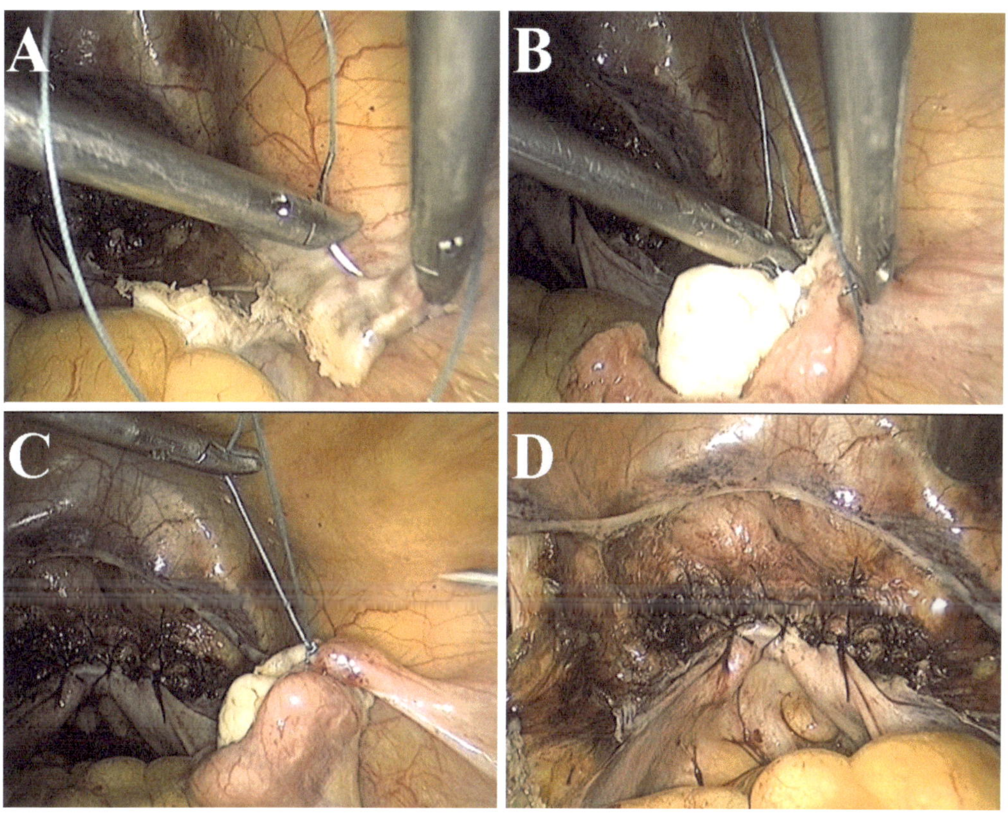

Fig. 15. (A to C) Fixation of the ovary to the round ligament on the right side using 2-0 Ethibond®. (D) Final appearance of the vaginal vault after homeostasis.

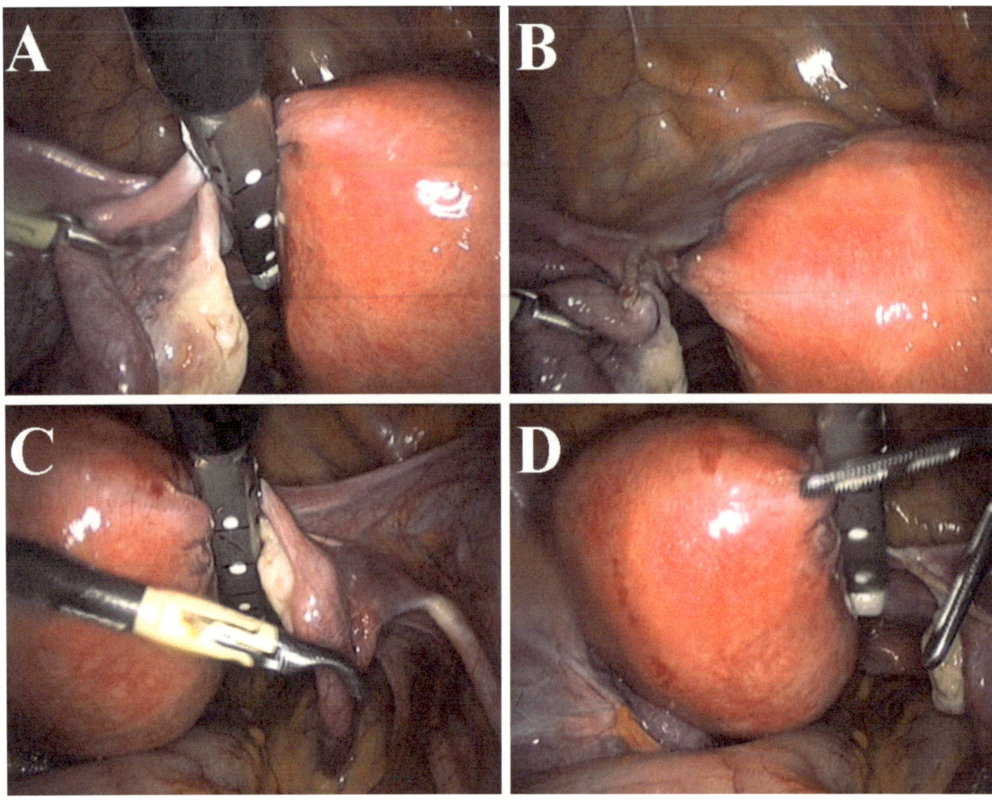

Fig. 16. Use of endoscopic linear cutting staplers for total laparoscopic hysterectomy.

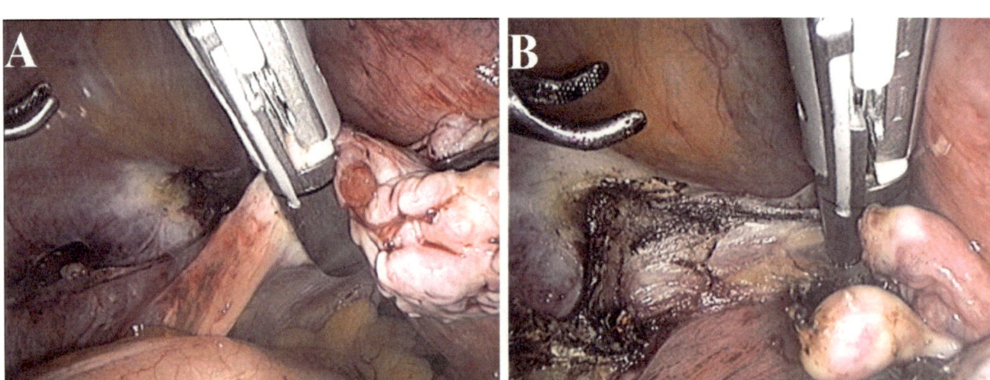

Fig. 17. Use of the LigaSure® Vessel Sealing for control of the infundibulopelvic ligament in total laparoscopic hysterectomy

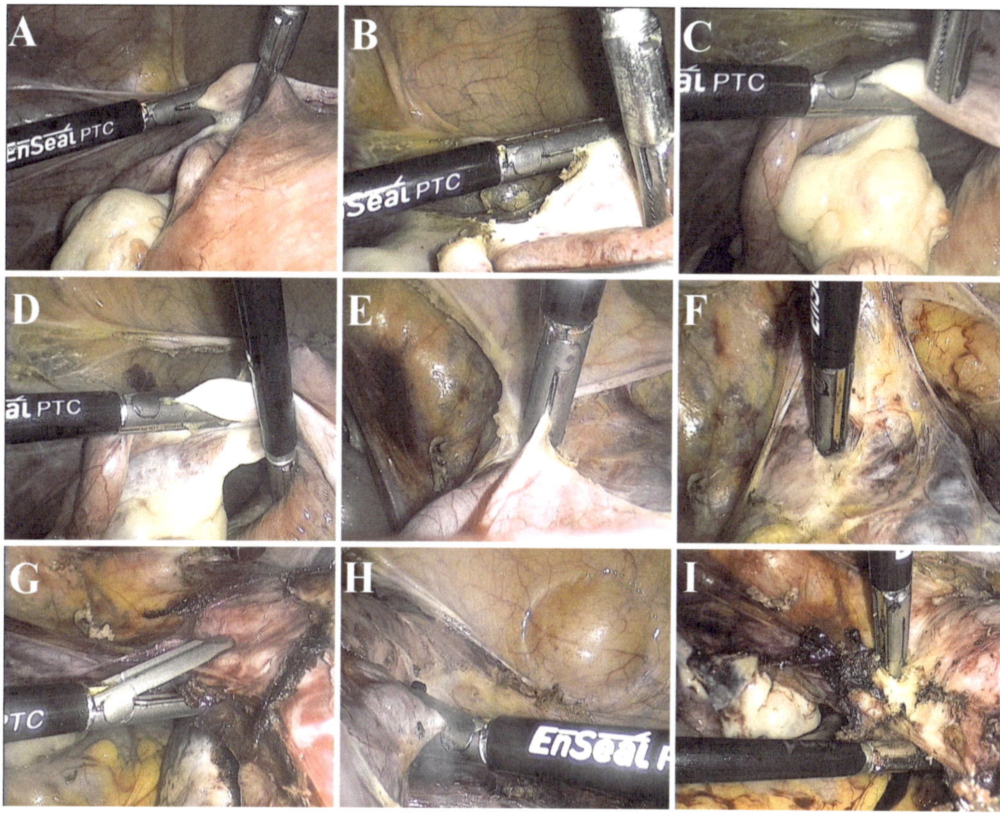

Fig. 18. Use of EnSeal® during total laparoscopic hysterectomy.

5. Surgical tricks

Some situations require further consideration: total laparoscopic hysterectomy in obese women and those with large uteri. The indications for removal of the ovaries and fallopian tubes are the same as in open surgery.

5.1 Bulky uterus

The access route to the achievement of hysterectomy in women with enlarged uteri is still controversial (Claerhout et al., 2005). A uterus is usually considered large when its size exceeds 12 weeks of gestation (average 280g) (Daraï et al., 2001). Despite the fact that a large uterus can be removed vaginally or laparoscopically, most gynecologists prefer to perform surgery by laparotomy. Randomized studies comparing open and laparoscopic hysterectomy for large uteri have shown the benefits of minimally invasive surgery with respect to blood loss, length of hospital stay and postoperative pain (Ferrari et al., 2000; Marana et al., 1999; Schütz et al., 2002; Sesti et al., 2008). However, disadvantages include longer surgical time (Ferrari et al., 2000; Johnson et al., 2006) and the significant learning curve, which has direct bearing on the frequency of major complications (Mäkinen et al., 2001).

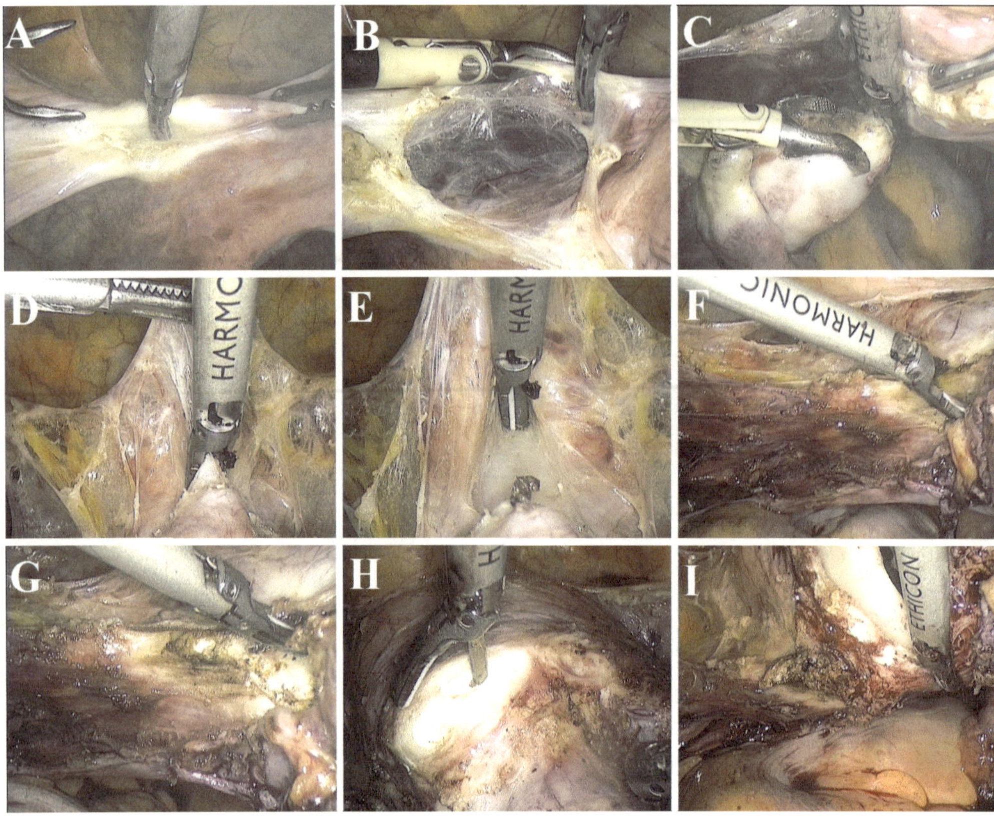

Fig. 19. Use of Ultracision® harmonic scalpel in total laparoscopic hysterectomy.

The size of the uterus seems to be an important factor for the occurrence of intraoperative bleeding and postoperative complications during laparoscopic hysterectomy, especially when performed for uteri larger than 500g (Bonilla et al., 2007). Some authors suggest the use of selective uterine artery coagulation at its origin during the laparoscopic procedure in large uteri to avoid or reduce intraoperative bleeding (Roman et al., 2008).
Laparoscopic hysterectomy for enlarged uteri has been studied by several authors. Wattiez et al (2002a) compared women undergoing total laparoscopic hysterectomy for uteri > 300g and ≤ 300g, and only the operative time was higher in the first group (156 vs. 108 minutes; $p<0.001$). There was no difference in the drop of hemoglobin levels, the need for analgesia and the time hospital stay between groups. In 2007, Bonilla et al. (2007) evaluated the impact of uterine weight in total abdominal and laparoscopic hysterectomy for benign diseases. The patients were divided into three groups according to the uterine weight (< 200g, 201-500g and > 500g) and it was observed that the average length of hospital stay and the risk of bleeding, the transfusion requirements and the postoperative complications increased with increasing uterine volume. Laparoscopic surgery was strongly associated with decreased morbidity, reduced hospitalization time and less blood loss compared to open surgery. Using a cut off of 500g to define a bulky uterus, Wang et al. (2004) demonstrated a prolonged operative time (91.1 vs. 77.4 minutes; $p<0.01$) and a increased intraoperative blood loss (570 vs. 262ml; $p<$ 0001) during laparoscopic assisted vaginal hysterectomy for uteri of increased size. A recent study by Fanning et al. (2008) confirmed the feasibility of

performing laparoscopically assisted vaginal hysterectomy for uteri above 1000g. They were able to successfully carry out 14 of 15 procedures (93%), with an average uterine weight of 1090g, a surgical time of 210 minutes and a blood loss of 400ml.
To perform laparoscopic hysterectomy in patients with bulky uterus is necessary to use a uterine manipulator with a long tip to reach the uterine fundus, allowing the manipulation of the entire uterus. The placement of trocars more cranial allows a greater surgical field and greater mobility of the laparoscopic instruments. The use of 30 degrees laparoscope allows a greater range of visual fields, and facilitates some surgical steps during the procedure for enlarged uteri.

5.2 Obese women

The impact of obesity on the outcomes of laparoscopic hysterectomy is still controversial. Although some authors suggest that laparoscopic hysterectomy can be safely performed in women with overweight and obesity, others report an increased risk of longer surgeries, intraoperative bleeding (Heinberg et al., 2004) and conversion to laparotomy (Leonard et al., 2005; Sokol et al., 2003). Comparing obese and nonobese females who underwent total abdominal hysterectomy, Pitkin (1976) observed a high incidence of wound complications (risk of 7x compared with the nonobese control group), which was directly responsible for the increased febrile morbidity and need for prolonged hospitalization. Similarly, Obermair et al. (2005) reported a 48% incidence of wound infections after surgery in obese women operated by laparotomy for endometrial cancer. In 2006, O'Hanlan et al. (2006) compared patients with uterine cancer undergoing total laparoscopic hysterectomy according to body mass index. The patients were stratified into five groups (underweight, ideal weight, overweight, obese and morbidly obese) and no statistically significant difference in mean duration of surgery, blood loss and hospital stay as observed between groups. Pellegrino et al. (2009) did not identify any difference between obese and nonobese women undergoing laparoscopic radical hysterectomy for stage I endometrial cancer in terms of surgical time, and intraoperative and long-term complications. Only blood loss was significantly higher in obese patients.

5.3 Salpingectomy / bilateral oophorectomy

The bilateral oophorectomy at the time of hysterectomy for benign disease is commonly performed in order to prevent the subsequent development of ovarian cancer or ovarian pathology that may require additional surgery. Currently, bilateral oophorectomy is performed in 78% of women aged between 45 and 64 years who undergo hysterectomy, and a total of 300,000 prophylactic oophorectomies are performed in the United States each year (Parker etl a., 2009b). Estrogen deficiency resulting from oophorectomy in pre- and post-menopause has been associated with increased risk of coronary heart disease, stroke, hip fracture, parkinsonism, dementia, cognitive impairment, depression and anxiety. In general, removal of the ovaries at the time of hysterectomy should be carefully evaluated in women who are not in the high risk group for developing breast cancer or ovarian cancer (Hickey et al., 2010; Parker etl a., 2009b; Parker, 2010). The Nurses' Health Study evaluated 16,345 women who underwent hysterectomy with bilateral oophorectomy and 13,035 undergoing hysterectomy with ovarian conservation (Parker et al., 2009a). They observed a reduced risk of ovarian cancer and breast cancer in the group undergoing concomitant oophorectomy, but an increased risk of mortality, fatal and nonfatal coronary heart disease, and lung cancer. In no analysis was oophorectomy associated with increased survival.

Repasy et al. (2009) evaluated the impact of removal of the tubes at the time of hysterectomy on ovarian survival, noting that 35.5% of patients in whom the fallopian tubes were intact developed hydrosalpinx. However, there was cystic degeneration of orphan ovaries (absence of the Fallopian tube) earlier than in the group with preservation of the tube (50 vs. 84.2 months; p=0.031). The authors' conclusion was that the removal of the tube during hysterectomy decreases the incidence of development of pelvic masses in the future, but it causes earlier cystic degeneration in remaining ovaries.

6. Postoperative care

The patient is given a regular diet 6 hours after the procedure. If the postoperative course is uneventful, patients can be discharged on the first postoperative day. They must be advised to avoid vaginal intercourse for 40 days.
Postoperative consultations are performed within 7 days to remove the dressings and 40 days to evaluate the healing of the vaginal vault.

7. Impact of the technique on modern practice

7.1 Complications

A hysterectomy is a safe procedure with a low mortality rate, estimated at 0.12 to 0.34 per 1000 surgeries (Falcone & Walters, 2008). Complications directly related to the laparoscopic approach include those related to the positioning of the Verees needle and trocars (bleeding, bowel injury), those related to pneumoperitoneum insufflation, hernia at the fascial defect created by the trocar and need to convert to open surgery. Other complications are related to the surgical procedure itself and are basically the same, regardless of the approach used for the hysterectomy, such as bleeding, urinary and bowel injuries, anesthetic problems, pulmonary thromboembolism, postoperative infection (urinary, pulmonary, surgical), problems in the vagina (hematoma, abscess and dehiscence), etc.
The VALUE study (Vaginal Abdominal Laparoscopic Uterine Excision) was a prospective nonrandomized study that evaluated the severe complications in 37,295 women undergoing abdominal (67%), vaginal (30%) and laparoscopically assisted vaginal hysterectomy (3%) (McPherson et al., 2004). The overall rate of severe complications was 3.5%, including visceral injury, bleeding, death, myocardial infarction, thromboembolic disease, stroke and organ failure. The risk was higher in patients undergoing surgery for fibroids (OR 1.34), in those with comorbidities (OR 1.47) and those subjected to laparoscopic surgery (OR 1.92). The laparoscopic procedures doubled the risk of complications compared to abdominal hysterectomy (6.1% vs. 3.6%).
The eVALuate study (Garry et al., 2004a) comprised two parallel randomized controlled trials: one comparing laparoscopic hysterectomy with abdominal hysterectomy and another comparing laparoscopic to vaginal. Laparoscopy was associated with a higher rate of major complications than laparotomy (11.1% vs. 6.2%; p=0.02). The conversion to laparotomy was included as a major complication, and when this was excluded, there was no statistically significant difference between the two types of access. When comparing the laparoscopic and vaginal access, no difference in complications was observed (however, this study arm did not reach the minimum required number of patients for treatment). The study confirmed some advantages of laparoscopy as less pain, shorter hospital stay, faster postoperative recovery, and better quality of life in the short term when compared with laparotomy. The disadvantages included the increased operative time and the highest rate of injuries to the urinary tract.

In a meta-analysis, laparoscopy was associated with increased risk of urinary tract lesions compared with abdominal hysterectomy (OR 2.61) (Johnson et al., 2005). When lesions of the ureters and bladder were considered separately, there was no increased risk of ureteral injury with laparoscopy. Laparoscopy was associated with fewer infections (OR 0.32), fewer episodes of fever (OR 0.65), less blood loss (mean difference 45.3ml) and smaller drop in hemoglobin (0.55g/l) compared with abdominal hysterectomy. Similar findings were noted comparing vaginal and abdominal hysterectomy. There was no difference in the fistula formation, urinary dysfunction, sexual dysfunction or patient satisfaction comparing all the access routes for hysterectomy. No difference was observed in the need for blood transfusion, occurrence of pelvic hematoma, infection of the vagina, urinary tract infection and thromboembolic events.

A total of 10,110 hysterectomies were analyzed in Finland during 1996 (Mäkinen et al., 2001), including 5,875 abdominal, 1,801 vaginal and 2,434 laparoscopic, noting an overall rate of complications (including major and minor) of 17.2%, 23.3% and 19%, respectively. Lesions of the ureter occurred predominantly in the laparoscopic group (0.2%, 0% and 1.1% respectively), whereas the intestinal lesions were more frequent in the vaginal group (0.2%, 0.5% 0.4%, respectively). The intra-operative bleeding requiring surgical intervention or blood transfusion during surgery was more common with vaginal hysterectomy (3.1% compared with 2.1% in abdominal hysterectomy). Infections (wound, intra-abdominal, vaginal, urinary tract, fever of unknown origin, etc.) were the most frequent complications, with an incidence of 10.5%, 13% and 9% in the abdominal, vaginal and laparoscopic hysterectomy groups, respectively.

The recent series of Donnez et al. (2009) which included 3,190 laparoscopic hysterectomies showed no increased rates of major complications when laparoscopic hysterectomy is performed by experienced surgeons. There was no difference in the rate of ureteral injury after vaginal (0.33%) and laparoscopic hysterectomy (0.25%). Bladder injuries occurred in 0.44% of women undergoing vaginal hysterectomy and 0.31% in those undergoing laparoscopic hysterectomy.

Some studies have observed that the incidence of vaginal vault dehiscence after laparoscopic hysterectomy is higher than after hysterectomy abdominal (Rivlin et al., 2010) In the case of total laparoscopic hysterectomy, the vagina is sutured using absorbable sutures. A study that reviewed 7,286 hysterectomies found an incidence of dehiscence of the vaginal vault of 4.93% after laparoscopic hysterectomy, 0.29% after vaginal hysterectomy and 0.12% after abdominal hysterectomy. The relative risk compared with vaginal and abdominal was 21 and 53.2, respectively, which was statistically significant (Hur et al., 2007). There are no prospective studies comparing methods of vaginal vault closure and the subsequent risk of dehiscence, partly due to the infrequent occurrence of this complication. In the absence of data that can clarify these findings, recommendations for colpotomy and the vaginal vault closure include: minimizing energy use in the vaginal dome, ensuring adequate depth at the time of vaginal suture, and paying attention to meticulous surgical technique, including hemostasis.

Another reported complication after laparoscopic hysterectomy is adnexal torsion. The prevalence of this complication was 7.91 per 1,000 cases and occurred approximately 2.64 years after laparoscopic hysterectomy in Mashiach et al. (2004)' study. To avoid this complication, we perform adnexal fixation (ovary and fallopian tube to the round ligament) at the time of laparoscopic hysterectomy as a routine measure.

7.2 Conversion

Risk factors for conversion in laparoscopic surgery include body mass index, history of previous laparotomy, suspected malignancy, presence of adhesions, technical difficulties, complex cases, surgeon experience and uterine weight (Sokol et al., 2003). Risk factors for conversion during laparoscopic hysterectomy in the first 5 years of experience included (Leonard et al., 2005): increased body mass index (adjusted OR 1.09, 95% CI 1.01 to 1.18), length of the uterus on transvaginal ultrasound of 8 to 10cm (adjusted OR 4.01, 95% CI 1.54 to 10.45), uteri greater than 10 cm in length on transvaginal sonography (adjusted OR 9.17, 95% CI 2.74 to 30.63), lateral myoma measuring more than 5cm on transvaginal sonography (adjusted OR 3.57, 95% CI 0.97 to 13.17) and history of previous surgery or pelvis infection as a basis for adhesions or scarring (adjusted OR 2.92, 95% CI 1.23 to 6.94).

7.3 Learning curve

Observational and retrospective studies have shown a lower rate of complications and conversion to laparotomy with increasing surgeon experience, thus demonstrating a learning curve for the procedure.

In the study by Mäkinen et al. (2001), surgeons who performed more than 30 laparoscopic hysterectomies had lower rates of complications of the ureter, bladder and bowel compared with less experienced colleagues. Ghomi et al. (2007) showed that after the initial experience of 30 cases the surgical time of laparoscopic supracervical hysterectomy decreased significantly. Ascher-Walsh & Capes (2007) observed a significant reduction in surgical time (from 201.4 minutes to 137.2 minutes, $p<0.001$) comparing the first 2 cases and the last two cases of laparoscopic supracervical hysterectomy performed by senior residents.

In 2002, Wattiez et al. (2002b) compared the frequency of complications of total laparoscopic hysterectomy during 1989-1995 (n = 695) and 1996-1999 (n = 952). The rate of major complications decreased from 5.6% to 1.3%. There was also significant reduction of excessive bleeding (1.9% vs. 0.1%) and the need for blood transfusion (2.2% vs. 0.1%) in the second period. The rate of urinary complications was 2.2% in the first period (10 lacerations of the bladder, 4 ureteric injuries and 1 vesico-vaginal fistula) and 0.9% in the second period (6 lesions of the bladder, 2 ureteral lacerations and 1 vesico-vaginal fistula), which was statistically significant ($p<0.005$). A single case of intestinal injury and intestinal obstruction occurred in the first period. The rate of conversion to laparotomy was 4.7% in the first period and 1.4% in the second period. The surgical time was reduced from 115 minutes in the first period to 90 minutes in the second period ($p<0.005$). Likewise, Brummer et al. (2008) observed that the overall incidence of major complications in laparoscopic hysterectomy in the period 1992-1999 (n = 13,885) was 1.8% and in 2000-2005 (n = 13,942) decreased to 1 %. During the same period, the urinary tract injuries decreased from 1.4% to 0.7% and specifically, lesions of ureter decreased from 0.9% to 0.3%.

8. Recommendations and conclusions

The benefits of minimally invasive hysterectomy (laparoscopic or vaginal) are undeniable when compared with open surgery. The exploration of the abdomino-pelvic cavity and the ability to perform a safe oophorectomy represent some advantages of laparoscopy over the vaginal route. Specific indications for each surgical technique remain uncertain. However, the proposal is not that laparoscopic hysterectomy replace vaginal hysterectomy but serve to increase the therapeutic armamentarium of the gynecologist surgeon to perform minimally invasive surgery for a wide range of indications, obviating the need for an abdominal hysterectomy in the presence of adnexal tumors, pelvic adhesions, endometriosis, previous pelvic surgeries, bulky uteri and obese patients.

9. References

American College of Obstetricians and Gynecologists. ACOG Committee Opinion. (2005). Appropriate use of laparoscopically assisted vaginal hysterectomy. *Obstet Gynecol,* 105, 4, (Apr 2005), pp. (929-930), ISSN 0029-7844.

Ascher-Walsh, CJ. & Capes, T. (2007). An evaluation of the resident learning curve in performing laparoscopic supracervical hysterectomies as compared with patient outcome: five-year experience. *J Minim Invasive Gynecol,* 14, 6, (Nov-Dec 2007), pp. (719-723), ISSN 1553-4650.

Bojahr, B., Tchartchian, G. & Ohlinger, R. (2009). Laparoscopic supracervical hysterectomy: a retrospective analysis of 1000 cases. *JSLS,* 13, 2, (Apr-Jun 2009), pp. (129-134), ISSN 1086-8089.

Bonilla, DJ., Mains, L., Whitaker, R., Crawford, B., Finan, M. & Magnus, M. (2007). Uterine weight as a predictor of morbidity after a benign abdominal and total laparoscopic hysterectomy. *J Reprod Med,* 52, 6, (Jun 2007), pp. (490-498), ISSN 0024- 7758.

Bourdel, N., Tran, X., Botchorhisvili, R., Pouly, JL., Canis, M. & Mage, G. (2009). Laparoscopic hysterectomy in 10 steps. *J Chir (Paris),* 146, 5, (Out 2009), pp. (483-491), ISSN 0021-7697.

Brummer, TH., Seppälä, TT. & Härkki, PS. (2008). National learning curve for laparoscopic hysterectomy and trends in hysterectomy in Finland 2000-2005. *Hum Reprod,* 23, 4, (Apr 2008), pp. (840-845), ISSN 1460-2350.

Chapron, C., Laforest, L., Ansquer, Y., Fauconnier, A., Fernandez, B., Bréart, G. & Dubuisson, JB. (1999). Hysterectomy techniques used for benign pathologies: results of a French multicentre study. *Hum Reprod,* 14, 10, (Out 1999), PP. (2464-2470), ISSN 1460-2350

Cipullo, L., De Paoli, S., Fasolino, L. & Fasolino, A. (2009). Laparoscopic supracervical hysterectomy compared to total hysterectomy. *JSLS,* 13, 3, (Jul-Sep 2009), pp. (370-375), ISSN 1086-8089.

Claerhout, F. & Deprest, J. (2005). Laparoscopic hysterectomy for benign diseases. *Best Pract Res Clin Obstet Gynaecol,* 19, 3, (Jun 2005), pp. (357-375), ISSN 1521-6934.

Clayton, RD. (2006). Hysterectomy. *Best Pract Res Clin Obstet Gynaecol,* 20, 1, (Feb 2006), pp. (73-87), ISSN 1521-6934.

Daraï, E., Soriano, D., Kimata, P., Laplace, C. & Lecuru, F. (2001). Vaginal hysterectomy for enlarged uteri, with or without laparoscopic assistance: randomized study. *Obstet Gynecol,* 97, 5 Pt 1, (May 2001), pp. (712-716), ISSN 0029-7844.

David-Montefiore, E., Rouzier, R., Chapron, C., Daraï, E. & Collegiale d'Obstétrique et Gynécologie de Paris-Ile de France. (2007). Surgical routes and complications of hysterectomy for benign disorders: a prospective observational study in

French university hospitals. *Hum Reprod*, 22, 1, (Jan 2007), pp. (260-265), ISSN 1460-2350.

Donnez, O., Jadoul, P., Squifflet, J. & Donnez, J. (2009). A series of 3190 laparoscopic hysterectomies for benign disease from 1990 to 2006: evaluation of complications compared with vaginal and abdominal procedures. *BJOG*, 116, 4, (Mar 2009), pp. (492-500), ISSN 1471-0528.

Ellström Engh, MA., Jerhamre, K. & Junskog, K. (2010). A randomized trial comparing changes in sexual health and psychological well-being after subtotal and total hysterectomies. *Acta Obstet Gynecol Scand*, 89, 1, (2010), pp. (65-70), ISSN 1600-0412.

Falcone, T. & Walters, MD. (2008). Hysterectomy for benign disease. *Obstet Gynecol*, 111, 3, (Mar 2008), pp. (753-767), ISSN 0029-7844.

Fanning, J., Fenton, B., Switzer, M., Johnson, J. & Clemons, J. (2008). Laparoscopic-assisted vaginal hysterectomy for uteri weighing 1000 grams or more. *JSLS*. 12, 4, (Oct-Dec 2008), pp. (376-379), ISSN 1086-8089.

Ferrari, MM., Berlanda, N., Mezzopane, R., Ragusa, G., Cavallo, M. & Pardi, G. (2000). Identifying the indications for laparoscopically assisted vaginal hysterectomy: a prospective, randomised comparison with abdominal hysterectomy in patients with symptomatic uterine fibroids. *BJOG*, 107, 5, (May 2000), pp. (620-625), ISSN 1471-0528.

Garry, R., Fountain, J., Mason, S., Hawe, J., Napp, V., Abbott, J., Clayton, R., Phillips, G., Whittaker, M., Lilford, R., Bridgman, S. & Brown, J. (2004a). The eVALuate study: two parallel randomised trials, one comparing laparoscopic with abdominal hysterectomy, the other comparing laparoscopic with vaginal hysterectomy. *BMJ*, 328, 7432, (Jan 2004), p. (129), ISSN 1468-5833.

Garry, R., Fountain, J., Brown, J., Manca, A., Mason, S., Sculpher, M., Napp, V., Bridgman, S., Gray, J. & Lilford. R. (2004b). EVALUATE hysterectomy trial: a multicentre randomised trial comparing abdominal, vaginal and laparoscopic methods of hysterectomy. *Health Technol Assess*, 8, 26, (Jun 2004), pp. (1-154), ISSN 1366-5278.

Ghomi, A., Hantes, J. & Lotze, EC. (2005). Incidence of cyclical bleeding after laparoscopic supracervical hysterectomy. *J Minim Invasive Gynecol*, 12, 3, (May-Jun 2005), pp. (201-205), ISSN 1553-4650.

Ghomi, A., Littman, P., Prasad, A. & Einarsson, JI. (2007). Assessing the learning curve for laparoscopic supracervical hysterectomy. *JSLS*, 11, 2, (Apr-Jun 2007), pp. (190-194), ISSN 1086-8089.

Gimbel, H., Settnes, A. & Tabor, A. (2001). Hysterectomy on benign indication in Denmark 1988-1998. A register based trend analysis. *Acta Obstet Gynecol Scand*, 80, 3, (Mar 2001), pp. (267-272), ISSN 1600-0412.

Heinberg, EM., Crawford, BL 3rd., Weitzen, SH. & Bonilla, DJ. (2004). Total laparoscopic hysterectomy in obese versus nonobese patients. *Obstet Gynecol*, 103, 4, (Apr 2004), pp. (674-680), ISSN 0029-7844.

Helström L. Sexuality after hysterectomy: a model based on quantitative and qualitative analysis of 104 women before and after subtotal hysterectomy. *J Psychosom Obstet Gynaecol*, 15, 4, (Dec 1994), pp. (219-229), ISSN 1743-8942.

Hickey, M., Ambekar, M. & Hammond, I. (2010). Should the ovaries be removed or retained at the time of hysterectomy for benign disease? *Hum Reprod Update*, 16, 2, (Mar-Apr 2010), pp. 131-141, ISSN 1460-2369.

Hur, HC., Guido, RS., Mansuria, SM., Hacker, MR., Sanfilippo, JS. & Lee, TT. (2007). Incidence and patient characteristics of vaginal cuff dehiscence after different modes of hysterectomies. *J Minim Invasive Gynecol*, 14, 3, (May-Jun 2007), pp. (311-317), ISSN 1553-4650.

Johnson, N., Barlow, D., Lethaby, A., Tavender, E., Curr, L. & Garry, R. (2005). Methods of hysterectomy: systematic review and meta-analysis of randomised controlled trials. *BMJ*, 330, 7506, (Jun 2005), p. (1478), ISSN 1468-5833.

Johnson, N., Barlow, D., Lethaby, A., Tavender, E., Curr, E. & Garry, R. (2006). Surgical approach to hysterectomy for benign gynaecological disease. *Cochrane Database Syst Rev*, 19, 2, (Apr 2006), p. (CD003677), ISSN 1469-493X.

Kluivers, KB., Johnson, NP., Chien, P., Vierhout, ME., Bongers, M. & Mol, BW. (2008). Comparison of laparoscopic and abdominal hysterectomy in terms of quality of life: a systematic review. *Eur J Obstet Gynecol Reprod Biol*, 136, 1, (Jan 2008), pp. (3-8), ISSN 0028-2243.

Leonard, F., Chopin, N., Borghese, B., Fotso, A., Foulot, H., Coste, J., Mignon, A. & Chapron C. (2005). Total laparoscopic hysterectomy: preoperative risk factors for conversion to laparotomy. *J Minim Invasive Gynecol*, 12, 4, (Jul-Aug 2005), pp. (312-317), ISSN 1553-4650.

Mäkinen, J., Johansson, J., Tomás, C., Tomás, E., Heinonen, PK., Laatikainen, T., Kauko, M., Heikkinen, AM. & Sjöberg, J. (2001). Morbidity of 10 110 hysterectomies by type of approach. *Hum Reprod*, 16, 7, (Jul 2001), pp. (1473-1478), ISSN 1460-2350.

Marana, R., Busacca, M., Zupi, E., Garcea, N., Paparella, P. & Catalano, GF. (1999). Laparoscopically assisted vaginal hysterectomy versus total abdominal hysterectomy: a prospective, randomized, multicenter study. *Am J Obstet Gynecol*, 180, 2 Pt 1, (Feb 1999), pp. (270-275), ISSN 0002-9378.

Mashiach, R., Canis, M., Jardon, K., Mage, G., Pouly, JL. & Wattiez, A. (2004). Adnexal torsion after laparoscopic hysterectomy: description of seven cases. *J Am Assoc Gynecol Laparosc*, 11, 3, (Aug 2004), pp. (336-339), ISSN 1074-3804.

McPherson, K., Metcalfe, MA., Herbert, A., Maresh, M., Casbard, A., Hargreaves, J., Bridgman, S. & Clarke, A. (2004). Severe complications of hysterectomy: the VALUE study. *BJOG*, 111, 7, (Jul 2004), pp. (688-694), ISSN 1471-0528.

Milad, MP., Morrison, K., Sokol, A., Miller, D. & Kirkpatrick, L. (2001). A comparison of laparoscopic supracervical hysterectomy vs laparoscopically assisted vaginal hysterectomy. *Surg Endosc*, 15, 3, (Marc 2001), pp. (286-268), ISSN 1432-2218.

Nieboer, TE., Johnson, N., Lethaby, A., Tavender, E., Curr, E., Garry, R., van Voorst, S., Mol, BW. & Kluivers, KB. (2009). Surgical approach to hysterectomy for benign gynaecological disease. *Cochrane Database Syst Rev*, 8, 3, (Jul 2009), p. (CD003677), ISSN 1469-493X.

Obermair, A., Manolitsas, TP., Leung, Y., Hammond, IG. & McCartney, AJ. (2005). Total laparoscopic hysterectomy versus total abdominal hysterectomy for obese women with endometrial cancer. *Int J Gynecol Cancer*, 15, 2, (Mar-Apr 2005), pp. (319-324), ISSN 1525-1438.

O'Hanlan, KA., Dibble, SL. & Fisher, DT. (2006). Total laparoscopic hysterectomy for uterine pathology: impact of body mass index on outcomes. *Gynecol Oncol*, 103, 3, (Dec 2006), pp. (938-941), ISSN 0090-8258.

Parker, WH., Broder, MS., Chang, E., Feskanich, D., Farquhar, C., Liu, Z., Shoupe, D., Berek, JS., Hankinson, S. & Manson, JE. (2009a). Ovarian conservation at the time of hysterectomy and long-term health outcomes in the nurses' health study. *Obstet Gynecol*, 113, 5, (May 2009), pp. (1027-1037), ISSN 0029-7844.

Parker, WH., Jacoby, V., Shoupe, D. & Rocca W. (2009b). Effect of bilateral oophorectomy on women's long-term health. *Womens Health (Lond Engl)*, 5, 5, (Sep 2009), pp. (565-576), ISSN 1745-5065.

Parker, WH. (2010). Bilateral oophorectomy versus ovarian conservation: effects on long-term women's health. *J Minim Invasive Gynecol*, 17, 2, (Mar-Apr 2010), pp. (161-166), ISSN 1553-4650.

Pellegrino, A., Signorelli, M., Fruscio, R., Villa, A., Buda, A., Beretta, P., Garbi, A. & Vitobello, D. (2009). Feasibility and morbidity of total laparoscopic radical hysterectomy with or without pelvic limphadenectomy in obese women with stage I endometrial cancer. *Arch Gynecol Obstet*, 279, 5, (May 2009), pp. (655-660), ISSN 1432-0711.

Pitkin, RM. (1976). Abdominal hysterectomy in obese women. *Surg Gynecol Obstet*, 142, 4, (Apr 1976), pp. (532-536), ISSN 0039-6087.

Reich, H., DeCaprio, J. & McGlynn, F. (1989). Laparoscopic hysterectomy. *J Gynecol Surg*, 5, (1989), pp. (213-216), ISSN 1042-4067

Repasy, I., Lendvai, V., Koppan, A., Bodis, J. & Koppan, M. (2009). Effect of the removal of the Fallopian tube during hysterectomy on ovarian survival: the orphan ovary syndrome. *Eur J Obstet Gynecol Reprod Biol*, 144, 1, (May 2009), pp. (64-67), ISSN 0028-2243.

Rivlin, ME., Meeks, GR. & May, WL. (2010). Incidence of vaginal cuff dehiscence after open or laparoscopic hysterectomy: a case report. *J Reprod Med*, 55, 3-4, (Mar-Apr 2010), pp. (171-174), ISSN 0024- 7758.

Roman, H., Zanati, J., Friederich, L., Resch, B., Lena, E. & Marpeau, L (2008). Laparoscopic hysterectomy of large uteri with uterine artery coagulation at its origin. *JSLS*, 12, 1, (Jan-Mar 2008), pp. (25-29), ISSN 1086-8089.

Schindlbeck, C., Klauser, K., Dian, D., Janni, W. & Friese, K. (2008). Comparison of total laparoscopic, vaginal and abdominal hysterectomy. *Arch Gynecol Obstet*, 277, 4, (Apr 2008), pp. (331-337), ISSN 1432-0711.

Schütz, K., Possover, M., Merker, A., Michels, W. & Schneider, A. (2002). Prospective randomized comparison of laparoscopic-assisted vaginal hysterectomy

(LAVH) with abdominal hysterectomy (AH) for the treatment of the uterus weighing >200 g. *Surg Endosc*, 16, 1, (Jan 2002), pp. (121-125), ISSN 1432-2218.

Sesti, F., Calonzi, F., Ruggeri, V., Pietropolli, A. & Piccione, E. (2008). A comparison of vaginal, laparoscopic-assisted vaginal, and minilaparotomy hysterectomies for enlarged myomatous uteri. *Int J Gynaecol Obstet*, 103, 3, (Dec 2008), pp. (227-231), ISSN 0020-7292.

Sokol, AI., Chuang, K. & Milad, MP. (2003). Risk factors for conversion to laparotomy during gynecologic laparoscopy. *J Am Assoc Gynecol Laparosc*, 10, 4, (Nov 2003), pp. (469-473), ISSN 1074-3804.

Sokol, AI. & Green, IC. (2009). Laparoscopic hysterectomy. *Clin Obstet Gynecol*, 52, 3, (Sep 2009), pp. (304-312), ISSN 1532-5520.

Vaisbuch, E., Goldchmit, C., Ofer, D., Agmon, A. & Hagay Z. (2006). Laparoscopic hysterectomy versus total abdominal hysterectomy: a comparative study. *Eur J Obstet Gynecol Reprod Biol*, 126, 2, (Jun 2006), pp. (234-8), ISSN 0028-2243.

Velemir, L., Azuar, AS., Botchorishvili, R., Canis, M., Jardon, K., Rabischong, B., Pouly, JL. & Mage, G. (2009). Optimizing the role of surgeons assistants during a laparoscopic hysterectomy. *Gynecol Obstet Fertil*, 37, 1, (Jan 2009), pp. (74-80), ISSN 1297-9589.

Walsh, CA., Walsh, SR., Tang, TY. & Slack, M. (2009). Total abdominal hysterectomy versus total laparoscopic hysterectomy for benign disease: a meta-analysis. *Eur J Obstet Gynecol Reprod Biol*, 144, 1, (May 2009), pp. (3-7), ISSN 0028-2243.

Wang, CJ., Yen, CF., Lee, CL., Tashi, T. & Soong, YK. (2004). Laparoscopically assisted vaginal hysterectomy for large uterus: a comparative study. *Eur J Obstet Gynecol Reprod Biol*, 115, 2, (Aug 2004), pp. (219-223), ISSN 0028-2243.

Warren, L., Ladapo, JA., Borah, BJ. & Gunnarsson, CL. (2009). Open abdominal versus laparoscopic and vaginal hysterectomy: analysis of a large United States payer measuring quality and cost of care. *J Minim Invasive Gynecol*, 16, 5, (Sep-Oct 2009), pp. (581-588), ISSN 1553-4650.

Wattiez, A., Soriano, D., Fiaccavento, A., Canis, M., Botchorishvili, R., Pouly, J., Mage, G. & Bruhat, MA. (2002a). Total laparoscopic hysterectomy for very enlarged uteri. *J Am Assoc Gynecol Laparosc*, 9, 2, (May 2002), pp. (125-130), ISSN 1074-3804.

Wattiez, A., Soriano, D., Cohen, SB., Nervo, P., Canis, M., Botchorishvili, R., Mage, G., Pouly, JL., Mille, P. & Bruhat, MA. (2002b). The learning curve of total laparoscopic hysterectomy: comparative analysis of 1647 cases. *J Am Assoc Gynecol Laparosc*, 9, 3, (Aug 2002), pp. (339-345), ISSN 1074-3804.

Whiteman, MK., Hillis, SD., Jamieson, DJ., Morrow, B., Podgornik, MN., Brett, KM. & Marchbanks, PA. (2008). Inpatient hysterectomy surveillance in the United States, 2000-2004. *Am J Obstet Gynecol*, 198, 1, (Jan 2008), pp. (34.e1-7), ISSN 0002-9378.

Wilcox, LS., Koonin, LM., Pokras, R., Strauss, LT., Xia, Z. & Peterson, HB. (1994). Hysterectomy in the United States, 1988-1990. *Obstet Gynecol*, 83, 4, (Apr 1994), pp. (549-555), ISSN 0029-7844.

Wu, JM., Wechter, ME., Geller, EJ., Nguyen, TV. & Visco, AG. (2007). Hysterectomy rates in the United States, 2003. *Obstet Gynecol*, 110, 5, (Nov 2007), pp. (1091-1095), ISSN 0029-7844.

Part 12

Vaginal Aplasia

18

Balloon Vaginoplasty: A Revolutionary Approach for Treating Vaginal Aplasia

Atef M.M. Darwish
Woman's Health University Center, Assiut, Egypt

1. Introduction

Vaginal aplasia is a rare anomaly that carries psychologic, physical and sexual problems to the female and her partner. Whereas a number of vaginoplasty methods have been developed, refined, and modified, no state-of-the-art surgical approach has been established. This is due to a number of factors including regional differences, surgeon experience and preference for a method, and patient choice. The goal of vaginoplasty is to develop a space between the bladder and the rectum suitable for satisfactory intercourse for both partners.
This review will discuss in details the common available procedures of vaginoplasty with stress on the evident pros and cons of each technique. Thereafter, it will discuss the new era of balloon vaginoplasty whether done laparoscopically or via the retropubic space. Every procedure will be discussed meticulously with excellent illustrations. Some tables to compare different techniques will be provided. In short, a step by step educational approach will be delivered to the readers to start practicing such simplified procedures in their own hospitals.

2. Background

Vaginal aplasia (figures 1-3) is a rare anomaly occurring in approximately 15,000 to 10,000 births (1). It carries an emotional, sexual, and social embarrassing effect on those women (2, 3). Previously, those cases are neglected by the general gynecologists and sent to be treated by very limited specialized centers all over the word. Thanks to continuous refinement and innovation of reconstructive surgical techniques, some of those women could be able to conceive (4–6). Even if this anomaly is associated with uterine aplasia, there is a hope for uterine transplantation within the coming few years (7, 8) because of successful animal transplantation (9, 10) and competent organ cryopreservation (11). These modern achievements pushed interested centers to refine their procedures and offer those cases the best available care.
Mayer-Rokitansky-Kuster-Hauser syndrome (MRKHS) is a subtype of vaginal agenesis comprising congenital absence of vagina and a variety of Mullerian duct anomalies, with aplasia of the uterus being the most common feature. In general, these patients have normally functioning ovaries, which are often located at the pelvic brim (figure 3). Anomalies of the urinary tract and the skeleton are frequently associated with MRKHS (12).

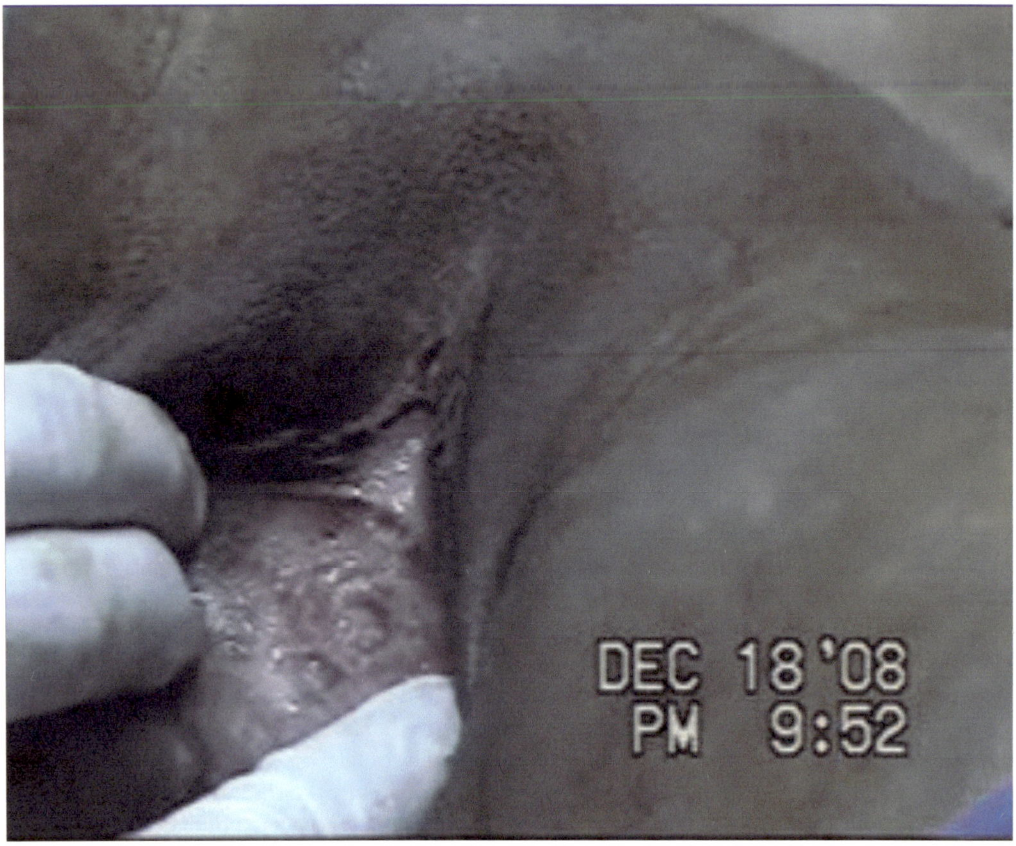

Fig. 1. Clinical appearance of vaginal aplasia.

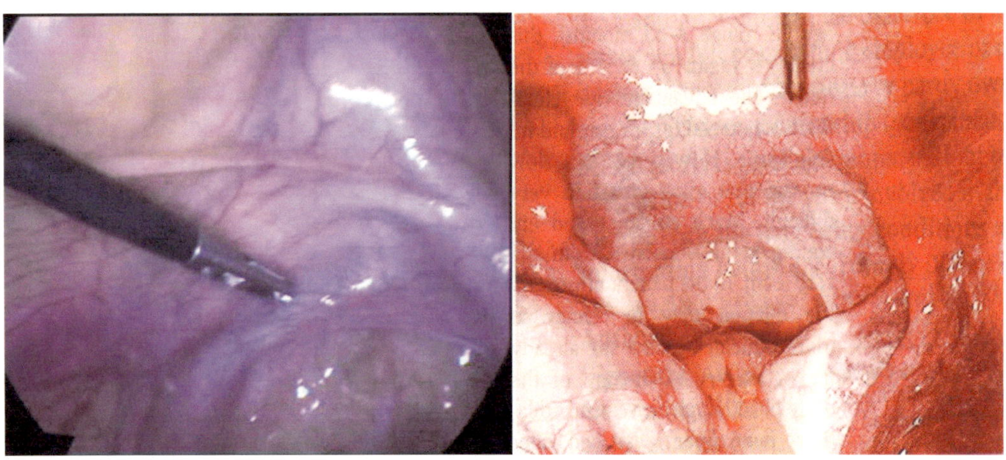

Fig. 2. Laparoscopic appearance of vaginal aplasia

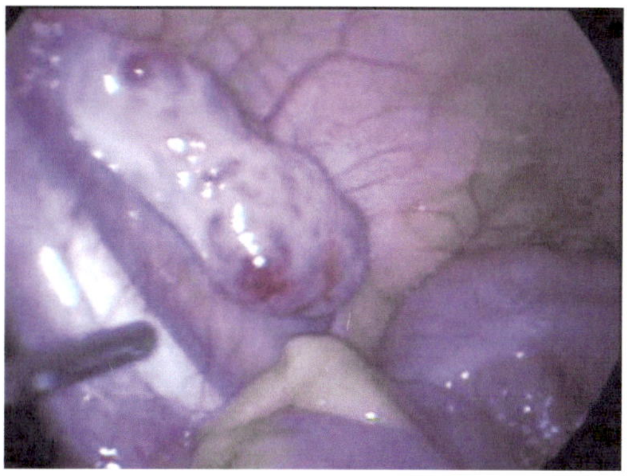

Fig. 3. Abnormal localization of the ovaries in MRKH syndrome.

3. Therapeutic options of vaginoplasty

Numerous surgical and nonsurgical procedures with varying degrees of success have been described for correction of the condition, but none have proved to be universally accepted. As this chapter is planned to focus on balloon vaginoplasty, I just quote some references on the common techniques of vaginoplasty (13-29). A lot of the published work on vaginoplasty demonstrates the feasibility of a particular procedure, highlights its possible advantages, and expresses the skills of the surgeons. The question now is not whether the procedure is feasible, but whether the approach is superior and beneficial to a particular patient, cost effective for the community at large, and more importantly easily performed by the general gynecologists without sophisticated instrumentation. The following algorism (figure 4) summarizes broadly the different methods of vaginoplasty.

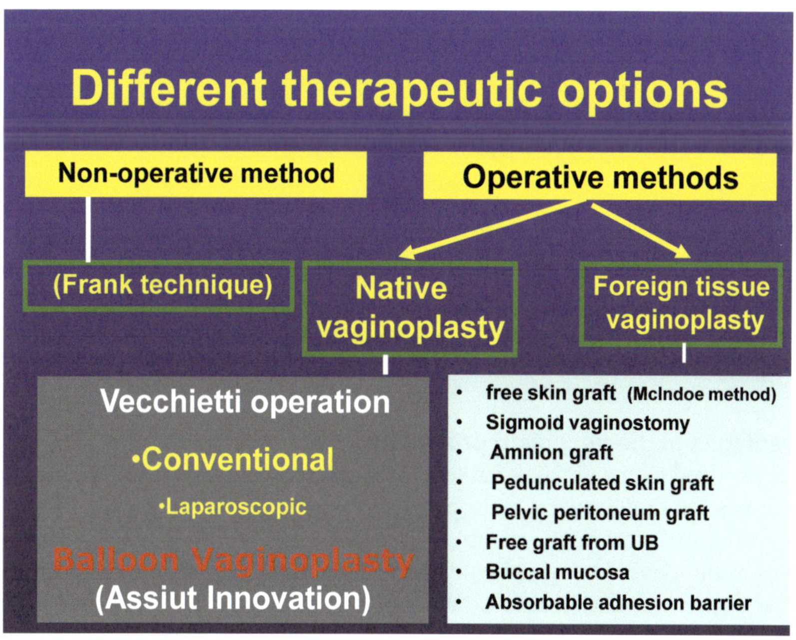

Fig. 4. Classification of vaginoplasty techniques.

3.1 Conventional surgery

Gynecologic surgeons or gynecologic endoscopists of average experience would find most of the published surgical techniques of vaginoplasty sophisticated and difficult to perform, and both cost and effectiveness must be considered conjointly when evaluating new surgical procedures. Given the rarity of the condition and the number of available methods, outcome data can be difficult to obtain (30). The traditional operative techniques (31) have major disadvantages, including prolonged recovery time and significant scarring (32). These techniques require lengthy, often embarrassing self-catheterization, which can be painful, and they may yield a vagina of only limited length (33). Many centers prefer Vecchietti's neovaginoplasty because of its low perioperative morbidity and quicker recovery period (34). These conventional surgical procedures are tedious, time consuming, and require a higher level of surgical expertise.

3.2 Laparoscopic approach

As described by Cooper et al. (35), laparoscopic neovagina can be created by drawing an olive into the vaginal grove and applying continuous tension via sutures passed at laparoscopy to a tensioning device on the anterior abdominal wall (35) using different instrument sets (36).

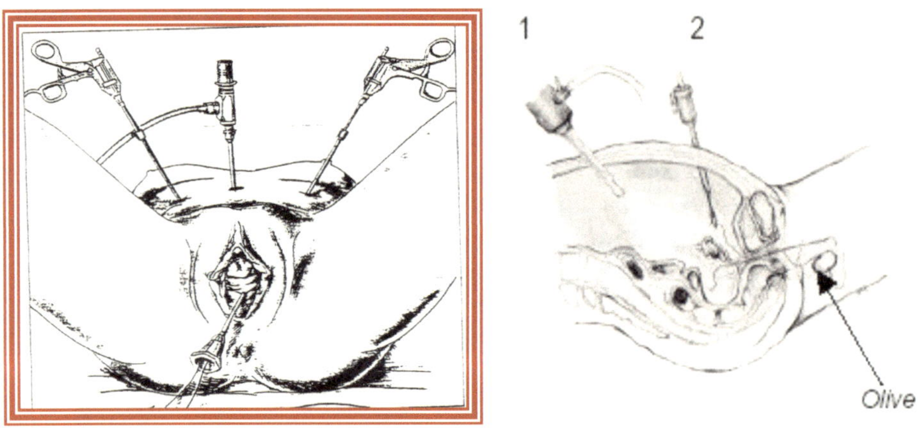

Fig. 5. Laparoscopic Vecchietti procedure

However, there are risks inherent in the most difficult step, passing the thread-bearing cutting needle from the abdominal wall to the retrohymenal fossa, through the vesicorectal space (37). It is important to ensure bladder and rectal integrity (38). Ultrasonographic control may increase safety (39).

3.3 Disadvantages of the Vecchietti procedure:

It requires specialized teams utilizing sophisticated instrumentation, however, and it is tedious to perform. It has the drawbacks of requiring daily traction for 8 to 10 days. Moreover, it lifts the posterior urethrovesical angle, making it more obtuse, with the possible consequence of causing stress incontinence later on (the posterior traction on the urethral supports also placing the patient at higher risk for stress incontinence). Furthermore, a change in the pelvic floor balance has been suspected (40). Another problem with the Vecchietti vaginoplasty is the use of a special abdominal traction device for a few days (41).

Other laparoscopic procedures are more complicated and tedious, such as the Davydov procedure (32) or sigmoid colpoplasty (42,43). Soong (44) described a laparoscopically assisted neovaginoplasty in which laparoscopic dissection of the rectovesical space is followed by traction of the pelvic peritoneum by a vaginal clamp and insertion of a vaginal stent for 1 week (45). The latter is not a pure laparoscopic approach and appears to be time consuming, although Soong did not comment on the operative time.

3.4 Advantages of laparoscopic approach

Apart from the common well established advantages of laparoscopic surgery over the conventional surgery, laparoscopy permits identification of the pelvic peritoneum as well as the proper site for the summit of the neovagina using the most mobile portion to form the vaginal fornix. Laparoscopy significantly facilitates this procedure, reduces operating time and risks, and makes the operation available to a wide range of surgeons skilled in laparoscopy (46).

3.5 Missing data in the previous studies:

The question is not whether the procedure is feasible, but whether the approach is superior and beneficial to a particular patient, cost effective for the community at large, and more importantly easily performed by the general gynecologists without sophisticated instrumentation. These guidelines constructed the frame of our institutional research on neovaginoplasty in recent years.

Examples and characteristics	Vaginoplasties with grafts	Vaginoplasties without grafts
	Free skin graft (the McIndoe method) - Sigmoid vaginostomy - Amnion graft - Pedunculated skin graft - Pelvic peritoneum graft - Free UB graft - Grafts from the buccal mucosa	The Vecchietti operation [7], which can be Conventional Laparoscopic balloon vaginoplasty Nonanatomic access to the vaginal dimple The posterior urethrovesical angle is lifted, which makes it more obtuse A change in the balance of the pelvic floor has been suggested

Table 1.

4. Balloon vaginoplasty innovation

This concept is developed at Assiut University (Egypt) by our team in 2007. Its main goal is to introduce a simplified approach that can be done by many gynecologists all over the world. As any innovation, it quickly passed through sequential steps of modifications to get the best available safe as well as effective approach.

4.1 Advantages of native balloon vaginoplasty over foreign tissue vaginoplasty

Cancer of the neovagina created by exogenous tissue, for example, bowel, skin graft, vulvar skin flaps, rectus abdominis (myocutaneous) flaps, or inverted penile skin, has been documented at younger ages than cancer of the native vagina (47). Tissue dysplasia can be expected because the tissue is suddenly subjected to new contacts or stresses (47). Therefore, recent interest has focused on dilatation as a treatment of choice (48,49). Most of the international centers promote the use of vaginal dilators (50). The success rate is reported to be up to 81% after vaginal dilatation (51). This can be attributed to the inherent nature of the vagina in the form of a high capability of elasticity and dispensability. Vaginal maximal tissue elongation is proved to be higher than that of normal skin (49). It seems logical that dilatation or other surgical procedures based on proper understanding of the nature of this organ would be preferred over techniques based on the idea of replacement of the vagina by skin, amniotic membrane, sigmoid, or otherwise. Moreover, replacement techniques would lead to scar formation. The prevalence of dyspareunia increases after transvaginal reconstructive pelvic surgeries (52). This concept stands behind the increased popularity of the conventional or laparoscopic Vecchietti operation as it is devoid of vaginal scars. Of peculiar advantages of balloon vaginoplasty particularly retropubic balloon vaginoplasty is the possibility of surgical intervention for recurrent or failed cases done by other procedures. Herein, I'll summarize the different techniques of balloon vaginoplasty.

1. **Laparoscopic balloon vaginoplasty after dissection of the rectovesical pouch (53):**

Under general endotracheal anesthesia, a standard laparoscopy evaluation is performed with two auxiliary 5-mm suprapubic portals. Dissection of the peritoneum covering the vesicorectal pouch is performed. A piece of gauze is inserted inside the rectum and is gently manipulated by a nurse in different directions, as directed by the surgeon. A metal catheter is inserted into the bladder, which is moved according to the directions of the surgeon. Gentle, sharp dissection of the vesicorectal space is done until a free area in between is achieved. Dissection then should be progressed until near the vaginal skin. The left 5-mm suprapubic trocar is extracted, followed by advancement of a blunt-ended grasper to make a gentle dissection of the peritoneum until reaching the dissected area. A 18F silicone Foley catheter is advanced extraperitoneally to replace the left-side blunt-ended grasper up to the dissected area. From the right side, blunt-ended grasping forceps are pushed into the rectovesical space. Vaginally, a snip is made on top of it, followed by advancement of another grasper to pick up the tip of the catheter vaginally. The balloon is inflated with 6 cm3 saline while the catheter is advanced upward; tension is maintained by applying two disposable umbilical cord clamps on the stretched catheter. To avoid skin ischemia or pain at the site of traction, a sterile dressing is insinuated beneath the clamps. To be fitted, a small hole is made at the center of the dressing before its application below the clamps. Maximal tension is achieved by continuous traction before applying the clamps (Fig. 6). The integrity

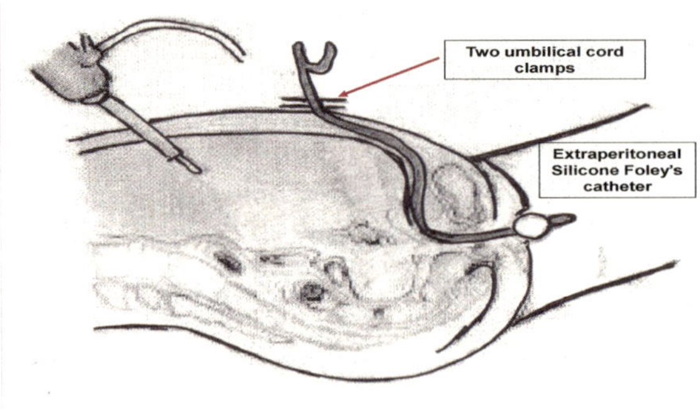

Fig. 6. Lateral view of the extrapeeritoneal catheter

of the bladder is easily checked by gentle testing using the blunt tip of a metal catheter. All laparoscopic instruments are extracted without any suturing. A Foley catheter is inserted into the urethra.

Disadvantages:

Despite being extraperitoneal, nevertheless, this procedure requires a considerable experience of laparoscopic surgery to dissect rectum from the bladder safely.

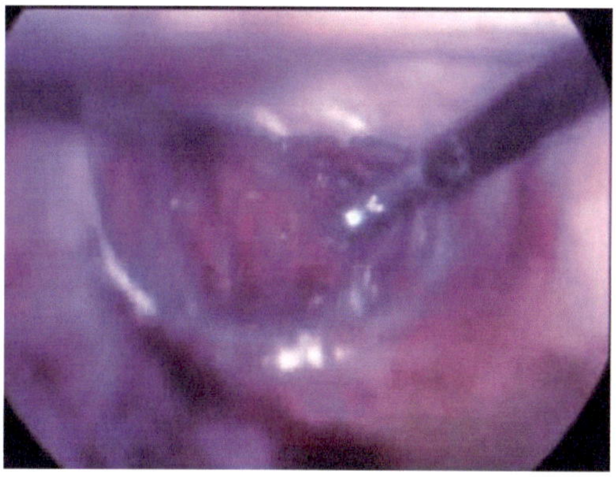

Fig. 7. Dissection of rectovesical space.

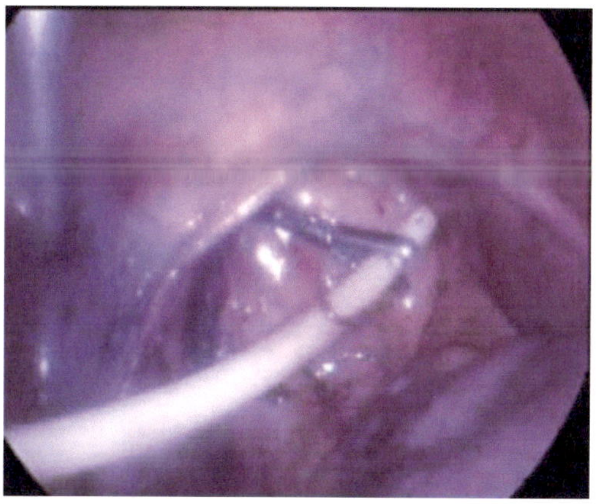

Fig. 8. Extraction of the catheter via the vaginal dimple.

2. **Laparoscopic balloon vaginoplasty without dissection of the rectovesical pouch (54,55)**

A silicon coated balloon catheter is manipulated by a specially designed inserter, which is passed transperitoneally and through the pelvic floor where the balloon is positioned at the vaginal dimple. An upward, gradual (1-2cm/day) traction is applied on the catheter stem from the abdominal side for one week. A concomitant increase in balloon capacity (5ml every other day) to increase the width of the neovagina is also done. Sexual relations are recommended as early as one week after surgery.

Disadvantages:

Despite being an easy procedure, it is a blind and intraperitoneal approach. Practically, an extraperitoneal approach is proved to be effective and carries no risk of coiling of some loops of intestine or peritoneal irritation.

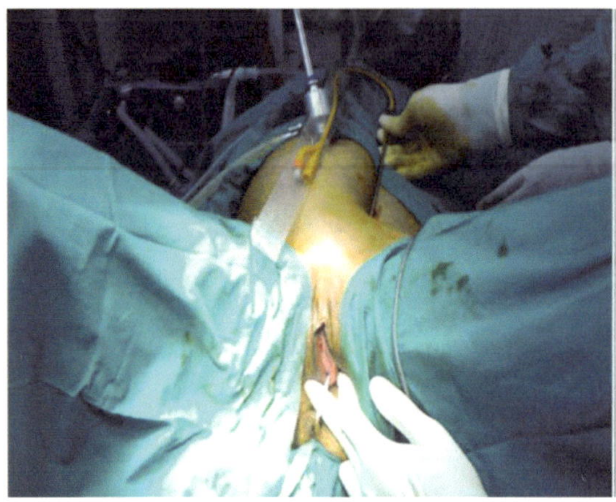

Fig. 9. Insertion of a specialty designed inserter.

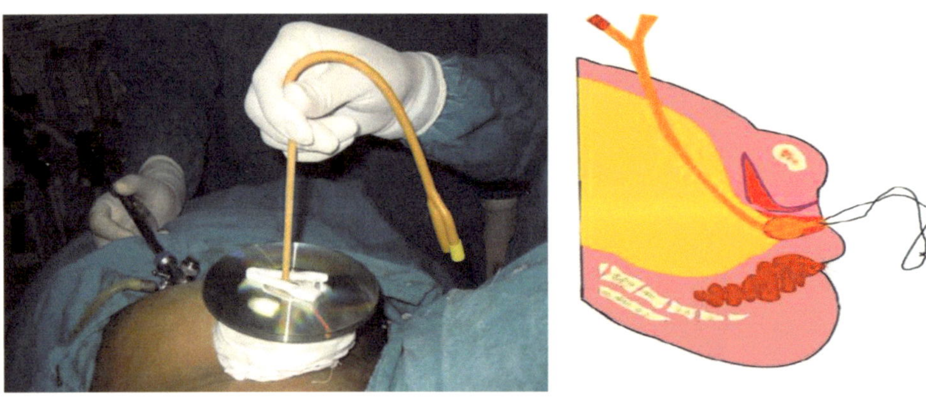

Fig. 10. Postoperative view.

3. Modified laparoscopically assisted BV (56,57):

The procedure starts with diagnostic laparoscopy (video). After full evaluation of intraabdominal and intrapelvic structures, the telescope is directed toward the pelvic floor. A suction irrigation cannula is introduced through the ancillary abdominal puncture and pushed firmly against the pelvic floor in the region of the pouch of Douglas (Figure 11). Simultaneously, using palpation, the tip of the cannula is introduced transperineally through the vaginal dimple, positioning it so that it presses at a central point of the dimple. The surgeon's right hand held the cannula from the abdominal side, and the left hand guides the pressed tip of the cannula from the perineal side. Next, a conventional surgical needle, its curve attenuated, is threaded with a long, double-stranded silk suture (DSSS) and passed through the vaginal dimple at the point where the cannula tip is positioned. The needle perforates the pelvic floor, and as it appears at the pouch of Douglas, the cannula is removed and a laparoscopic grasper/needle-holder is inserted so that the needle could be extracted through the ancillary abdominal puncture (Figure 12). Then, the needle is removed from the DSSS, and the suture is threaded into the opening of an 18-gauge silicon coated Foley's catheter. Traction is exerted on the DSSS from the perineal side until the catheter is pulled back through the abdominal port to the pelvic floor and through the pelvic floor to the dimple (Figure 13). This step is greatly facilitated by exerting counter traction on the catheter, stretching it to decrease its caliber especially while it is moved through the pelvic floor, since the channel created by the needle is very narrow. After the balloon-bearing end of the catheter appears at the dimple, it is inflated with 15 mL of saline. Traction is exerted from the abdominal side until the balloon moved up, carrying the stretched dimple above the introitus. Catheter placement in past procedures relied on a unique catheter inserter, but the catheter can be manipulated into position using a suction irrigation cannula and a surgical needle. Traction on the catheter is maintained without the supporting plate that had been expressly made for that purpose. Traction on the catheter should be maintained using a supportive plate. It may be made of stainless steel and sterilized by autoclave, closely resembles a DVD disk. In the first method, a thick, multilayered dressing is tightly wrapped around the catheter, until a cylinder, at least 5 cm high and 10 cm wide, is formed perpendicular to the abdomen. The outermost layer of the dressing is encircled with

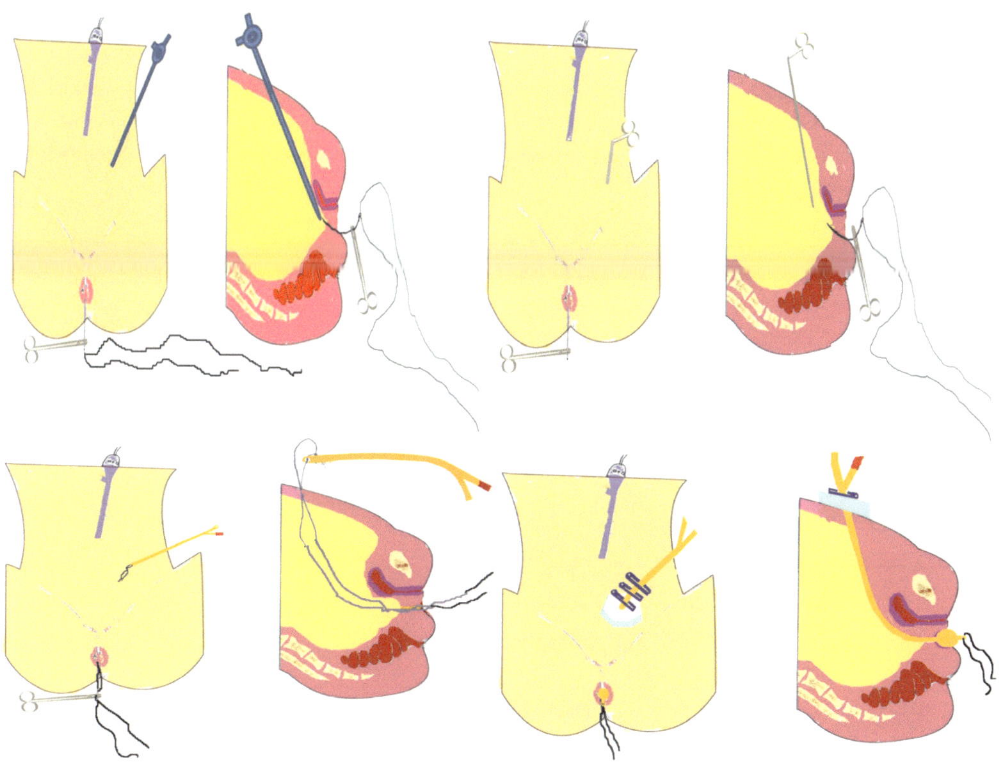

Fig. 11.-14. Modified laparoscopic intraperitoneal balloon vaginoplasty.

adhesive tape to guard against unraveling (Figure 14). In addition, the cord clamp would be well supported away from the abdominal wall, thus preventing pressure necrosis. An alternative supporting plate made of 3 DVDs joined together with silicon and sterilized with ethylene oxide can be used. It is placed around the catheter and over a dressing so that it distributed the force from traction over a wide surface area, preventing pressure sloughing of the abdominal skin. Postoperative care is the same as that previously described for BV and included controlled traction and distension, prevention of infection, continued psychosocial support, and emphasis on early resumption of sexual activity; patients are instructed to use a condom and gentamicin cream during the first 10 days after discharge.

Disadvantages:

It seems to be non applicable by the general gynecologists as it is an intraperitoneal approach with a risk of subsequent intestinal coiling, risky as they reported a case of rectal injury out of three cases (33.3%) added to the risks of laparoscopy particularly if the patient has a scar of correctiob of other malformations or pelvic surgery.

5. Space of Retzius (figure 15)

In 1858, Retzius described the eponymous space, situated anterior and lateral to the urinary bladder (prevesical space) (58). It is the space between the symphysis, the bladder, and the anterior abdominal wall. It is bordered anteriorly by the pelvic bone; posteriorly by the endopelvic fascia (the urogenital, pubocervical, and pelvic fascia, which cover the bladder and the urethra); and laterally by the obturator muscle. It contains loose connective tissue and fat and affords the surgeon access to the bladder without opening the peritoneal cavity. It is an optimal extraperitoneal approach well addressed in the field of urogynecology. Access though it would eliminate laparoscopy and its complications. Moreover, because of its proximity, it seems logical to access the vaginal dimple through it rather than through the auxiliary laparoscopic portals.

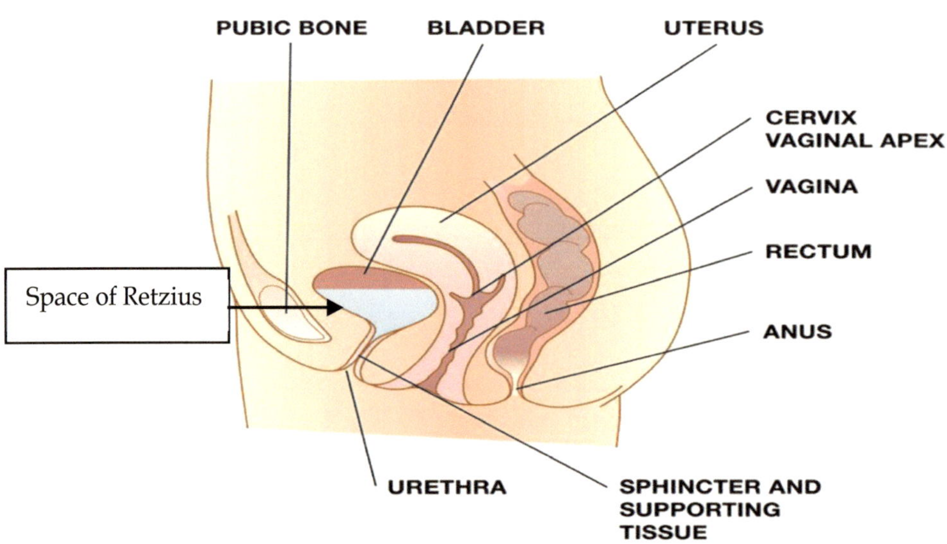

Fig. 15.

6. Retropubic fine needle vaginoplasty (59)

Patients are prepared as usual for any simple gynecologic operation. Under IV propophol anesthesia, the bladder is evacuated followed by insertion of a rigid catheter guide (bladder stylet) loaded inside a urethral catheter. It aims to mobilize the bladder neck away from the tip of the needle when it passes into the retropubic space. A 7 mm suprapubic incision is made just lateral to the midline in the suprapubic area 2 cm above the symphysis pubis in the same manner as tension free traction (TVT) operation for treating genuine stress incontinence (60). A fine single lumen egg retrieval needle with its stainless handle tightly fitted to a cut distal end of a Foley catheter is used. We prefer Swemed Sense needle (Virtolife Sweden AB, Kungsbacka, Sweden) which has a reduced distal end of 0.9 mm OD while the rest of the needle has 1.4 mm OD (Figure 16). An additional advantage of this needle is good malleability that allows bending of the needle during insertion to adapt the curve of space of Retzius (Figure15). The bended needle is inserted through the suprapubic incision directed towards the space of Retzus with simultaneous mobilization of the bladder inwards and laterally into the ipsilateral side with the bladder stylet. To help the needle reach the correct place in the center of the vaginal dimple, a small incision in the vaginal dimple is made which is used to allow the introduction of the operator's contraletral index finger to guide the tip of the fine needle. Once the tip of the needle appears, the bladder catheter is removed followed by cystoscopic examination. If the bladder is intact, the needle is advanced with some force to allow the fitted catheter to bypass the anterior abdominal wall layers. Once the balloon is seen from the vaginal side, it is disconnected from the needle, inflated with 6-8 cc of saline, and pulled upwards (figure 16). Traction is maintained by applying two alternating umbilical cord plastic clamps on its part adjacent to the anterior abdominal wall. To avoid skin ischemia, an intervening layer of sterile gauze is placed underneath a stainless steel fenestrated plate (Figure 17). To avoid retention effect of the balloon, a urethral catheter is inserted and fixed. After a short postoperative interval, before discharge, the patient is instructed to maintain antibiotic coverage and to take a non-steroidal anti-inflammatory drug whenever required. She is taught how to evacuate and care for the urine collection bag, make frequent proper vaginal douches using bovidone Iodine 10%, and apply sterile vulval dressings to guard against ascending infection. Three days later, she has to come to the office for more traction on the catheter which is maintained using a third umbilical clamp. The abdominal and the uretheral catheters are removed on day 8.

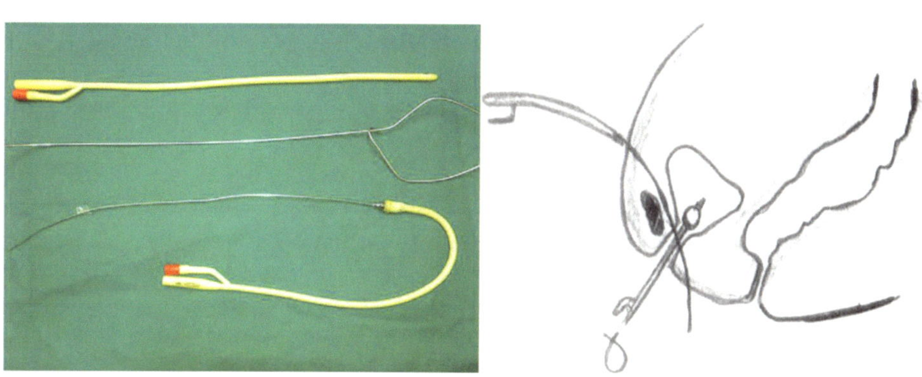

Fig. 16. Instrumentation and a diagram of fine needle vaginoplasty

Disadvantages:

Despite being simple, it is a relatively unsafe as the needle is passed blindly towards the vaginal dimple sometimes after several trials. There is a risk of needle puncture of the surgeon's fingers. Moreover, the needle is malleable and unstable during its perforation of the retropubic space. Lastly, the vaginoabdominal approach is more comfortable than abdominovaginal approach used during the fine needle procedure.

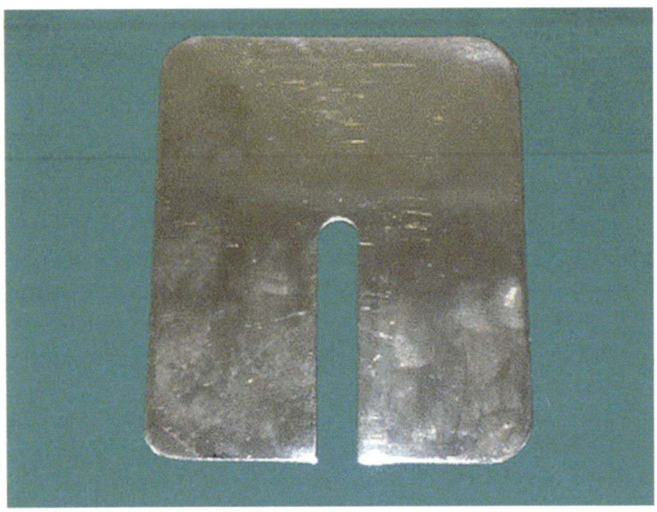

Fig. 17. Stainless steel fenestrated plate

7. Transretropubic traction vaginoplasty (TRT) (60)

Using an olive rather than balloon but goes along the road of balloon vaginoplasty that's why I preferred to include it here.
Idea: In the course of a few days, a plastic olive placed on the vaginal dimple is lifted by a mesh tape inserted through the space of Retzius and anchored to the anterior abdominal wall. The upward traction exerted on the vaginal dimple is sufficient to create a neovagina.

Steps

The patients are prepared for the TRT vaginoplasty as for any simple gynecologic surgical procedure. Under general anesthesia, bladder evacuation is followed by the insertion of a urethral catheter, through which a rigid guide (or bladder stylet) is then passed. This step is taken to mobilize the bladder neck away from the tip of the needle when it passed into the retropubic space. A 7-mm incision is then made on both sides in the suprapubic area, 2 cm from the midline and 2 cm above the symphysis pubis, as if to install tension-free vaginal tape to treat stress urinary incontinence (61). A sharp, curved needle especially designed with a wide eye attached to a plastic handle (Fig. 18) is used to perforate the vaginal dimple bilaterally, just 1 cm below the bladder neck. A strip of mesh composed of a knitted polypropylene monofilament (Pro Mesh (Ethicon, Somerville, NJ, USA), 1 cm in width and 30 cm in length, is stretched and passed through the eye of the needle. A 2 x 3 cm, fenestrated plastic olive is threaded like a bead on the tape. The needle is inserted through the vaginal dimple skin without prior incision, directed upwards and slightly laterally toward the space of Retzius, with simultaneous mobilization of the bladder inwards and laterally on the same side with the bladder stylet. After which, the needle is directed slightly medially toward the suprapubic incision on the same side. Once the tape is seen through the incision, the needle is withdrawn while the tape is clamped with a forceps. The bladder catheter is then removed and a cystoscopic examination performed. If the bladder is intact, the same steps are repeated on the other side. Traction on the tape is maintained by placing a plastic umbilical cord clamp on each end of the mesh tape. A layer of sterile gauze is placed underneath a fenestrated plate of stainless steel to avoid skin ischemia. A urethral catheter is inserted to prevent urinary retention from the pressure applied by the plastic olive.

After a short postoperative interval, before discharge, the patient is instructed to take an antibiotic medication for 1 week and a nonsteroidal anti-inflammatory drug (NSAID) whenever required. She is also taught how to void her bowels, care for her urine collection bag, frequently cleanse her vagina with a 10% povidone iodine solution, and apply sterile vulvar dressings to guard against ascending infection. She returned to the office 3 days later to increase the traction to the tape, and the new traction is maintained using an additional umbilical clamp on each side. If the patient is afraid of experiencing pain from the traction, she is given an intravenous injection of an NSAID 15 minutes before the procedure. The tape, plastic olive, and uretheral catheter are removed on the eighth day after the procedure. During an examination, a medium-sized speculum is inserted into the vagina and the vaginal length is measured and recorded. The patient is encouraged to start sexual intercourse on that day. She presented to the office every 2 weeks for the next 2 months for evaluations. Each spouse is privately asked about dyspareunia and sexual satisfaction at each visit. The husbands are also asked about penetration. A score of 100 is used for satisfaction and penetration. It is a simple scoring chart designed at our institution after the visual analog scale for pelvic pain. After the 2-month follow-up, the couple presented to the clinic only when they had operation-related complaints.

Advantages: TRT vaginoplasty seems to be superior as it does not depend on endoscopy, does not require dissecting the rectovesical space or the vaginal dimple, and is performed relatively quickly. Moreover, the risk of stress incontinence is still present in patients undergoing balloon vaginoplasty because of the posterior traction exerted on the vaginal dimple (62).

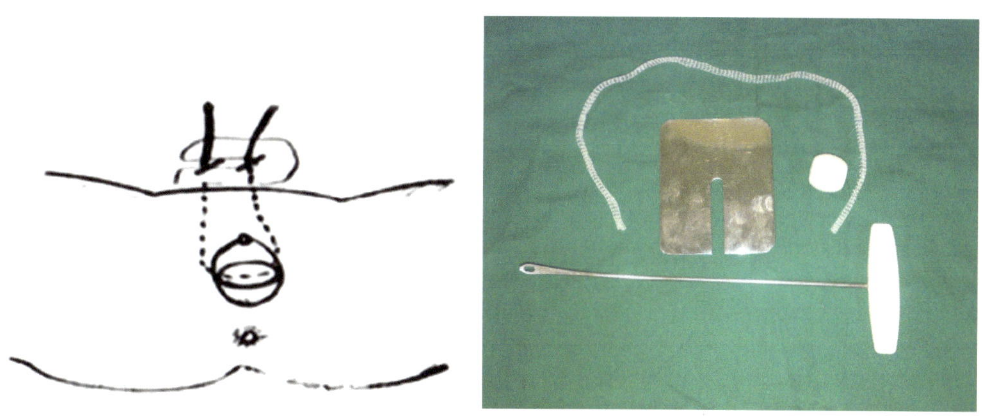

Fig. 18. TRT vaginoplasty

Disadvantages: a bit sophisticated and these instrumentations are not available in all operating rooms. Moreover, we reported exaggerated patient discomfort and repeated complaints particularly during traction on day 3. In the following table, I'll summarize the differences between some vaginoplasty techniques.

	Transretropubic (TRT) vaginoplasty	Laparoscopic Veccheitti vaginoplasty	Laparoscopic balloon vaginoplasty (53)
Admission	No need	In-patient for 8 days	No need
Increased postoperative pain	Exaggerated once on day 3	Mild daily stretching of the threads	Mild once on day 3
Slipping of traction device	None	reported	None
Ripping	None	possible	None
General anesthesia	Once	Twice	Once
laparoscopic expertise	Usually not needed	Nearly level III	Nearly level II
Instrumentation	Less sophisticated and reproducible	Sophisticated	Less sophisticated and reproducible
Laparoscopy	Usually not needed	needed	needed
Relation to peritoneum	Extraperitoneal	Intraperitoneal or extraperitoneal	Extraperitoneal
Postoperative stress incontinence	Not possible as it improves posterior vesicourethral angle	Possible and reported (61)	Possible but not reported

Table 2.

8. Transretropubic balloon vaginoplasty approach (63)

The patients are prepared for the operation as for any simple gynecologic surgical procedure. Under spinal anesthesia, bladder evacuation is followed by the insertion of a urethral catheter, through which a rigid guide (or bladder stylet, figure 1) is then passed. This step is taken to mobilize the bladder neck away from the tip of the needle when it passed into the retropubic space. A 5- mm incision is then made on the midline in the suprapubic area, 2 cm above the symphysis pubis. A especially designed sharp, curved needle with a wide eye attached to a plastic handle (Fig. 19) is used to perforate the vaginal dimple centrally, just 1 cm below the bladder neck. The needle is inserted through the vaginal dimple skin without prior incision, directed cephalically upwards and slightly laterally toward the space of Retzius, with simultaneous mobilization of the bladder inwards and laterally on the same side utilizing the bladder stylet. In all cases, the perforation is controlled by perioperative ultrasonographic examination of the space of Retzius. Thereafter, the needle is directed slightly medially toward the suprapubic incision in the midline. Once the fenstrum of the needle is seen through the incision, the distal end of a silicone Foley catheter is fixed to it by a double strengthened Vicryl 2 sutures. Thereafter, the needle is withdrawn downwards and the Vicryl suture is cut leaving the distal end of the Foley catheter outside the vaginal dimple which is immediately filled with 4-6 cc of saline to avoid excessive pain. The bladder catheter is then removed and a cystoscopic examination is performed. Upward traction on the catheter is maintained by placing a plastic umbilical cord clamp on its abdominal side. A layer of sterile gauze is placed underneath a fenestrated plate of stainless steel to avoid skin ischemia (Fig. 19). A urethral catheter is inserted to prevent urinary retention from upward traction the inflated balloon. Operative time is recorded for all case. After a short postoperative interval of few hours, before discharge, the patient is instructed to take an antibiotic medication for 1 week and a nonsteroidal anti-inflammatory drug (NSAID) whenever required. She is also taught how to void her bowels, care for her urine collection bag, frequently cleanse her vagina with a 10% povidone iodine solution, and apply sterile vulvar dressings to guard against ascending infection. She returned to the office 3 days later to increase the upward traction and the size to the balloon by reinflation with extra 3-4 cc of saline and the new traction is maintained using a new umbilical clamp. The suprapubic and uretheral catheters are removed on the 8th day after the procedure.

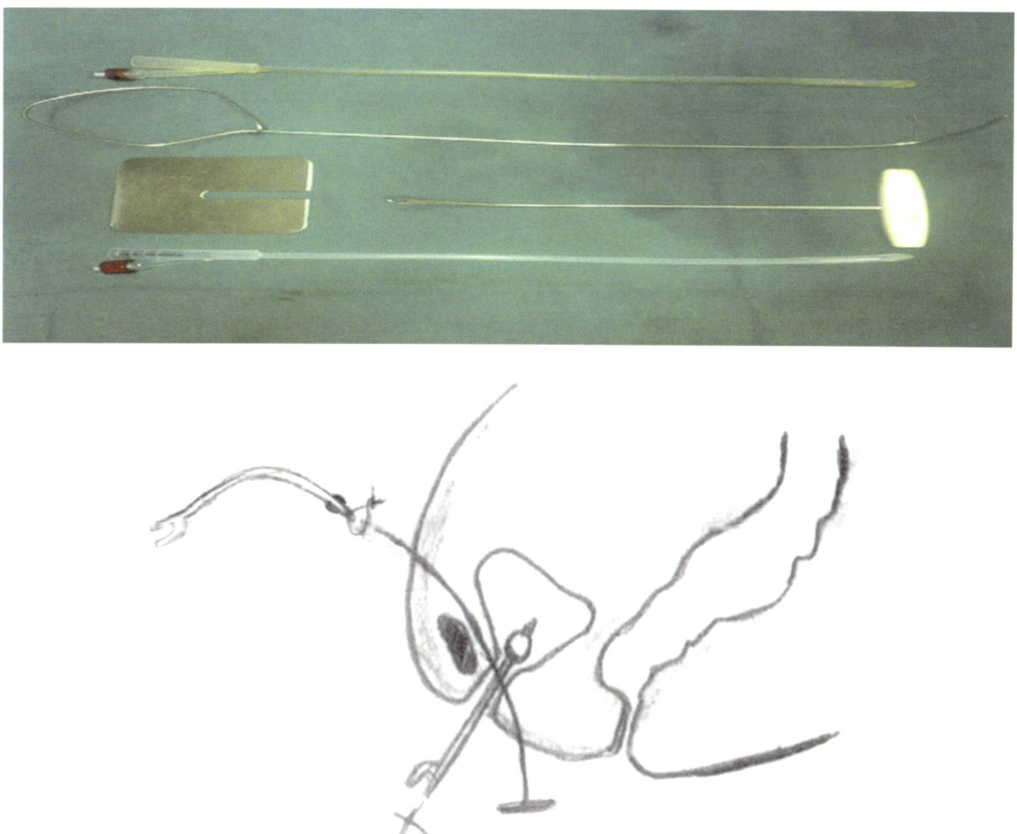

Fig. 19. Transretropubic balloon vaginoplasty: instrumentation and a diagram.

9. Modified retropubic vaginoplasty(64-66)

Through a small supra pubic puncture, the catheter inserter is passed from above into the retropubic space just behind the pubic bone and guided to the center of the vaginal dimple.

Then, a cystoscopic examination is performed to ensure bladder and uretheral integrity. This is followed by gradual controlled distention of the balloon and traction on the catheter stem as described in laparoscopic balloon vaginoplasty.
Drawbacks: this is a relatively unsafe procedure as the inserter is about 5 mm in caliber and there is no safety issue to protect the urethra from injury during perforation. Non usage of a bladder stylet is another disadvantage as it is used for contralateral displacement of the urethra away from the perforation site. Again, they used perforation from the abdominal site which is considered difficult and unguided if compared with perforation from the vaginal side. Another technical problem of their procedure is the absence of a fenestrum to easily carry threads to the vaginal side.

10. Which balloon vaginoplasty should I use?

After this detailed discussion of the published studies on balloon vaginoplasty, I would recommend retropubic balloon vaginoplasty (63) due to the following causes:
Transretropubic balloon vaginoplasty is a simple, fast, safe and available extraperitoneal procedure. It can be easily done by any gynecologist having basic knowledge of the anatomy of the retropubic space. Not only does it save time for the gynecologists, but it also saves a lot of money for the patient and the community as well.
A recent study on laparoscopic balloon vaginoplasty by ElSaman et al reported a case of rectal injury out of three cases (33.3%). This possibility is remote if the retropubic approach is utilized. Being an extraperitoneal approach makes retropubic balloon vaginoplasty very suitable for cases with extensive intraperitoneal adhesions or with history of intestinal surgery. Moreover, due to its proximity, it seems logic to access the vaginal dimple through it rather than the laparoscopic portals. Retropubic balloon vaginoplasty disturbs neither the urethral support nor the urethrovesical angle. It may even add support to the bladder neck, although for a short period. This technical point is considered as an additional advantage of the retropubic approach over transabdominal conventional or even laparoscopic vaginoplasty. Retropubic balloon vaginoplasty is a good example of minimally-invasive surgery for vaginal aplasia, an anomaly currently corrected with very sophisticated techniques utilizing foreign tissues such as peritoneum, skin, sigmoid, or amnion grafts. Selection of the retropubic space and performing the procedure in the same way as tension-free tape (TVT) for treating stress incontinence is assuring regarding safety and is confirmed by absence of complications in our pilot study. It seems that this transretropubic balloon vaginoplasty is superior to transretropubic vaginoplasty using a tape and an olive in terms of shorter mean operative time (8.5 vs. 26.5min) due to single perforation of the space of Retzius, elimination of the exaggerated intolerable pain on traction on the tape that required analgesics in all cases of the previous study, and utilization of the silicone balloon with easier traction due to elastic recoil character and changeable balloon size. Clearly, this procedure is much cheaper than transretropubic vaginoplasty.
A modified retropubic vaginoplasty has been recently published by ElSaman et al. The authors used an inserter carrying threads at its distal end and passed from the suprapubic side towards the vaginal dimple. This instrument is short and straight unlike the long curved needle used in this study. Moreover, their procedure is blind and completely unsafe as this instrument has a wide caliber with a high possibility of urethral injury. Out of three cases, they reported one case of urethral damage (33.3%) that required catheterization for 8 days. Another technical problem of their procedure is the absence of a fenestrum to easily carry threads to the vaginal side.

11. References

[1] Evans PN, Poland NL, Boving RL: Vaginal malformations. Am J Obstet Gynecol 1981;141:910-920.

[2] Poland ML, Evans TN. Psychologic aspects of vaginal agenesis. J Reprod Med. 1985;30(4):340-4.

[3] Morgan EM, Quint EH. Assessment of sexual functioning, mental health, and life goals in women with vaginal agenesis. Arch Sex Behav. 2006;35(5):607-18.

[4] Prapas Y., Papanicolaou A., Prapas N., Goutzioulis M., Papanicolaou N. Term pregnancy after vaginal transplantation in a case of vaginal agenesis with a functional uterus. Acta Europaea fertilitatis 1993;24 (2), 77-78.

[5] Paniel B, Haddad B. Utero-vaginal aplasia and pregnancy. Journal de Gynecologie Obstetrique et Biologie de la Reproduction1994; 23 (5), 626-628.

[6] Moura M D, Navarro P, Nogueira A. Pregnancy and term delivery after neovaginoplasty in a patient with vaginal agenesis . International Journal of Gynecology and Obstetrics 2000; 71 (3),215-21.

[7] Brannstrom M, Wranning CA. Uterus transplantation: How far away from human trials? Acta Obstet Gynecol Scand. 2008;87(11):1097-1100.

[8] Gosden RG. Ovary and Uterus Transplantation. Reproduction. 2008 Aug 26, in press.

[9] Wranning CA, Akhi SN, Kurlberg G, Brannstrom M. Uterus transplantation in the rat: Model development, surgical learning and morphological evaluation of healing. Acta Obstet Gynecol Scand. 2008;87(11):1239-1247.

[10] Dahm-Kähler P, Wranning C, Lundmark C, Enskog A, Mölne J, Marcickiewicz J et al.. Transplantation of the uterus in sheep: methodology and early reperfusion events. J Obstet Gynaecol Res. 2008;34(5):784-93.

[11] Dittrich R, Beckmann MW, Mueller A, Binder H, Hoffmann I, Maltaris T. Uterus Cryopreservation: Maintenance of Uterine Contractility by the Use of Different Cryoprotocols. Reprod Domest Anim. 2008 Oct 13, in press.

[12] Ulrich U, Schrickel J, Dorn C, Richter O, Lewalter T, Lu¨deritz B, Rhiem K. Mayer-von Rokitansky-Ku¨ster-Hauser syndrome in association with a hitherto undescribed variant of the Holt-Oram syndrome with an aorto-pulmonary window. Hum Reprod 2004;19:1201–3.

[13] Croak AJ, Gebhart JB, Klingele CJ, Lee RA, Rayburn WF. Therapeutic strategies for vaginal Mullerian agenesis. J Reprod Med 2003;48:395-401.

[14] Wierrani F, Grunberger W. Vaginoplasty using deepithelialized vulvar transposition flaps: the Grunberger method. J Am Coll Surg 2003;196:159-162.

[15] Noguchi S, Nakatsuka M, Sugiyama Y, Chekir C, Kamada Y, Hiramatsu Y. Use of artificial dermis and recombinant basic fibroblast growth factor for creating a neovagina in a patient with Mayer-Rokitansky-Kuster-Hauser syndrome. Hum Reprod 2004;19:1629-1632.

[16] Motoyama S, Laoag-Fernandez JB, Mochizuki S, Yamabe S, Maruo T. Vaginoplasty with Interceed absorbable adhesion barrier for complete squamous epithelialization in vaginal agenesis. Am J Obstet Gynecol 2003;188:1260-1264.

[17] Jackson ND, Rosenblatt PL. Use of Interceed Absorbable Adhesion Barrier for vaginoplasty. Obstet Gynecol 1994;84:1048-1050.

[18] Dietrich JE, Hertweck SP, Traynor MP, Reinstine JH. Laparoscopically assisted creation of a neovagina using the Louisville modification. Fertil Steril 2007;88:1431-1434.

[19] Cai B, Zhang JR, Xi XW, Yan Q, Wan XP. Laparoscopically assisted sigmoid colon vaginoplasty in women with Mayer-Rokitansky-Kuster-Hauser syndrome: feasibility and short-term results. Bjog 2007;114:1486-1492.

[20] Bailez MM. Laparoscopy in uterovaginal anomalies. Semin Pediatr Surg 2007;16:278-287.

[21] Michala L, Cutner A, Creighton SM. Surgical approaches to treating vaginal agenesis. Bjog 2007;114:1455-1459.

[22] Rock JA, Schlaff WD. The obstetric consequences of uterovaginal anomalies. Fertil Steril 1985;43:681-692.

[23] Mc IA. The treatment of congenital absence and obliterative conditions of the vagina. Br J Plast Surg 1950;2:254-267.

[24] Buttram VC, Jr., Gibbons WE. Mullerian anomalies: a proposed classification. (An analysis of 144 cases). Fertil Steril 1979;32:40-46.

[25] Andryjowicz E, Qizilbash AH, DePetrillo AD, O'Connell GJ, Taylor MH. Adenocarcinoma in a cecal neovagina--complication of irradiation: report of a case and review of literature. Gynecol Oncol 1985;21:235-239.

[26] Rotmensch J, Rosenshein N, Dillon M, Murphy A, Woodruff JD. Carcinoma arising in the neovagina: case report and review of the literature. Obstet Gynecol 1983;61:534-536.

[27] Williams EA. Congenital Absence of the Vagina: a Simple Operation for Its Relief. J Obstet Gynaecol Br Commonw 1964;71:511-512.

[28] Fedele L, Bianchi S, Frontino G, Fontana E, Restelli E, Bruni V. The laparoscopic Vecchietti's modified technique in Rokitansky syndrome: anatomic, functional, and sexual long-term results. Am J Obstet Gynecol 2008;198:377 e371-376.

[29] Fedele L, Busacca M, Candiani M, Vignali M. Laparoscopic creation of a neovagina in Mayer-Rokitansky-Kuster-Hauser syndrome by modification of Vecchietti's operation. Am J Obstet Gynecol 1994;171:268-269.

[30] Mizia K, Bennett MJ, Dudley J, Morrisey J. Mu¨llerian dysgenesis: a review of recent outcomes at Royal Hospital forWomen. Aust NZJ Obstet Gynaecol 2006;46:29–31.

[31] Laffargue F, Giacalone PL, Boulot P, Vigouroux B, Hedon B, Benos P. A laparoscopic procedure for the treatment of vaginal aplasia. Br J Obstet Gynaecol 1995;102:565–7.

[32] Ismail IS, Cutner AS, Creighton SM. Laparoscopic vaginoplasty: alternative techniques in vaginal reconstruction. BJOG 2006;113:340–3.

[33] Lotan G, Mashiach R, Halevy A. Total endoscopic vaginal reconstruction in a case of Mayer-Rokitansky-Kuster-Hauser syndrome. J Laparoendosc Adv Surg Tech A 2005;15:435–8.

[34] Charvat M, Horejsi J, Teslik L. Laparoscopic neovaginoplasty—a modification of the Vecchietti operation. Ceska Gynekol 2001;66:247–51.

[35] Cooper MJ, Fleming S, Murray J. Laparoscopic assisted Vecchietti procedure for the creation of a neovagina. J Obstet Gynaecol Res 1996;22:385–8.

[36] Fedele L, Bianchi S, Berlanda N, Fontana E, Bulfoni A, Borruto F. Laparoscopic creation of a neovagina with the laparoscopic Vecchietti operation: comparison of two instrument sets. Fertil Steril 2006;86:429–32.

[37] Fedele L, Bianchi S, Dorta M, Zanconato G, Raffaelli R. Laparoscopic creation of a neovagina in women with pelvic kidney. J Am Assoc Gynecol Laparosc 1999;6:327–9.

[38] Giacalone PL, Laffargue F, Faure JM, Deschamps F. Ultrasound-assisted laparoscopic creation of a neovagina by modification of Vecchietti's operation. Obstet Gynecol 1999;93:446–8.

[39] Giacalone PL, Laffargue F, Bousquet F, Faure JM, Deschamps F. Creation of a neovagina using ultrasonography-assisted laparoscopy (modified Vecchietti technique). J Gynecol Obstet Biol Reprod 1998;27:514–6.

[40] Bianchi M, Sola V, Ricci P, Pomes C. Late postoperative urinary stress incontinence after a laparoscopic-assisted Vecchietti procedure for neovagina creation in a patient with Rokitansky syndrome: successful treatment with the TVT-O technique. J Minim Invasive Gynecol 2007;14(1):116–8.

[41] Jansen FW, Kolkman W, Bakkum EA, de Kroon CD, Trimbos-Kemper TC, Trimbos JB. Complications of laparoscopy: an inquiry about closed- versus open-entry technique. Am J Obstet Gynecol 2004;190(3):634–8.

[42] Ohashi S, Ikuma K, Koyasu Y, Tei K, Kanno H, Akashi A, Haque SM. Laparoscopic reconstruction of vagina using sigmoid autograft. Surg Endosc 1996;10:1019–21.

[43] Crouch NS, Creighton SM. Sigmoid colpoplasty for vaginal agenesis. Fertil Steril 2004;81:1721.

[44] Soong YK. Laparoscopically assisted neovaginoplasty. In: Tulandi T, ed. Atlas of laparoscopic and hysteroscopic techniques for gynecologists. London: Saunders, 1999. Chapter 24.

[45] Adamian LV, Zurabiani ZR, Kiselev SI, Khashukoeva AZ. Laparoscopy in surgical treatment of vaginal aplasia: laparoscopy-assisted colpopoiesis and perineal hysterectomy with colpopoiesis. Int J Fertil Menopausal Stud 1996;41:40–5.

[46] Adamian LV, Zurabiani ZR, Kiselev SI, Khashukoeva AZ. Laparoscopy in surgical treatment of vaginal aplasia: laparoscopy-assisted colpopoiesis and perineal hysterectomy with colpopoiesis. Int J Fertil Menopausal Stud 1996;41:40–5.

[47] Schober JM. Cancer of the neovagina. J Pediatr Urol 2007;3:167–70.

[48] Liao L, Doyle J, Crouch NS, Creighton SM. Dilation as treatment for vaginal agenesis and hypoplasia: a pilot exploration of benefits and barriers as perceived by patients. J Obstet Gynaecol 2006;26:144–8.

[49] Ismail-Pratt IS, Bikoo M, Liao LM, Conway GS, Creighton SM. Normalization of the vagina by dilator treatment alone in Complete Androgen Insensitivity Syndrome and Mayer-Rokitansky-Kuster-Hauser Syndrome. Hum Reprod 2007;22:2020–4.

[50] Laufer MR. Congenital absence of the vagina: in search of the perfect solution. When, and by what technique, should a vagina be created? Curr Opin Obstet Gynecol 2002;14:441–4.

[51] Abramov Y,Webb A, Miller J, Alshahrour A, Botros S, Goldberg R, et al. Biomechanical characterization of vaginal versus abdominal surgical wound healing in the rabbit. Am J Obstet Gynecol 2003;194:1472–7.

[52] Abramov Y, Gandhi S, Botros S, Goldberg R, ShermanW, Rurak M, et al. Do alterations in vaginal dimensions after reconstructive pelvic surgeries affect the risk for dyspareunia? Am J Obstet Gynecol 2005;192:1573–7.

[53] Atef M.M. Darwish. A simplified novel laparoscopic formation of neovagina in cases of Mayer-von Rokitansky-Kuster-Hauser syndrome Fertil Steril. 2007;88(5):1427-30.

[54] El Saman AM, Fathalla MM, Nasr AM, Youssef MA. Laparoscopically assisted balloon vaginoplasty for management of vaginal aplasia. Int J Gynecol Obstet 2007;98:134–7.

[55] El Saman AM, Zakheraha MS, Nasra AM, Fathalla MM. Distension versus traction in laparoscopically assisted balloon vaginoplasty for management of vaginal aplasia. Int J Gynecol Obstet 2007;98:134–7.

[56] El Saman AM, Fathalla MM, Zakherah MS, Shaaban OM, Nasr A. Modified balloon vaginoplasty: the fastest way to create a natural: minor changes in technique eliminate the need for customized instruments. Am J Obstet Gynecol. 2009; 201(5):546 e1-5.

[57] El Saman AM, Ismael AM, Zakherah MS, Nasr A, Tawfik RM, Bedaiwy MA.Enhancement balloon vaginoplasty for treatment of blind vagina due to androgen insensitivity syndrome. Fertil Steril. 2011 Feb;95(2):779-82

[58] Mirilas P, Colborn GL, McClusky DA 3rd, Skandalakis LJ, Skandalakis PN, Skandalakis JE. The history of anatomy and surgery of the preperitoneal space. Arch Surg 2005;140:90–4.

[59] Darwish AM. Fine needle vaginoplasty: a simplified novel approach for correction of vaginal aplasia. Fertil Steril. 2010 Jun;94(1):309-12.

[60] Darwish AM. Transretropubic traction vaginoplasty for correction of vaginal aplasia. Int J Gynaecol Obstet. 2009 Dec;107(3):262-5

[61] Bent AE. Sling and bulking agent placement procedures. Rev Urol 2004;6 (Suppl 5):S26–46.

[62] Bianchi M, Sola V, Ricci P, Pomes C. Late postoperative urinary stress incontinence after a laparoscopic-assisted Vecchietti procedure for neovagina creation in a patient with Rokitansky syndrome: successful treatment with the TVT-O technique. J Minim Invasive Gynecol 2007;14(1):116–8.

[63] Darwish AM, Mohammad AM. A new era for treating vaginal aplasia using transretropubic balloon vaginoplasty approach. Fertil Steril. 2011 Mar 1;95(3):1104-8.

[64] El Saman AM. Retropubic balloon vaginoplasty for management of Mayer-Rokitansky-Kuster-Hauser syndrome. Fertil Steril 2009.

[65] El Saman AM. Combined retropubic balloon vaginoplasty and laparoscopic canalization: a novel blend of techniques provides a minimally invasive treatment for cervicovaginal aplasia. Am J Obstet Gynecol 2009;201:333 e331-335

[66] El Saman AM. Retropubic balloon vaginoplasty for management of Mayer-Rokitansky-Küster-Hauser syndrome. Fertil Steril. 2010 Apr;93(6):2016-9.)

Part 13

Pelvic Pain

19

Myofascial Dysfunction and Its Relationship to Laparoscopy

John Jarrell
University of Calgary, Calgary, AB, Canada

1. Introduction

The specific objective of this review is to describe the elements of myofascial dysfunction particularly as they relate to visceral disease of the pelvis and how the awareness of myofascial dysfunction might affect the management of certain visceral diseases by the procedure of laparoscopy. The specific areas to be reviewed are among the most common gynecological conditions - chronic pelvic pain and endometriosis.

Although diagnostic and operative laparoscopy has brought about significant improvements to women's health, there is growing concern that this procedure might be over-utilized. Increased rates of the procedure may influence the health of women in a deleterious manner as there are significant complications associated with the procedure. This is then a cautionary chapter that seeks to provide the clinician with tools to appreciate the presence of myofascial dysfunction and its ramifications.

2. Case history

Miss C.M. is a 24 year old woman who presents with the development of severe chronic pelvic pain in the right and left lower quadrant of the abdomen for approximately one year. The pain began as a cyclic pain which resulted in an operative laparoscopy during which she had a number of areas of endometriosis cauterized in the *cul de sac*. The pain seemed to abate for a number of months but came back suddenly and progressed to the point she was unable to work. She experienced painful urination, painful defecation and a complete inability to have penetrative sexual relations. She was advised to have a hysterectomy. Before the procedure was undertaken a second opinion was requested.

At the second opinion, the examination demonstrated *cutaneous allodynia* in the lower abdomen and two myofascial trigger points in the right and left lower quadrants (Figure 1). When the myofascial trigger points were compressed the woman's pain was replicated. Pain radiated into her chest and back in a manner similar to the sudden onset of her pain. When released, the pain dissipated. Examination of the perineum showed *cutaneous allodynia* of the perineum and was also associated with a trigger point in the perineal body that allowed only a single digit examination. Digital examination of the *cul de sac* and uterus did not demonstrate tenderness to motion or pressure. Using a Von Frey Electroanesthesiometer, reduction in pain thresholds was recorded in the right (56 gm)and left lower (45 gm) quadrants and in particular the perineal body (26 gm) where normal tissues were >100 gm.

This chapter is directed to an evaluation of this common clinical situation.

3. Benefits of laparoscopy

Diagnostic and operative laparoscopy has added significantly to the management of many surgical conditions[1-4]. These have extended to improved management of certain gynecological conditions [5-7]. In addition to diagnosis, laparoscopy has evolved to more invasive procedures to include ovarian cystectomy, oophorectomy, assisted hysterectomy, total hysterectomy, radical hysterectomy and pelvic and paraaortic lymph node dissection [8-15]. There is general acceptance that the procedure has immense benefits for the management of acute pain conditions such as those related to the management of ovarian torsion, ovarian cyst hemorrhage and the diagnosis of pelvic inflammatory disease[16-18]. Laparoscopic surgery has resulted in reduced hospital admissions, and operating time thereby increasing efficiencies in health service provision[19;20].

4. Laparoscopy for chronic pelvic pain

Although marked benefits for some conditions are substantial the same cannot be said for its use in the diagnosis and treatment of chronic pelvic pain. This condition is very common

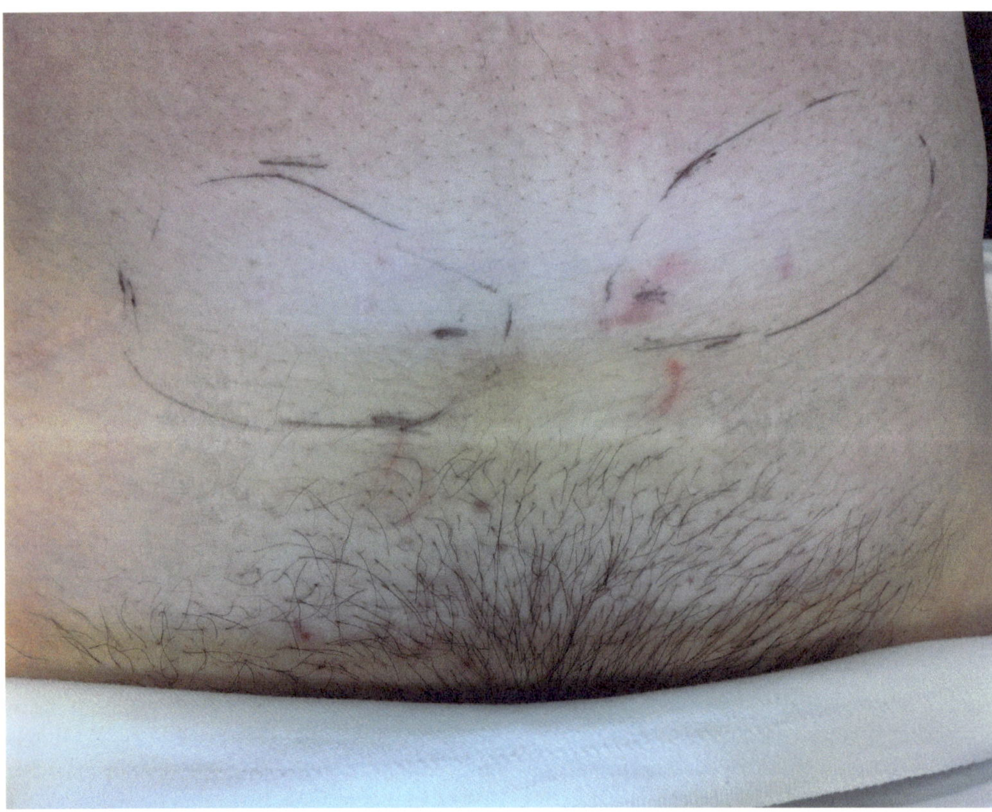

Fig. 1. This photograph demonstrates the presence of cutaneous allodynia in the lower abdomen of a young woman presenting with recurrent pain following a laparoscopic cautery of endometriosis. Within the highly repetitive areas of cutaneous allodynia re two myofascial trigger points indicated by dots. Pressure on the dots completely reproduces the woman's pain.

among women and is responsible for significant disability and personal suffering[21]. Much of the distress of the condition is associated with a difficulty in "being believed". The condition is defined as pain in the abdomen, pelvis or lower back lasting six months. However, the concept that there is an operational definition for the condition has been challenged[22]. The absence of a pattern that permits categorization of the condition in terms of pain duration, location, co morbidities has been identified as a barrier to appropriate research [22].

Despite this important limitation, there have been a large number of studies with a variety of results that have explored the relationship of chronic pelvic pain and laparoscopy. In some cases, the benefits have been identified as the diagnosis of chronic pelvic inflammatory disease. Although often not noted, these benefits seem to be associated with the first laparoscopy[23-28]. More recently, reports have indicated that the ability to identify a pathological condition are not as high as previously reported[29]. It has been estimated that 25-40% of women having laparoscopies for chronic pain conditions do not have a reliable diagnosis identified[29;30]. Among the identifiable conditions associated with chronic pelvic pain, one condition is readily identified as a potential cause in 65% of cases and one third of these will have endometriosis[31]. Additional causes identified are reported to be pelvic inflammatory disease, ovarian cysts, hernias, pelvic congestion syndrome, ovarian remnant syndrome, post-operative peritoneal inclusion cysts and endosalpingeosis[31]. The remainder appears to have no obvious cause of the pain and can extend to a total of 40% of cases. These "negative" procedures are often quite upsetting to patients looking for a specific problem that can be solved in the manner associated with the treatment of acute illness.

5. Laparoscopy for endometriosis

One of the major indications in gynecology for diagnosis and treatment through the means of laparoscopy is directed to the management of endometriosis[32]. Space does not permit a comprehensive review of this condition but a brief summary will introduce its relationship to laparoscopy and myofascial dysfunction[33-35]. Endometriosis is a developmental abnormality in which there is endometrium-like tissue in ectopic locations of the pelvis and rarely in other areas of the body and requires pathological review for the confirmations of diagnosis[36]. It has been reported that the disease can occur in any area of the body with the exception of the spleen. The condition is associated with pain and infertility although these associations are not always present. In some cases of severe disease, there is no pain whatsoever while in other women, small amounts of endometriosis are associated with severe pain and disability[37]. Also, the presence of endometriosis does not preclude infertility as the disease is not uncommonly identified at the time of sterilization[38]. The condition is common and is seen in approximately 15% of women in the reproductive age group. It is increasingly being recognized in adolescents and appears to decrease after the menopause although here are exceptions to this.

Although there is a classification of the stages of endometriosis by the American Fertility Society, this classification is seen as helpful in the area of fertility but of a lesser benefit to pain considerations[39;40]. More recently the disease is classified with respect to four categories: peritoneal in location, nodular and invasive, ovarian endometriomas and uterine adenomyosis[41-44]. This latter condition represents a developmental abnormality in which the abnormal endometrial location is within the actual wall of the uterus. The epidemiology of the condition indicates risk factors to be delayed pregnancy, pelvic pain, pelvic mass, early menarche and frequent menses[43;45-47].

Pain from endometriosis has been largely associated with the ectopic endometrium[40]. This tissue produces agents that can stimulate nocicepetive pain and drugs that inhibit inflammatory activity are often of benefit. The traditional approach to specific therapy has been to reduce estrogen as it stimulates the growth of the tissue. From a medical therapeutic perspective this has involved the use of progesterone, danazol and GnRH agonists that result in an ovarian suppression and a reduction in ovarian estrogen release[48].

Prior to laparoscopy the surgical approach meant removal of the ovaries and uterus often in young women thereby eliminating their fertility. In recent years laparoscopy has afforded another approach. The operative removal of endometriosis at the time of laparoscopy has remained controversial. There has been several randomized controlled trial of the excision of endometriosis compared to sham surgery during operative laparoscopy. This approach was heralded as a highly effective prior to the randomized trials[49]. The randomized studies vary in terms of pain assessment and tend to be small in size and in some cases there is evidence of effectiveness [50;51]. In another study, pain was measured during the entire menstrual cycle and was tested prior to and quarterly post-operatively for a year and there was no difference in pain between the excision group and the sham operated group. Most of the cases had early disease, identified as stage 1 or 2 by the American Fertility Society and peritoneal in location. Long term follow- up of the study indicated there was no difference in the time to the next operation undertaken for pelvic pain by survival analysis[53]. One of the interesting features was the observation that the level of pain from the first Pre-operative assessment predicted the time of subsequent surgery. Although this might seem self evident it has not been reported previously. In relation to the excision of endometriomas of the ovary, there is evidence of effectiveness[54]

There is a growing concern that the operations undertaken for endometriosis are not directed to the actual problem of pain[55]. This has been reviewed from the perspective of the limitations of surgery recently[56]. Also, there are recent reports that indicate the source of the pain which has been assumed to be the ectopic sites of endometriosis may in fact not represent the sole source of the pain[33;57]. The data that raise these concerns can be summarized as follows:

In addition to these studies of pain physiology, there is evidence from clinical utilization studies that operative laparoscopy is heavily used in the management of problems associated with endometriosis and adhesions. A review of the diagnostic and operative laparoscopies was undertaken in the Province of Alberta, Canada between the years 1994 and 2007[58]. The data were collected on individual women over these years so that the frequency of repeated surgery on one woman could be assessed and then aggregated for the span of the study. The results indicated there was a significant repeat rate of surgery among 24,473 women (Figure 2). In addition, a statistical process control chart indicated the repeat rates were out of statistical control for both diagnostic and operative procedures for the years 1999-2000 (Figure 3)[59]. The interpretation is that there was a bias to operate during these years as it is highly unlikely that there was a sudden change in the rate of disease. Also, as there is a cut off in this study by the years 1999 and 2007 it is recognized these rates are limited as some women would have had procedures before and after these dates.

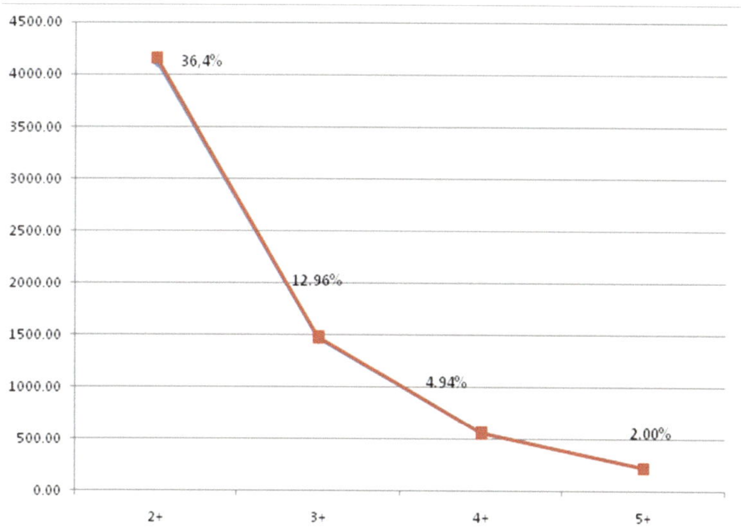

Fig. 2. The rates of repeated operative laparoscopy among 24473 women with operative laparoscopies undertaken between the years 1994-2007 in The Province of Alberta Canada where virtually all operative laparoscopies are collected in this database as the province has a comprehensive health insurance Program[60]

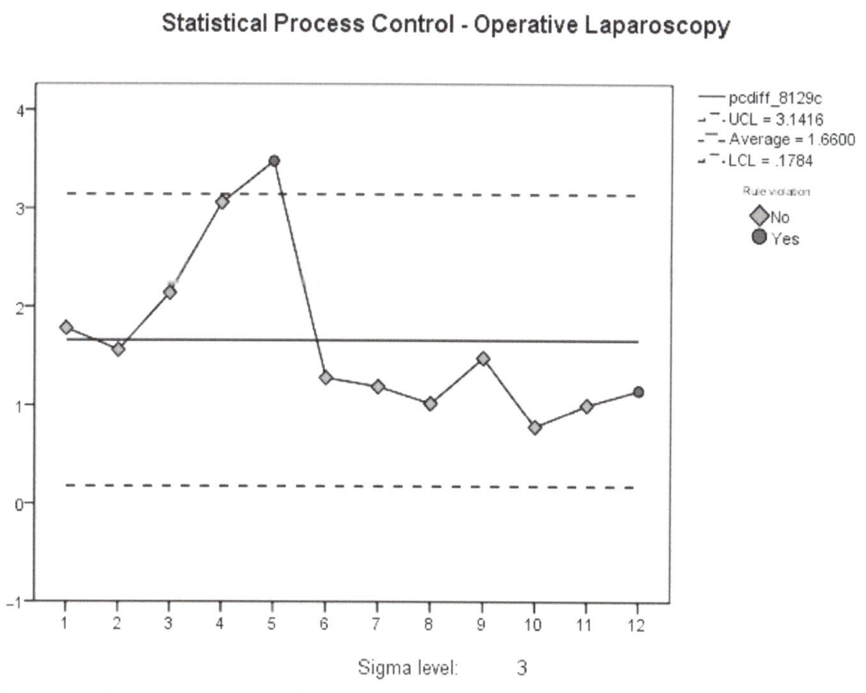

Fig. 3. Statistical Process Control Charts of the aggregated annual rates of repeat laparoscopies on a fiscal basis from 1994-2007 among 24000 women. The charts indicate the rates are "out of control" or represent a "special cause" where the probability of occurrence is <0.001[59]

6. Myofascial dysfunction

Pain associated with muscle and fascia actually has a long history, going back to the seminal work of Sir Henry Head who recognized there were tender areas on the skin that consistently appeared in relation to disorders of the underlying viscera[61]. He called these Head zones and they were the basis for the recognition of the dermatomes. More recently these areas of pain were associated with both injury and trauma and were called trigger points. These are small areas of persistent contracture of muscle fibers that can cause severe pain and disability but are not generally appreciated among medical specialties with the exception of rehabilitation medicine. Since 1945 there have only been 1191 references in PubMed although there has been a significant increase in recent years. Recent reviews of myofascial pain and its relationship to trigger points have indicated the areas remains very complex[62;63]. Interest in the physiology of trigger points in relations to brain activity as well as muscle physiology is expanding[64-67].

Myofascial pain syndrome is a muscle condition that has the characteristics of having local and referred pain originating in a myofascial trigger point[68]. This term describes a nodule or band of muscle that can produce intense pain when spontaneously or when stimulated. There are two aspects of the trigger point: a motor component that is palpable and a sensory component that produces pain locally and in an area of referred pain. The diagnosis of the presence of a trigger point is based on the palpation of a tender nodule or band that reproduces the patient's symptoms and can be confirmed if there is a local twitch response as a result of manipulation of the taut band[68]. The pain is often referred to distant locations such as the back, chest or legs when considering pelvic trigger points.

Investigations of myofascial trigger points have focused on alterations in the synaptic cleft of the neuromuscular junction, the spinal cord and the brain response to myofascial pain[68-70]. The trigger point has been characterized as a local area of sensory and motor activity. The motor activity is based on the presence of the nodule or taut band. The area not maintained by persistent a motor activity as there are no motor action potentials present. Instead there are a variety of altered electrical observation that can be made including spontaneous small voltage activity, and spike discharges[71]. More recent studies have indicated that electrophysiological responses are commonly found when an electrode is placed in the trigger point for therapy[72]. There are also evoked changes in electrical activity in association with the local twitch response. These changes are not eliminated by an upper cord transaction indicating there is a spinal arc involved in their maintenance. Spontaneous discharges fropm a trigger point in the rabbit can be inhibited with phentolamine, an a blocker indicating the potential role of the sympathetic nervous system in the maintenance of these electrical discharges[73].

The sensory component of the trigger point is based on changes in the intracellular environment. There is an increased synaptic level of acetylcholine activity, local ischemia as evidenced by biochemical changes of a lowered pH, and an increased concentration of Substance P, CGRP, bradykinin, serotonin, prostaglandins and potassium[74]. These areas act to stimulate nociceptors that are present in muscle tissue. Local ischemia has been identified as the cause of pain and is a result of the metabolic crisis that occurs in these areas.

Clinically the causes of myofascial trigger points have focused primarily on primary or secondary causes. The primary causes are identified as single or recurrent episodes of micro or macrotrauma or from muscle overload[75]. Overuse, postural stress and altered mechanics can produce trigger points in the neck and back. Secondary causes have included cervical whiplash, migraine headache, temporomandibular pain, frozen shoulder, radicular pain, postlaminectomy syndrome and viscero-somatic pain[76]. This chapter is directed to the application of the secondary trigger points associated with disorders of the viscera that produce pain.

7. Visceral causes of myofascial pain

There are a number of conditions that have resulted in myofascial trigger points. Diseases of the gall bladder have produced shoulder pain and trigger points in the right upper quadrant of the abdomen. Angina-like pain can be produced on the chest from cardiac ischemia and can lead to diagnostic confusion. Flank pain and trigger points can be produced by ureterolithiasis. One of the characteristics of these trigger points is that they may dissipate after the original condition has resolved but they may also remain for significant periods of time[77;78].

The most common cause of myofascial pain has been trauma but in recent years there is an appreciation that visceral disease can produce somatic muscle pain and myofascial trigger points[79;80]. Examples in which there is an interaction of the viscera with somatic tissues include somatic hyperalgesia[81;82], trophic changes in tissue[83;84]. In the rat, intense stimulation of the intrauterine cavity is associated with neurogenic extravasation of administered dye in the region of the dermatomes innervating the pelvic[85]. In visceral pain as well as migraine, there are reports that in addition to myofascial trigger points, there is a development of cutaneous allodynia in the respective dermatomal regions[86;87].

On important aspect of the physiology of viscero-somatic pain referral has been undertaken in relation to the gall bladder. Diseases of the gall bladder were found to produce changes in pain thresholds in the skin, subcutaneous tissues and muscle, reduction in muscle thickness and cutaneous allodynia on the side of the gall bladder when compared to the contralateral side[83]. There was a direct negative correlation between the number of colicky aspects and the measurement of pain threshold.

These findings are also relevant in relation to the pelvis. The pelvic viscera include the uterus, ovaries, Fallopian tubes, pelvic peritoneum, bladder and rectum. Disorders such as endometriosis can potentially affect all of these structures. Disorders such as interstitial cystitis and irritable bowel syndrome are also disorders that affect the visceral tissues. It is now known the viscera contain nociceptors. It is now being recognized that visceral pain is a specific syndrome associated with alterations in the pelvic structures [88]. As an example of human research related to visceral pain, the administration of capsaicin, an activator of the heat sensitive receptor TRPV1[89] to the intestinal stomata of volunteers with ileostomy or colostomy resulted in dramatic changes in the referral of pain and the temperature of the same areas of skin[90].

8. Visceral pain in the pelvis

These changes have been studied in the abdomen and pelvis of women with chronic pelvic pain. A cross-sectional study of women with chronic pelvic pain for at least six months was done that included an assessment of the number of areas of myofascial pain, including the abdomen, perineum, *levator ani* and *obturator internus* muscles. This number was assessed in terms of clinical variables of age, gravidity, parity, pain duration number of laparoscopies and laparotomies. The duration of pain and number of laparoscopies significantly predicted the number of areas of trigger points[91]. These findings would suggest that in a similar mechanism to the gall bladder, the extent of pain is an important factor in the genesis of chronic pelvic pain due to myofascial trigger points[83]. Also, the presence of laparoscopy as a predictor of the number of areas of trigger points could be considered another proxy for the duration of pain but it also suggests that the surgical procedure itself might affect ongoing pain experience.

It is recognize that the diagnosis of chronic pelvic pain can be very misleading[22]. To attempt to partially address this, a cross-sectional study of bedside testing of *cutaneous allodynia*, myofascial trigger points and reduced pain thresholds is being undertaken among women presenting with a variety of apparent causes to determine if these tests were helpful in the identification of visceral disease[92]. The subjects are categorized in a manner that is appropriate to a clinician involved in chronic pain - those with previously documented visceral disease, those with no clinical evidence of visceral disease, including those women with no prior laparoscopy.

Briefly, *cutaneous allodynia* is tested among women with chronic pelvic pain by the use of a simple cotton-tipped applicator or culture stick[93]. The stick is drawn down the abdomen from the mid-clavicular line on both sides of the abdomen and the woman is asked if there is a sudden change in the sensation or a sudden painful sensation. The areas can be small or large. They are commonly associated with the region where the lower anterior branches of the lumbar cutaneous nerves enter the *rectus abdominis* muscle, just above the pubic triangle bilaterally. These areas can also be large to involve the regions of the T11-L1 dermatomes or small and localized as shown in Figure 3. The test is highly reproducible and has significant inter-rater validity.

A test for myofascial dysfunction involves the palpation of a myofascial trigger point that is usually located within the area of *cutaneous allodynia*. These areas appear as a small knot in the muscle although they often feel closer to the skin as a small lipoma. When pressed they cause severe pain and referred pain into unusual locations such as the chest, back and legs. When the pressure is released, the pain decreases. Women commonly can direct the examining finger to the exact site.

The identification of reduced pain thresholds was undertaken using the Von Fry Anesthesiometer[95;96]. This instrument has a variety of threshold adaptors but for these tests a 90 gram threshold was selected. Women were tested for pain in the deltoid muscle as an internal control for central pain an then in the right and left upper quadrant, right and left lower quadrants and the perineal body for a measure of intra-pelvic sensitivity.

The results of these tests indicate at least on a preliminary basis, an ability to differentiate women with pre-existing or concurrent visceral disease from women without such a condition. The most significant test to be undertaken was the simple use of a cotton-tipped applicator, a device that is available in every clinician's office. Although the discrimination of these groups may not be perfect, it is an approach that is recognizable from clinicians.

The clinical importance of these preliminary findings is that they may identify an important potential confounder in the clinical determination of the cause of pain, particularly the recurrent pain associated with women presenting with recurrent pain following operative laparoscopy. It is entirely possible that the reasons for many of the "negative" laparoscopies associated with chronic pelvic pain may be due to high frequencies of myofascial dysfunction. Traditionally, clinicians have been trained in gynecology to undertake a clinical examination for a pelvic mass. The bimanual examination is one that places a lot of stress on the abdominal wall exactly over the most common areas of trigger points. It also places a great deal of pressure on the perineum and the vaginal barrel that is the product of the tone of the *levator ani* muscles. It is instructive to note the pressures that are identified as causing pain are quite small. In some cases the weight of pressure causing pain in the lower abdomen and perineum can be as low as 15 grams - the weight of two Canadian one dollar coins. It is entirely possible that pressure placed in these areas can be appreciated as disorders of the adnexa, resulting in further laparoscopic surgery of no particular benefit to the woman. Arguably, this is the case with our case presentation.

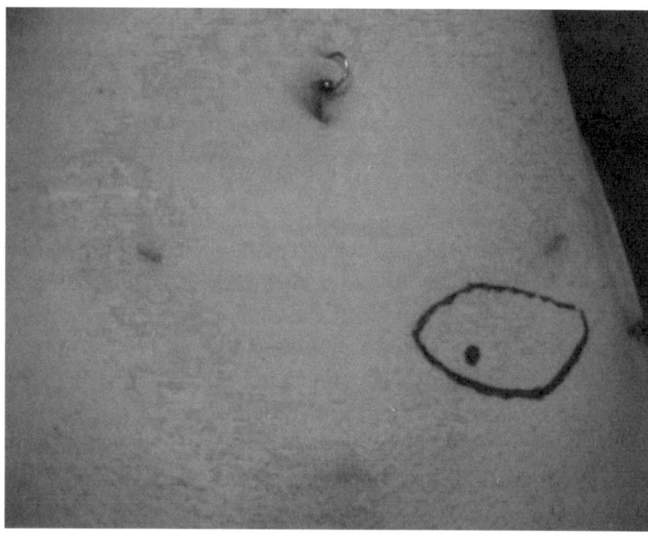

Fig. 3. A demonstration of *cutaneous allodynia* containing a myofascial trigger point in a woman complaining of persistent pain in the left lower quadrant of the abdomen following an operative laparoscopy that treated the presence of endometriosis on the left ovary. The persistent pain was resolved by management of the trigger point - exercise, pressure, stretching and occasional trigger point injections.

Briefly in the evaluation of a woman with chronic pelvic pain, the presence of *cutaneous allodynia* has a significant ability to detect the presence of visceral disease. This documentation indicates that in addition to further medical interventions, an important aspect of care should be undertaken. In many cases, this will represent an alternative to further laparoscopic surgery.

9. Alternatives to laparoscopy

Women with chronic pelvic pain will benefit from multidisciplinary care. There is Level 1 Evidence of its effectiveness. The approach is based on the shift from the traditional acute medical model directed to a "cure" to the recognition that cures in chronic pain are extremely rare and the more appropriate approach is to manage pain in a rehabilitative sense. The elements of such rehabilitation are first and foremost education in the change in concept that is not always accepted by the woman seeking care. Women who seek the cure at all costs have been identifies as pre-contemplative to the rehabilitative model and unlikely to benefit from this type of management. Similarly catastrophic thinking or approaches to the pain have been recognized as risk factors for failure. In addition to education, cognitive behavioral therapy has Level 1 Evidence of effectiveness. This involves self monitoring of pain, pacing activities carefully and ensuring a restorative sleep pattern is possible. Smoking is strongly discouraged.

Myofascial pain is often effectively managed by physiotherapy self exercise and muscle injections with local anesthetic or botulinum toxin[97]. One must be cautious in the use of botulinum toxin in the abdomen as cases of its migration into the hip casuing temporary difficulties in ambulation have occurred. It is highly effective however in the perineum where it improves aspects of sexual function. Use in the *levator ani* and *obturator internus* muscles is also effective in this regard, particularly for pain that follows intercourse for several days or pain associated with orgasm. Medical management is directed to the suppression of menstrual bleeding with oral contraceptives, GnRH agonists or medicated intrauterine contraceptive devices[98;99]. The medicated intrauterine contraceptive device has been identified as a particularly effective treatment when inserted at the time of operative laparoscopy for endometriosis[99].

Management also assists at times with pain relief that some times requires opiate medication to permit a reduction in hyperalgesia to allow physiotherapists access to areas of myofascial tenderness. Psychological assessment is critical in the approaches to managing stress and the early detection of depression that occurs in approximately 50% of women with chronic pain. Depression is an important barrier to clinical improvement[100]. Occupational therapy is involved in the assessment of capability in working and ergonomic assessments of the worksites[101]. One of key concepts is the development of self directed management of pain[102]. Group therapy can be extremely beneficial in providing access to approaches to intimacy for women who have sexual pain[103]. Groups directed to generating pelvic muscle stretch and strengthening of core muscles are also beneficial[104].

10. Summary

While laparoscopy has demonstrative evidence of effectiveness in many situations, its position in relation to chronic conditions requires additional consideration. Viscero-somatic pain referral is very common. It can be identified in association with endometriosis, pelvic inflammatory disease and other pelvic visceral diseases. It can be identified with simple bedside tests, the most helpful being the recognition of cutaneous allodynia with a simple culture stick. Its recognition help to identify alternative mechanisms of pain and potentially reduced unnecessary surgery.

11. References

[1] T. M. Young-Fadok et al., "Benefits of Laparoscopic-Assisted Colectomy for Colon Polyps: a Case-Matched Series," *Mayo Clin.Proc.* 75, no. 4 (2000): 344-348.

[2] J. F. Smith et al., "Risks and Benefits of Laparoscopic Cholecystectomy in the Community Hospital Setting," *J Laparoendosc.Surg.* 1, no. 6 (1991): 325-332.

[3] W. Schwenk et al., "Short Term Benefits for Laparoscopic Colorectal Resection," *Cochrane Database Syst Rev*, no. 3 (2005): CD003145.

[4] M. A. Memon and R. J. Fitzgibbons, Jr., "Assessing Risks, Costs, and Benefits of Laparoscopic Hernia Repair," *Annu.Rev Med* 49 (1998): 95-109.

[5] V. Mais et al., "Laparoscopic Versus Abdominal Myomectomy: a Prospective, Randomized Trial to Evaluate Benefits in Early Outcome," *Am J Obstet Gynecol* 174, no. 2 (1996): 654-658.
[6] R. Garry, "The Benefits and Problems Associated With Minimal Access Surgery," *Aust.N Z.J Obstet Gynaecol.* 42, no. 3 (2002): 239-244.
[7] S. Dueholm, H. Zingenberg, and G. Sandgren, "[The Risks and Benefits of Laparoscopic Sterilization]," *Ugeskr.Laeger* 147, no. 47 (1985): 3780-3783.
[8] F. Zullo et al., "Minilaparoscopic Ovarian Drilling Under Local Anesthesia in Patients With Polycystic Ovary Syndrome," *Fertil.Steril.* 74, no. 2 (2000): 376-379.
[9] P. M. Yuen et al., "A Randomized Prospective Study of Laparoscopy and Laparotomy in the Management of Benign Ovarian Masses," *Am J Obstet Gynecol* 177, no. 1 (1997): 109-114.
[10] T. Schollmeyer et al., "Chronic Isolated Torsion of the Left Fallopian Tube: a Diagnostic Dilemma," *Arch.Gynecol Obstet* 277, no. 1 (2008): 87-90.
[11] M. H. Cheng et al., "Laparoscopic Plication of Partially Twisted Ovary With Massive Ovarian Edema," *J Chin Med Assoc.* 69, no. 5 (2006): 236-239.
[12] S. Sadik, B. Uran, and T. Ozaydin, "Laparoscopic-Assisted Vaginal Hysterectomy and Bilateral Salpingo-Oophorectomy With Suturing Technique," *J Am Assoc.Gynecol Laparosc.* 2, no. 4 (1995): 437-440.
[13] J. T. Liang et al., "Laparoscopic Prophylactic Oophorectomy Plus N3 Lymphadenectomy for Advanced Rectosigmoid Cancer," *Ann.Surg.Oncol.* 14, no. 7 (2007): 1991-1999.
[14] S. P. Puntambekar et al., "Laparoscopic Total Radical Hysterectomy by the Pune Technique: Our Experience of 248 Cases," *J Minim.Invasive.Gynecol* 14, no. 6 (2007): 682-689.
[15] M. Malzoni et al., "Feasibility, Morbidity, and Safety of Total Laparoscopic Radical Hysterectomy With Lymphadenectomy: Our Experience," *J Minim.Invasive.Gynecol* 14, no. 5 (2007): 584-590.
[16] G. Augustin and M. Majerovic, "Non-Obstetrical Acute Abdomen During Pregnancy," *Eur.J Obstet Gynecol Reprod.Biol.* 131, no. 1 (2007): 4-12.
[17] U. Goktolga et al., "Isolated Torsion of Fallopian Tube in a Premenarcheal 12-Year-Old Girl," *J Obstet Gynaecol.Res* 33, no. 2 (2007): 215-217.
[18] I. Oji, A. Kitching, and K. Smith, "Severe, Acute Pain Following Application of Filshie Clips: a Case of Possible Viscero-Visceral Sensitization," *J Obstet Gynaecol.* 25, no. 4 (2005): 400-401.
[19] J. P. Gagne et al., "Advanced Laparoscopic Surgery in a Free-Standing Ambulatory Setting: Lessons From the First 50 Cases," *Surg.Innov.* 14, no. 1 (2007): 12-17.
[20] H. G. Gaitan, J. Eslava-Schmalbach, and P. I. Gomez, "Cost Effectiveness of Diagnostic Laparoscopy in Reproductive Aged Females Suffering From Non-Specific Acute Low Abdominal Pain," *Rev Salud Publica (Bogota.)* 7, no. 2 (2005): 166-179.
[21] K. Zondervan and D. H. Barlow, "Epidemiology of Chronic Pelvic Pain," *Baillieres Best.Pract.Res Clin.Obstet Gynaecol.* 14, no. 3 (2000): 403-414.
[22] R. E. Williams, K. E. Hartmann, and J. F. Steege, "Documenting the Current Definitions of Chronic Pelvic Pain: Implications for Research," *Obstet.Gynecol.* 103, no. 4 (2004): 686-691.
[23] Lira S. Carranza et al., "[The Laparoscopic Findings in Patients With Chronic Pelvic Pain and Dysmenorrhea]," *Ginecol.Obstet Mex.* 62 (1994): 82-84.

[24] P. Vercellini et al., "Laparoscopy in the Diagnosis of Chronic Pelvic Pain in Adolescent Women," *J Reprod.Med* 34, no. 10 (1989): 827-830.
[25] G. Priou et al., "[The Diagnostic Value of Celioscopy in the Evaluation of Chronic Pelvic Pain. Apropos of 184 Cases]," *J Gynecol Obstet Biol.Reprod.(Paris)* 13, no. 4 (1984): 395-402.
[26] A. J. Kresch et al., "Laparoscopy in 100 Women With Chronic Pelvic Pain," *Obstet Gynecol* 64, no. 5 (1984): 672-674.
[27] M. Redecha et al., "[Laparoscopic Findings in Women With Chronic Pelvic Pain]," *Bratisl.Lek.Listy* 101, no. 8 (2000): 460-464.
[28] C. M. Bahary and I. G. Gorodeski, "The Diagnostic Value of Laparoscopy in Women With Chronic Pelvic Pain," *Am.Surg.* 53, no. 11 (1987): 672-674.
[29] A. P. Newham, Z. M. van der Spuy, and F. Nugent, "Laparoscopic Findings in Women With Chronic Pelvic Pain," *S.Afr.Med J* 86, no. 9 Suppl (1996): 1200-1203.
[30] F. M. Howard, "The Role of Laparoscopy in the Chronic Pelvic Pain Patient," *Clin.Obstet Gynecol* 46, no. 4 (2003): 749-766.
[31] F. M. Howard, "The Role of Laparoscopy As a Diagnostic Tool in Chronic Pelvic Pain," *Baillieres Best.Pract.Res Clin.Obstet Gynaecol.* 14, no. 3 (2000): 467-494.
[32] G. H. Eltabbakh and N. A. Bower, "Laparoscopic Surgery in Endometriosis," *Minerva Ginecol.* 60, no. 4 (2008): 323-330.
[33] R. C. Reiter and J. C. Gambone, "Nongynecologic Somatic Pathology in Women With Chronic Pelvic Pain and Negative Laparoscopy," *J.Reprod.Med.* 36, no. 4 (1991): 253-259.
[34] J. E. Carter, "A Systematic History for the Patient With Chronic Pelvic Pain," *JSLS.* 3, no. 4 (1999): 245-252.
[35] J. F. Jarrell, "The Weight of Chronic Pelvic Pain," *J.Obstet.Gynaecol.Can.* 26, no. 5 (2004): 453-456.
[36] G. L. Marchino et al., "Diagnosis of Pelvic Endometriosis With Use of Macroscopic Versus Histologic Findings," *Fertil.Steril.* 84, no. 1 (2005): 12-15.
[37] D. L. Chatman and E. A. Zbella, "Biopsy in Laparoscopically Diagnosed Endometriosis," *J Reprod.Med* 32, no. 11 (1987): 855-857.
[38] P. Vercellini, L. Bocciolone, and P. G. Crosignani, "Is Mild Endometriosis Always a Disease?," *Hum.Reprod.* 7, no. 5 (1992): 627-629.
[39] M. Canis et al., "Classification of Endometriosis," *Baillieres Clin.Obstet Gynaecol.* 7, no. 4 (1993): 759-774.
[40] F. M. Howard, "Endometriosis and Mechanisms of Pelvic Pain," *J Minim.Invasive.Gynecol* 16 (2009): 540-550.
[41] I. Brosens, J. Donnez, and G. Benagiano, "Improving the Classification of Endometriosis," *Hum.Reprod.* 8, no. 11 (1993): 1792-1795.
[42] C. Chapron et al., "Deeply Infiltrating Endometriosis: Pathogenetic Implications of the Anatomical Distribution," *Hum.Reprod.* 21, no. 7 (2006): 1839-1845.
[43] X. Liu et al., "Patterns of and Risk Factors for Recurrence in Women With Ovarian Endometriomas," *Obstet Gynecol* 109, no. 6 (2007): 1411-1420.
[44] O. Yeniel et al., "Adenomyosis: Prevalence, Risk Factors, Symptoms and Clinical Findings," *Clin.Exp.Obstet Gynecol* 34, no. 3 (2007): 163-167.
[45] S. W. Guo and Y. Wang, "The Prevalence of Endometriosis in Women With Chronic Pelvic Pain," *Gynecol Obstet Invest* 62, no. 3 (2006): 121-130.

[46] N. Sinaii et al., "Differences in Characteristics Among 1,000 Women With Endometriosis Based on Extent of Disease," *Fertil.Steril.* (2007).

[47] M. H. Moen and B. Schei, "Epidemiology of Endometriosis in a Norwegian County," *Acta Obstet Gynecol Scand.* 76, no. 6 (1997): 559-562.

[48] E. S. Surrey, "The Role of Progestins in Treating the Pain of Endometriosis," *J Minim.Invasive.Gynecol* 13, no. 6 (2006): 528-534.

[49] D. B. Redwine, "Remote Recollection of Preoperative Pain in Patients Undergoing Excision of Endometriosis," *J Am Assoc.Gynecol Laparosc.* 1, no. 2 (1994): 140-145.

[50] C. J. Sutton et al., "Prospective, Randomized, Double-Blind, Controlled Trial of Laser Laparoscopy in the Treatment of Pelvic Pain Associated With Minimal, Mild, and Moderate Endometriosis," *Fertil.Steril.* 62, no. 4 (1994): 696-700.

[51] K. D. Jones, P. Haines, and C. J. Sutton, "Long-Term Follow-Up of a Controlled Trial of Laser Laparoscopy for Pelvic Pain," *JSLS.* 5, no. 2 (2001): 111-115.

[52] J. Jarrell et al., "Laparoscopy and Reported Pain Among Patients With Endometriosis," *J Obstet.Gynaecol.Can.* 27, no. 5 (2005): 477-485.

[53] J Jarrell et al., "Women's Pain Experience Predicts Future Surgery for Pain Associated With Endometriosis," *JOGC* in press (2008).

[54] R. Hart et al., "Excisional Surgery Versus Ablative Surgery for Ovarian Endometriomata: a Cochrane Review," *Hum.Reprod.* 20, no. 11 (2005): 3000-3007.

[55] P. Stratton and K. J. Berkley, "Chronic Pelvic Pain and Endometriosis: Translational Evidence of the Relationship and Implications," *Hum.Reprod Update.* (2010).

[56] P Vercellini et al., "The Effect of Surgery for Symptomatic Endoometriosis:the Other Side of the Story," *Hum.Reprod.Update.* 15, no. 2 (2009): 177-188.

[57] MLS Montenegro et al., "Abdominal Myofascial Pain Syndrome Must Be Considered in the Differential Diagnosis of Chronic Pelvic Pain," *Europ J Obstet Gynecol Repr Biol* 147 (2009): 21-24.

[58] J. Jarrell, "Diagnostic and Operative Laparoscopy in Alberta 1994-2006," *JOGC accepted, 2008* (2008).

[59] J Jarrell, "Annual Repeat Laparoscopic Surgery: A Marker of Practice Variation," *AM J Medical Quality* 25, no. 5 (2009): 378-383.

[60] J Jarrell, "Diagnostic and Operative Laparoscopy in Alberta 1994-2006," *J Obstet Gynaecol.Can.* 30, no. 11 (2008): 1045-1049.

[61] Head H, "On Disturbances of Sensation With Especial Reference to the Pain of Visceral Disease," *Brain* 17 (2010): 339-480.

[62] E. Vazquez-Delgado, J. Cascos-Romero, and C. Gay-Escoda, "Myofascial Pain Syndrome Associated With Trigger Points: a Literature Review. (I): Epidemiology, Clinical Treatment and Etiopathogeny," *Med Oral Patol.Oral Cir.Bucal.* 14, no. 10 (2009): e494-e498.

[63] E. Vazquez-Delgado, J. Cascos-Romero, and C. Gay-Escoda, "Myofascial Pain Associated to Trigger Points: A Literature Review. Part 2: Differential Diagnosis and Treatment," *Med Oral Patol.Oral Cir.Bucal.* (2010).

[64] D. M. Niddam, "Brain Manifestation and Modulation of Pain From Myofascial Trigger Points," *Curr Pain Headache Rep.* 13, no. 5 (2009): 370-375.

[65] D. G. Simons, "New Views of Myofascial Trigger Points: Etiology and Diagnosis," *Arch.Phys.Med Rehabil.* 89, no. 1 (2008): 157-159.

[66] J. P. Shah and E. A. Gilliams, "Uncovering the Biochemical Milieu of Myofascial Trigger Points Using in Vivo Microdialysis: an Application of Muscle Pain Concepts to Myofascial Pain Syndrome," *J Bodyw.Mov Ther.* 12, no. 4 (2008): 371-384.
[67] J. P. Shah et al., "Biochemicals Associated With Pain and Inflammation Are Elevated in Sites Near to and Remote From Active Myofascial Trigger Points," *Arch.Phys.Med Rehabil.* 89, no. 1 (2008): 16-23.
[68] R. D. Gerwin, J. Dommerholt, and J. P. Shah, "An Expansion of Simons' Integrated Hypothesis of Trigger Point Formation," *Curr Pain Headache Rep.* 8, no. 6 (2004): 468-475.
[69] T. S. Kuan, "Current Studies on Myofascial Pain Syndrome," *Curr Pain Headache Rep.* 13, no. 5 (2009): 365-369.
[70] D. M. Niddam, "Brain Manifestation and Modulation of Pain From Myofascial Trigger Points," *Curr Pain Headache Rep.* 13, no. 5 (2009): 370-375.
[71] C. Z. Hong and D. G. Simons, "Pathophysiologic and Electrophysiologic Mechanisms of Myofascial Trigger Points," *Arch Phys Med Rehabil* 79, no. 7 (1998): 863-872.
[72] M. H. Rivner, "The Neurophysiology of Myofascial Pain Syndrome," *Curr Pain Headache Rep.* 5, no. 5 (2001): 432-440.
[73] J. T. Chen et al., "Phentolamine Effect on the Spontaneous Electrical Activity of Active Loci in a Myofascial Trigger Spot of Rabbit Skeletal Muscle," *Arch Phys Med Rehabil* 79, no. 7 (1998): 790-794.
[74] J. P. Shah et al., "Biochemicals Associated With Pain and Inflammation Are Elevated in Sites Near to and Remote From Active Myofascial Trigger Points," *Arch.Phys.Med Rehabil.* 89, no. 1 (2008): 16-23.
[75] A. H. Wheeler and G. W. Aaron, "Muscle Pain Due to Injury," *Curr Pain Headache Rep.* 5, no. 5 (2001): 441-446.
[76] R. D. Gerwin, "Classification, Epidemiology, and Natural History of Myofascial Pain Syndrome," *Curr Pain Headache Rep.* 5, no. 5 (2001): 412-420.
[77] L. Vecchiet, J. Vecchiet, and M. A. Giamberardino, "Referred Muscle Pain: Clinical and Pathophysiologic Aspects," *Curr Rev Pain* 3, no. 6 (1999): 489-498.
[78] L. Vecchiet and M. A. Giamberardino, "Referred muscle pain and hyperalgesia from viscera," in *Muscle Pain, Myofascial Pain and Fibromyalgia* (New York, NY: Haworth Medical
press, 1999), 61-69.
[79] L. Vecchiet, J. Vecchiet, and M. A. Giamberardino, "Referred Muscle Pain: Clinical and Pathophysiologic Aspects," *Curr.Rev Pain* 3, no. 6 (1999): 489-498.
[80] L. Vecchiet, J. Vecchiet, and M. A. Giamberardino, "Referred Muscle Pain: Clinical and Pathophysiologic Aspects," *Curr Rev Pain* 3, no. 6 (1999): 489-498.
[81] M. Stawowy et al., "Somatosensory Changes in the Referred Pain Area in Patients With Acute Cholecystitis Before and After Treatment With Laparoscopic or Open Cholecystectomy," *Scand.J Gastroenterol.* 39, no. 10 (2004): 988-993.
[82] M. A. Giamberardino, "Recent and Forgotten Aspects of Visceral Pain," *Eur.J Pain* 3, no. 2 (1999): 77-92.
[83] M. A. Giamberardino et al., "Relationship Between Pain Symptoms and Referred Sensory and Trophic Changes in Patients With Gallbladder Pathology," *Pain* 114, no. 1-2 (2005): 239-249.

[84] P. Procacci, M. Zoppi, and M. Maresca, "Clinical Approach to Visceral Sensation," *Prog.Brain Res* 67 (1986): 21-28.

[85] U. Wesselmann and J. Lai, "Mechanisms of Referred Visceral Pain: Uterine Inflammation in the Adult Virgin Rat Results in Neurogenic Plasma Extravasation in the Skin," *Pain* 73, no. 3 (1997): 309-317.

[86] D. Bevilaqua-Grossi et al., "Temporomandibular Disorders and Cutaneous Allodynia Are Associated in Individuals With Migraine," *Cephalalgia* 30, no. 4 (2010): 425-432.

[87] W. Janig and H. J. Habler, "[Physiology and Pathophysiology of Visceral Pain]," *Schmerz.* 16, no. 6 (2002): 429-446.

[88] U. Wesselmann, "Neurogenic Inflammation and Chronic Pelvic Pain," *World J.Urol.* 19, no. 3 (2001): 180-185.

[89] A. M. Drewes et al., "Gut Pain and Hyperalgesia Induced by Capsaicin: a Human Experimental Model," *Pain* 104, no. 1-2 (2003): 333-341.

[90] L. Arendt-Nielsen et al., "Viscero-Somatic Reflexes in Referred Pain Areas Evoked by Capsaicin Stimulation of the Human Gut," *Eur.J Pain* (2007).

[91] Jarrell J, "Gynecological Pain, Endometriosis, Visceral Disease and the Viscero-Somatic Connection," *J Muscskel Health* 16 (2008): 21-27.

[92] Jarrell J, Giamberardino MA, and Robert M, "Bedside Tests of Viscero-Somatic Pain," Obstetrics and Gynecology Submitted 2011

[93] Jarrell J, "Demonstration of Cutaneous Allodynia in Association With Chronic Pelvic Pain," *Journal of Visualized Experimentation* (9 A.D.).

[94] B. W. Fenton et al., "Quantification of Abdominal Wall Pain Using Pain Pressure Threshold Algometry in Patients With Chronic Pelvic Pain," *Clin J Pain* 25, no. 6 (2009): 500-505.

[95] A. Fischer, "Pressure Algometry Over Normal Muscles. Standard Values, Validity and Reproducibility of Pressure Threshold," *Pain* 30, no. 1 (1986): 115-126.

[96] Cairns BE et al., "Glutamate-Induced Sensitization of Rat Masseter Muscle Fibers. Neuroscience," *Neuroscience, 2002* 109 (2002): 389-399.

[97] Andres J. De et al., "A Double-Blind, Controlled, Randomized Trial to Evaluate the Efficacy of Botulinum Toxin for the Treatment of Lumbar Myofascial Pain in Humans," *Reg Anesth.Pain Med* 35, no. 3 (2010): 255-260.

[98] H. M. Fraser et al., "Long-Term Suppression of Ovarian Function by a Luteinizing-Hormone Releasing Hormone Agonist Implant in Patients With Endometriosis," *Fertil.Steril.* 53, no. 1 (1990): 61-68.

[99] P. Vercellini et al., "Comparison of a Levonorgestrel-Releasing Intrauterine Device Versus Expectant Management After Conservative Surgery for Symptomatic Endometriosis: a Pilot Study," *Fertil.Steril.* 80, no. 2 (2003): 305-309.

[100] D. Mirkin, C. Murphy-Barron, and K. Iwasaki, "Actuarial Analysis of Private Payer Administrative Claims Data for Women With Endometriosis," *J Manag.Care Pharm.* 13, no. 3 (2007): 262-272.

[101] C. Fenga et al., "[Chronic Pelvic Pain in Women and Prevalent Orthostatic Work. Preliminary Results of a Study on Health Staff of the Surgical Field]," *Minerva Ginecol.* 52, no. 3 (2000): 69-72.

[102] B. Glenn and J. W. Burns, "Pain Self-Management in the Process and Outcome of Multidisciplinary Treatment of Chronic Pain: Evaluation of a Stage of Change Model," *J.Behav.Med.* 26, no. 5 (2003): 417-433.

[103] A. Breton, C. M. Miller, and K. Fisher, "Enhancing the Sexual Function of Women Living With Chronic Pain: a Cognitive-Behavioural Treatment Group," *Pain Res Manag*. 13, no. 3 (2008): 219-224.

[104] A. Trampas et al., "Clinical Massage and Modified Proprioceptive Neuromuscular Facilitation Stretching in Males With Latent Myofascial Trigger Points," *Phys Ther Sport* 11, no. 3 (2010): 91-98.